# ADVANCES IN MALIGNANT MELANOMA – CLINICAL AND RESEARCH PERSPECTIVES

Edited by **April W. Armstrong**

**Advances in Malignant Melanoma – Clinical and Research Perspectives**
Edited by April W. Armstrong

**Published by InTech**
Janeza Trdine 9, 51000 Rijeka, Croatia



**Publishing Process Manager** Sandra Bakic

**Technical Editor** Teodora Smiljanic

**Cover Designer** InTech Design Team

Additional hard copies can be obtained from orders@intechopen.com

Advances in Malignant Melanoma – Clinical and Research Perspectives,
Edited by April W. Armstrong
p. cm.
ISBN 978-953-307-575-4

For EU product safety concerns:
IN TECH d.o.o., Prolaz Marije Krucifikse Kozulić 3, 51000 Rijeka, Croatia,
info@intechopen.com or visit our website at intechopen.com.

# Meet the editor

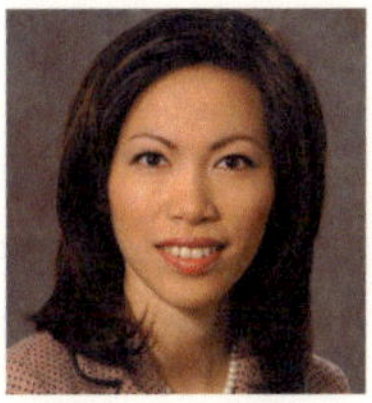

Dr. April W. Armstrong is Director of the Clinical Research Unit and Teledermatology Program at the Department of Dermatology. Dr. Armstrong completed training at Harvard Dermatology Residency Program and Harvard School of Public Health. While at Harvard, she also completed a one-year dermatopathology research fellowship with Dr. Martin Mihm focusing on the prognostic significance of tumor infiltrating lymphocytes in melanoma. Dr. Armstrong is actively engaged in clinical research as well as medical education, with an emphasis on telehealth and chronic inflammatory dermatoses. She believes that good clinical practice needs to be rooted in evidence-based medicine, and rigorous research forms the foundation for innovations in dermatology. Dr. Armstrong's research is supported by the Dermatology Foundation, National Psoriasis Foundation, California Healthcare Foundation, Agency for Healthcare Research and Quality, and the National Institute of Health.

# Contents

# Preface

This book titled *Advances in Malignant Melanoma - Clinical and Research Perspectives* represents an international effort to highlight advances in our understanding of malignant melanoma from both clinical and research perspectives. The authors for this book consist of an international group of recognized leaders in melanoma research and patient care, and they share their unique perspectives regarding melanoma epidemiology, risk factors, diagnostic and prognostic tools, phenotypes, treatment, and future research directions.

The book is divide into four sections: (1) Epidemiology and Risk Factors of Melanoma, (2) Clinical Phenotypes of Melanoma, (3) Investigational Treatments for Melanoma and Pigmentary Disorders, and (4) Advances in Melanoma Translational Research. This book does not attempt to exhaustively cover all aspects of the aforementioned areas of melanoma; rather, it is a compilation of the pearls and unique perspectives on the relevant advances in melanoma during the recent years.

**Section 1: Epidemiology and Risk Factors of Melanoma**

Professors Fisher and Hawryluk from the United States of America begin this book by an invigorating discussion of melanoma epidemiology, risk factors, and clinical phenotypes. The authors highlight increases in the incidence of melanoma in the Caucasian population and the overall relatively stable mortality rates. The incidence and mortality rates of melanoma are also framed in terms of geography and ethnicity using data worldwide. Professors Fisher and Hawryluk also examine intrinsic and extrinsic risk factors that predispose patients to melanoma development. . While mutations in either BRAF or NRAS are found in a significant majority of the most common cutaneous melanoma types, other phenotypes such as lentigo maligna melanoma have no known specific genetic mutation to date.

In the chapter"Increasing Incidences of Cutaneous Malignant Melanoma by Region Around the World", Dr. Godar from the United States of America analyzes the incidences of cutaneous malignant melanoma in the years 1980 and 2000 worldwide and factors that might contribute to development of melanoma, with an emphasis on the role of ultraviolet light.

In their chapter"Skin Pigmentation and Melanoma Risk", Professors D'Orazio, Marsch, Lagrew, and Veith from the United States review the link between melanoma and skin complexion, focusing on the genes that control innate and adaptive skin pigmentation and the mechanisms by which pigmentation differences may account for melanoma risk. Specifically, the authors highlighted how melanocortin 1 receptor (MC1R) signaling pathway may affect melanoma risk and the efficiency by which an individual can adaptively tan and repair UV-induced photolesions after UV exposure.

**Section 2: Clinical Phenotypes of Melanoma**

In the chapter"Desmoplastic Melanoma,"Professors Cheng and Armstrong from the United States of America review the current literature of desmoplastic melanoma with regards to its epidemiology, clinical presentations, histopathology, treatment, and prognosis.

In the chapter,"Melanoma during Pregnancy", Professors Popovic, Grgic, and Popovic from Serbia discuss melanomas that develop during pregnancy, an evolving and important topic in melanoma detection and management of this special population. The authors summarize the literature regarding epidemiology, prognostic factors, and mortality rates for in this population and highlight the importance of further research that will enable optimal management.

In the chapter"Familial Melanoma in Italy: a Review", Professors Funari, Menin, Elefanti, D'Andrea, and Scaini from Italy discuss familial melanoma in Italy, a country usually considered to have a low melanoma incidence. In Italy, there are geographical variations in melanoma incidence between the north and the south. In this chapter, the authors discussed high risk genes associated with familial melanoma, genetic counseling and testing for familial melanoma, CDKN2A unclassified variants, and mutational analysis of melanoma-predisposing genes in Italy.

In the chapter"Genetics of Uveal Melanoma", Professors van den Bosch, van Beek, Kiliç, Naus, Paridaens, and de Klein from the Netherlands discuss updates in cytogenetic and molecular genetic approaches to discoveries in uveal melanoma and implications for current and future management of patients with uveal melanoma.

**Section 3: Investigational Treatments for Melanoma and Pigmentary Disorders**

In the chapter"Targeting IGF-1 Based Melanoma Immunotherapy", Professor Duc from France discusses research using IGF-1 as target for melanoma immunotherapy. Specifically, Dr. Duc considers IGF-1 as target in melanoma immunotherapy, in vitro analyses of inhibited IGF-1 melanoma cells, in vivo effects of inhibited IGF-1 melanoma cells, and characterization of immune effectors stimulated by modified melanoma cells exhibiting inhibited IGF-1 expression.

In the chapter,"Melanin Hyperpigmentation Inhibitors from Natural Resources", Professors Matsuda, Murata, Itoh, Masuda and Naruto from Japan discuss melanogenesis and ways to influence this process with natural plant sources. They report a number of ingredients with an inhibitory effect on melanin hyperpigmentation. Specifically, the authors describe their screening strategy and studies on targeted melanin hyperpigmentation inhibitors from natural plant sources, such as Umbelliferae, Ericaceae, Rubiaceae, Piperaceae and Rutaceae plants.

**Section 4: Advances in Melanoma Translational Research**

In the chapter,"Caveolin-1 in Melanoma Progression,"Professors Lobos-González, Aguilar, Fernández, Sanhueza, and Quest from Chile discuss work from their laboratory focusing on a scaffolding protein called caveolin-1. This protein is implicated in a large number of cellular processes, including caveolae formation and vesicular transport, cholesterol transport, and the regulation of signal transduction. Initial reports also suggested that caveolin-1 might function as a tumor suppressor. In this chapter, the authors summarize the literature regarding the function of caveolin-1 in cancer development, mechanisms, and relevance of caveolin-1 in the development of melanomas.

In the chapter,"IMP3 and Malignant Melanoma", Professors Mentrikoski and Xu from the United States of America highlight challenges of distinguishing among melanocytic lesions based on histological morphologic criteria alone and the need for reliable diagnostic and prognostic biomarkers. The authors discussed their work in Insulin-like growth factor II (IGF-II) mRNA-binding protein 3 (IMP3), which functions to promote tumor cell proliferation by enhancing IGF-II protein expression. Specifically, the authors discuss the diagnostic value of IMP3 in the differential diagnosis of melanocytic lesions and in separating intranodal nevi from metastatic melanoma, as well as its prognostic value in malignant melanoma.

Finally, in the chapter"Effects of Social Stress on Immunomodulation and Tumor Development", Professors Vegas, Garmendia, Arregi and Azpiroz from Spain take us on an interesting journey through the field of psychoneuroimmunology as it relates to melanoma. Specifically, the authors discuss communication pathways between the central nervous system and the immune system, the relationship between social stress and cancer, the effect of social stress on melanoma tumor development, and psychosocial intervention and cancer progression.

**Conclusion**

We deeply appreciate your interest in this book. We hope that the contents of this book will inspire further research to advance our understanding of melanoma pathogenesis and to find promising novel treatments for this cancer.

**April W. Armstrong**
University of California Davis Health System
Sacramento, California
United States of America

# Part 1

# Epidemiology and Risk Factors of Melanoma

# 1

# Melanoma Epidemiology, Risk Factors, and Clinical Phenotypes

Elena B. Hawryluk and David E. Fisher
*Massachusetts General Hospital, Harvard University*
*United States of America*

## 1. Introduction

Malignant melanoma is an aggressive malignancy responsible for nearly 60% of death from skin cancers. Recent advancements in the biology and molecular genetics of melanoma are accompanied by an improved appreciation of the roles of both intrinsic and extrinsic risk factors in their contribution to disease. This chapter reviews the epidemiology, risk factors, and clinical phenotypes of melanoma.

## 2. Melanoma epidemiology

Over the past two decades we have observed increases in the incidence of malignant melanoma in the Caucasian population, while overall mortality rates have remained somewhat stable. The incidence and mortality of melanoma is considered in terms of geography and ethnicity using data from the United States and worldwide.

### 2.1 U.S. melanoma epidemiology

Melanoma trends in the United States were examined using data from the Surveillance, Epidemiology, and End Results (SEER) Program, a National Cancer Institute program that collects cancer and survival data from approximately 26% of the U.S. population. The SEER data revealed an increase in age-adjusted incidence rates of melanoma, which more than doubled among females and nearly tripled among males between 1973 and 1997 (Jemal *et al.*, 2001). After an additional 7 years of SEER data, it was found that among young adults (aged 15–39 years) there was an increase in melanoma incidence among young women, and the authors suggested a possible role of ultraviolet radiation exposure, as discussed in further detail below (Purdue *et al.*, 2008). Melanoma incidence has increased at 3.1% per year, with increases in tumors of all subtypes and thicknesses, and non-significant increases in melanoma mortality (Linos *et al.*, 2009). The median age of melanoma diagnosis is 60 years, with an age-adjusted incidence of 20.1 per 10,000 individuals, from 2003–2007 (SEER website, accessed 2011).

There are differences in melanoma incidence and mortality dependent upon ethnicity. The SEER data shows the highest incidence among Caucasians (19.1 females and 29.7 males per 100,000), followed by Hispanics (4.7 females and 4.4 males per 100,000), American Indians/Alaska Natives, Asian/Pacific Islanders, and Blacks (1.0 females and 1.1 males per 100,000)(SEER website, accessed 2011). Incidence data are depicted in Figure 1. Among U.S.

Hispanics and non-Hispanics from 2004–2006, it was noted that Hispanic melanoma patients had poorer prognostic characteristics (stage, tumor depth, and ulceration) at the time of diagnosis (Merrill *et al.,* 2011). Comparing the same ethnic groups over different regions of the country, male Hispanic Floridian patients had a 20% higher and non-Hispanic black Floridian patients had a 60% higher incidence of melanoma compared to non-Florida patients of the same gender and ethnicity (Rouhani *et al.,* 2010). The SEER data projected that, in 2010, there would be 68,130 new melanoma diagnoses and melanoma-related deaths among 8,700 men and women (SEER website, accessed 2011). The median age at death is 68 years, with the highest death rates among the U.S. Caucasian population (2.0 females and 4.5 males per 100,000), followed by American Indian/Alaska Natives, Hispanics, Blacks, and Asian/Pacific Islanders, from 2003–2007 (SEER website, accessed 2011). Overall mortality is depicted in Figure 1. African American patients with melanoma have poor overall survival outcomes, which were not explained by external factors such as treatment discrepancies or socioeconomic status (Zell *et al.,* 2008). One plausible contributor is the anatomic distribution of melanomas in patients of differing cutaneous pigmentation. Whereas melanomas are most likely to occur on typical cutaneous surfaces in Caucasians, they are proportionally more common (though of similar overall incidence) on acral (hairless) or mucosal surfaces among darkly pigmented individuals—surfaces commonly associated with thicker lesions at diagnosis.

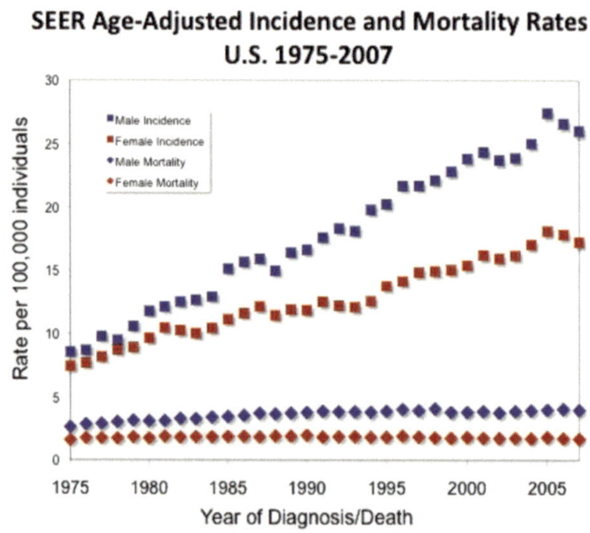


Fig. 1. Melanoma Incidence and Mortality Rates in the United States from 1975-2007. Data was extracted from the SEER database (SEER website, accessed 2011).

### 2.2 Global melanoma epidemiology

Data from a variety of countries and latitudes show similar trends in the incidence of melanoma. The role of geographic latitude on sun exposure was examined through pooled analysis of case-control studies including 5,700 melanoma cases (Chang *et al.,* 2009a; Chang *et al.,* 2009b). A meta-analysis of risk factors for cutaneous melanoma found that latitude is an important risk factor for melanoma (P=.031), and higher latitudes (distant from the equator) conferred an increased risk for sunburns (another melanoma risk factor), possibly due to intermittent intense sun exposure (Gandini *et al.*, 2005a). The role of sun and ultraviolet exposure will be explored in further detail below.

Epidemiological data on melanoma incidence is available from a number of countries. In Australia between 1990 and 2006, there was a stabilization of the thin melanoma rate, and the highest rates of melanomas occurred in the northern tropical regions; however, there was also an increase in the number of thick melanomas, particularly in the southern regions (Baade *et al.*, 2011). The authors speculated that the decrease in thick melanomas may be positively affected by early detection and skin awareness campaigns (Baade *et al.*, 2011). A 10-year study of melanoma in a central England population revealed an increase in thin melanoma, particularly among younger patients, and a slower increase in thick (>4mm) and intermediate (1.01–4mm) melanomas (Hardwicke *et al.*, 2011). In Northern Ireland, a seasonal variation of melanoma diagnosis timing suggested that incidence of cutaneous melanoma is highest in the summer; the trend was most prominent for women (Chaillol *et al.*, 2011). Analysis of malignant melanoma incidence in Turkey from 1988–2007 showed a median age of melanoma diagnosis of 52 years and statistically significant increases of melanoma incidence with increasing age (Tas, 2011).

Global data for melanoma is available from the World Health Organization (WHO), which states that the incidence of melanoma has been increasing over the past decades, with 132,000 melanomas occurring globally each year (WHO website, accessed 2011). The annual incidence increase varies among populations (estimated 3–7%), while overall mortality rates have been increasing at a lesser rate (Diepgen and Mahler, 2002; Lens and Dawes, 2004). From the mid-1950s through the mid-1980s, melanoma mortality rose among young and middle-aged adults in most of Europe, North America, Australia, and New Zealand (La Vecchia *et al.*, 1999). Between 1985 and 1995, there was a continued increase in mortality (though at lesser rates) in middle-aged men and declining mortality rates in middle-aged women in northern Europe, North America, Australia, and New England (La Vecchia *et al.*, 1999). Overall global increases in cutaneous malignant mortality were reported in 2000, based upon data from countries with a minimum time series of 30 years and 100 deaths annually in one sex from melanoma. This analysis revealed small decreases in mortality rates in Australia, Nordic countries, and the United States; lesser decreases in the United Kingdom and Canada; and ongoing increases in melanoma mortality rates in France, Italy, and Czechoslovakia (Severi *et al.*, 2000). Mortality also continued to increase among patients in Spain (Nieto *et al.*, 2003). Regional and worldwide campaigns to increase melanoma awareness have been launched, as survival is associated with thickness of lesion at the time of diagnosis.

### 2.3 Trends in melanoma epidemiology data

There exists some debate over the explanation for the observed trends in epidemiological measures, which suggest overall increases in disease incidence, with some stabilization of mortality rate over time. Likely there is some contribution associated with longer life expectancy and improved detection of cancer (Balducci and Beghe, 2001); however, the debate among experts continues as to whether there is a true increase in disease versus better detection with improved surveillance (Lamberg, 2002). It has been questioned whether the increased disease surveillance programs have succeeded to identify melanomas with more indolent behavior (Swerlick and Chen, 1996), as it is shown that the incidence of biopsy rates between 1986 and 2001 was associated with an increase in diagnosis of in situ and local melanomas, but not the incidence of advanced melanomas, in nine geographical areas of the United States (Welch *et al.*, 2005). More frequent thinner melanoma detection was also noted in Germany and France (Lasithiotakis *et al.*, 2006; Lipsker *et al.*, 2007). A large-scale prospective randomized survival-based study has not been carried out to prove benefit of skin cancer screening—although the requirement for such a study, or the ethics of being randomized to a non-screening arm, remains controversial.

While the expansion of skin screening programs may have increased the detection of relatively indolent melanomas, other studies have found that there are also increases in melanomas of all thicknesses (Linos *et al.*, 2009), so the detection of more histologically aggressive melanomas may be increasing as well. To address concern that the histological diagnosis of melanoma has drifted over time, with lesions classified more severely over time, a large 9-country review of pigmented lesions was conducted. This study examined diagnoses of pigmented lesions between approximately 1930 and 1980 and found only a 2.8% shift of melanoma cases from benign to malignant classification (van der Esch *et al.*, 1991), thus the increased disease incidence cannot be solely attributed to drift in histological interpretation. The debate over whether the increase in melanoma incidence reflects a true "melanoma epidemic" is also complicated by a number of biases and controversies, including surveillance intensity, length-time bias, diagnostic uncertainty, the cancer-relevant medico-legal climate, and problems related to data collection and recording (Swerlick and Chen, 1997; Florez and Cruces, 2004). Questions have been raised regarding a potential underreporting of melanoma over time, with estimates as high as 17% in the SEER database (Purdue *et al.*, 2008). Regardless of the interpretation of epidemiology measures, these studies have offered insights on trends in melanoma incidence and mortality, in addition to the intrinsic and extrinsic risk factors that are increasingly important in the management and prevention of future disease.

## 3. Melanoma risk factors

Melanoma risk factors include both intrinsic (genetic and phenotype) and extrinsic (environmental or exposure) factors. While intrinsic factors are inherent to the patient and cannot be modified, it is important to identify the at-risk population of patients. Conversely, extrinsic factors, from environment to behaviors, should be examined and minimized as possible, especially for the population with intrinsic increased melanoma risk. Major risk factors for melanoma include ultraviolet radiation exposure, family history, nevi (dysplastic, large number, or giant congenital nevi), increased age, fair skin phototype, occupation, and BMI (Rigel, 2010).

### 3.1 Intrinsic risk factors

Intrinsic melanoma risk factors are non-modifiable attributes that influence one's risk of melanoma, including age and gender, Fitzpatrick skin phototype (which is a gauge of one's skin color and burning or tanning response to sun exposure), and nevi pattern (quantity, size, clinical atypia, or dysplasia), which are readily apparent on examination. Also considered are the impacts of a patient's family history of melanoma, personal history of skin cancer, and underlying medical conditions including obesity, immunosuppression, cancer, and Parkinson's disease.

#### 3.1.1 Age and gender

Melanoma is among the most rapidly rising cancers in the United States, with highest melanoma risk among elderly males (Jemal *et al.*, 2001). There is a general increase in lifetime melanoma risk with advancing age for both men and women (Psaty *et al.*, 2010). Among patients with melanoma, the incidence of development of a second primary melanoma is 5.3% at 20 years and is also highest in older male patients (Goggins and Tsao, 2003). Older patients were found to have lentigo maligna melanoma more often than younger patients, with 75% occurring on the head and neck (Elwood *et al.*, 1987). Risk based upon sex is greater overall in males; however, incidence is higher in women until the age of 40 and then greater in males, with a ratio of 2:1 males: females by age 80 (Rigel, 2010). The SEER dataset shows the highest mortality among elderly males in all races from 1992-2007, with a mortality rate of 30.9 per 100,000 among males over age 85, in contrast to the highest female mortality rate of 12.4 per 100,000 for patients over age 85. Elderly males have disproportionately greater melanoma mortality, with mortality rates that are greater than double the female mortality rate when comparing all age groups over 55 years (SEER website, accessed 2011).

### 3.1.2 Skin phototype

An increased risk of melanoma has long been associated with characteristics of low Fitzpatrick skin phototype, such as pale skin, blond or red hair, freckles, and tendency to burn and tan poorly (Bataille and de Vries, 2008). The greatest risk is among patients with red hair or fair complexions, followed by those who burn easily, tan poorly, and freckle (Rigel, 2010). Fitzpatrick phototype I skin versus phototype IV imparts a relative risk of 2.09 of developing melanoma, with an increased relative risk for individual physical attributes such as fair skin color (2.06 versus dark), blue eye color (1.47 versus dark), red hair color (3.64 versus dark), and high density of freckles (relative risk of 2.10), as calculated by systematic meta-analysis of observational studies of melanoma risk factors (Gandini *et al.*, 2005b). A large prospective study from Norway and Sweden (>100,000 women) showed statistically significant risk of melanoma associated with hair color (red versus dark brown/black), in addition to other factors such as large body surface area (at least 1.79 m2) and number of large asymmetric nevi on legs (Veierod *et al.*, 2003), as reviewed below. The genetics associated with a clinical phenotype of red-haired patients with melanoma is discussed in further detail in Section 4.

### 3.1.3 Nevi

Dysplastic nevi are markers for increased melanoma risk, for both the individual and his or her family (Rigel, 2010). The presence of more than 50 common nevi, dysplastic nevi, or large nevi is associated with increased melanoma risk. Pooled studies involving 5,700 melanoma patients supported an increased risk with a nevus phenotype including greater whole body nevus counts, presence of clinically atypical nevi, or presence of large nevi, regardless of latitude (Chang *et al.*, 2009b). Their data showed a strongly increased risk with the presence of large nevi on the body and arms, and it suggested that an abnormal nevus phenotype is associated with melanomas on intermittently sun-exposed body sites (Chang *et al.*, 2009b). Clinically dysplastic nevi were associated with increased melanoma risk depending upon their number: One dysplastic nevus imparts 2-fold risk, while 10 or more dysplastic nevi impart a 12-fold increased risk of melanoma (Tucker *et al.*, 1997). Presence of a scar was identified as an independent risk factor for melanoma, as a scar may suggest the prior removal of a clinically atypical nevus at the site (Tucker *et al.*, 1997).

Nondysplastic nevi are also associated with increased melanoma risk when there are a large number of nevi and/or giant pigmented congenital nevi. The presence of large numbers of nondysplastic nevi confers a lesser risk than dysplastic nevi. Having many small nevi imparts approximately 2-fold increased risk, and the presence of both small and large nondysplastic nevi imparts a 4-fold risk (Tucker *et al.*, 1997). Congenital nevi were not associated with increased melanoma risk (Tucker *et al.*, 1997); however, giant pigmented congenital nevi (covering >5% body surface area) confer substantial melanoma risk (Swerdlow *et al.*, 1995).

### 3.1.4 Changing skin lesions

Changing skin lesions are associated with melanoma risk, as 75% of melanoma patients presented with a symptom or complaint associated with their melanoma lesion, most commonly "increase in size" (Negin *et al.*, 2003). Patient complaints that strongly associated with an increased Breslow depth of melanoma upon multivariate analysis include bleeding, pain, lump, itching, and change in size (Negin *et al.*, 2003).

### 3.1.5 Personal history of skin cancer

An important risk factor for melanoma is having a prior skin cancer, of either melanoma or non-melanoma type. Among patients diagnosed with a primary melanoma, 11.4% will develop a second primary melanoma within five years, and the risk is further increased if the patient also has a positive family history of melanoma or dysplastic nevi (Ferrone *et al.*, 2005). Risk of a second primary cutaneous melanoma among melanoma patients is found to be 6.01 per 1,000 person years after analysis of 20 years of follow-up in Queensland from 1982–2003 (McCaul *et al.*, 2008). Analysis of a Swiss registry found the 20-year incidence of second primary melanoma to be 5% (Levi *et al.*, 2005).

A retrospective study of patients with multiple primary melanomas identified several risk factors for multiple melanomas such as early age at diagnosis, dysplastic nevi (diagnosed clinically or histologically), family history of dysplastic nevi or melanoma, and history of dysplastic nevus with a family history of melanoma (Stam-Posthuma *et al.*, 2001). In a large prospective cohort study of Queensland patients, risk factors for development of a second cutaneous melanoma were found to be similar: high nevus count, high familial melanoma risk, fair skin, inability to tan, an *in situ* first primary melanoma, and male sex (Siskind *et al.*, 2011).

A prior diagnosis of non-melanoma skin cancer is generally indicative of a history of UV exposure, which is an extrinsic risk factor that will be discussed in detail below. Patients with a history of squamous cell carcinoma, basal cell carcinoma, or pre-malignant actinic keratoses are reported to have a relative risk of developing melanoma of 4.28–17 (Marghoob *et al.*, 1995; Gandini *et al.*, 2005b). Interestingly, other cutaneous neoplasms that don't associate as strongly with ultraviolet exposure have also been associated with an increased melanoma risk. Patients with mycosis fungoides carry a relative risk of 15.3 for development of melanoma, which may be related to immunosuppression or pathophysiology caused by the disease and/or associated therapies (Pielop *et al.*, 2003). In Merkel Cell Carcinoma, an increased risk for melanomas has not been established, though the high fatality and advanced age of Merkel Cell Carcinoma patients may reduce the opportunity to develop additional cancers (Howard *et al.*, 2006).

### 3.1.6 Family history of melanoma

A family history of melanoma has long been associated with increased melanoma risk; having a primary relative with melanoma imparts a relative risk of 1.74 of developing melanoma (Gandini *et al.*, 2005b). The highest risk occurs when a parent has multiple melanomas, with a relative risk of 61.78 (Hemminki *et al.*, 2003). The Familial Atypical Multiple Moles and Melanoma (FAMMM) syndrome describes a syndrome in which two or more primary relatives have multiple dysplastic nevi and a history of melanoma (Fusaro and Lynch, 2000). Often these patients carry mutations in the *CDKN2A* gene or the related pathway, as described below. Among melanoma prone-families followed prospectively, the cumulative risk of developing melanoma at a young age (before age 50) was 48.9% (Tucker *et al.*, 1993), and close surveillance is recommended. As described below, a family history of melanoma may arise from shared environmental risks, rather than purely genetically based risks.

### 3.1.7 Other personal medical history

A variety of medical conditions beyond a personal history of cutaneous carcinomas have reported associations with melanoma. Inherent diseases are described in this section, while associations with medical treatments are considered external risk factors and discussed in further detail below.

There may be an increased risk of melanoma with elevated body mass index, as a meta-analysis of 141 articles revealed a statistically significant positive association between increased BMI and malignant melanoma in men, though not as strong of an association that exists for esophageal, thyroid, colon, or renal cancers (Renehan *et al.*, 2008).

Both the immune system and DNA repair mechanisms are known to have important roles in protection from melanoma. Accordingly, in AIDS, there appears to be elevated risk of melanoma, which is highest among men who have sex with men, according to analysis of population-based U.S. AIDS and cancer registries in 2009 (Lanoy *et al.*, 2009). A history of organ transplantation carries increased melanoma risk, with melanoma occurring in 6% of adult transplant recipients and 14% of patients who received organ transplantation in childhood (Penn, 1996). However, non-melanoma skin cancers, particularly squamous cell carcinomas, present with higher frequency than melanomas after organ transplantation (Moloney *et al.*, 2006). Organ transplantation also carries a risk of transmission from the donor organ if the donor was previously affected with melanoma, and a diagnosis of melanoma requires careful consideration about whether to donate, or to revise the recipient patient's transplant immunosuppression regimen (Zwald *et al.*, 2010). Another population at increased risk of melanoma includes patients with xeroderma pigmentosum, who have defective DNA repair capability and are diagnosed with melanoma at a 5% rate. In these patients, 65% of their melanomas occurred on locations exposed to ultraviolet radiation such as the face, head, or neck (Kraemer *et al.*, 1987). Ultraviolet radiation is associated with gene mutations and increased melanoma risk as discussed in further detail below.

A number of non-cutaneous carcinomas have been shown to have associations with melanoma. Among women with a history of previous breast cancer, there is a standardized incidence ratio of 1.4 signifying an increased risk for cutaneous malignant melanoma among a Swiss Cancer Registry including 9,729 breast cancer patients followed over 24 years (Levi *et al.*, 2003). The Breast Cancer Linkage Consortium studied cancer risks in *BRCA* mutation carriers and found that *BRCA2* mutation carriers have an increased risk of developing malignant melanoma (2.58 relative risk) (The Breast Cancer Linkage Consortium, 1999), while *BRCA1* mutation carriers have an increased risk for colon cancer and prostate cancer, but no significant excesses in rates of cancers of other body sites (Ford *et al.*, 1994). Patients with a history of chronic lymphocytic leukemia or non-Hodgkin's lymphoma have an increased risk of melanoma, as malignant melanoma is among the most common presenting second cancer in both patient populations (Travis *et al.*, 1991; Travis *et al.*, 1992).

Associations with pancreatic carcinoma and renal cell carcinoma are explored based upon the discovery of gene mutations that are similar to those mutated in familial melanomas. In a study of familial pancreatic carcinoma families, 12% of these families carried a *CDKN2A* mutation (Lynch *et al.*, 2002). There is also an association of patients with melanoma and renal cell carcinoma, as both types of cancer carry an increased risk for the other. A study of 42 patients with both melanoma and renal cell carcinoma found a high frequency of positive melanoma family history, though the identification of only two *CDKN2A* mutant carriers in this series suggests that there may be a *CDKN2A*-independent genetic association involved (Maubec *et al., 2011*).

A putative association between Parkinson Disease and melanoma has been controversial and was perhaps based on the fact that both diseases involve cells that metabolize tyrosine via dopaquinone intermediates (albeit using distinct enzymes, tyrosine hydroxylase vs. tyrosinase). Literature review does not offer evidence that levodopa therapy is associated with development of malignant melanoma (Pfutzner and Przybilla, 1997). In 1978, levodopa therapy, a mainstay of Parkinson Disease management, was examined in a prospective query of 1,099 melanoma patients; at the time of presentation, only one patient had been taking levodopa (Sober and Wick, 1978). A family history of melanoma conferred an increased multivariate relative risk of developing Parkinson Disease among 157,036 individuals followed prospectively, with no associations between a family history of other major types of cancer or several environmental risk factors (Gao *et al.*, 2009). In addition, a recent study showed an increased melanoma risk in patients with Parkinson disease (prevalence was 2.24-fold higher than age and sex-matched SEER population data), and it was recommended that these patients be followed closely for skin changes over time (Bertoni *et al.*, 2010).

### 3.2 Extrinsic risk factors

In this section, external factors that are associated with melanoma risk are considered. Aspects of a patient's social history, such as their occupation, socioeconomic status, and marital status, have been shown to impact melanoma risk, though the mechanism for these interactions is not well understood. The risk of ultraviolet exposure is more readily explained, and data have accumulated regarding the effects of both natural and artificial ultraviolet radiation. Medications and chemical exposures can influence melanoma risk, and new studies have examined whether medications can play a role in modification of one's melanoma risk.

#### 3.2.1 Social history

Analysis of 29,792 cases of melanoma in California for trends involving socioeconomic status showed that individuals who lived in areas of highest socioeconomic status were at increased risk for melanoma (Linos *et al.*, 2009). Low socioeconomic status is also regarded as a poor predictor of melanoma outcomes and has been associated with disparities in utilization of sentinel lymph node biopsy (Zell *et al.*, 2008; Bilimoria *et al.*, 2009). Financial concerns were found to influence outcomes of disease in melanoma patients; a retrospective study found that perceived financial difficulty (compared to patients with an equivalent deprivation score) was related to recurrence risk, after adjusting for histological characteristics of the melanoma (Beswick *et al.*, 2008). Examination of SEER data of melanoma patients for the effect of marital status on melanoma stage, after controlling for a number of factors including histology, anatomic site, and socioeconomic status, suggested that unmarried patients had a higher risk of late-stage cutaneous melanoma diagnosis (McLaughlin *et al.*, 2010).

Occupation is associated with greater melanoma incidence in indoor workers and those with higher education, in addition to occupation-specific associations that have been observed utilizing cancer registries (Rigel, 2010). Analysis of cancer registries in England, Wales, and Sweden found the highest occupation-associated risk to be with airline pilots, finance and insurance brokers, professional accountants, dentists, inspectors, and supervisors in transport, with many of these professions sharing a high level of education (Vagero *et al.*, 1990). Among males in a California cancer database that listed fire fighter as their occupation, there was an increased risk of melanoma, in addition to increased risks of testicular cancer, brain, esophageal, and prostate cancers, compared to other types of cancer (Bates, 2007). Occupation-specific non-solar exposures impart increased melanoma risks for workers in the petroleum, printing, electronics, automobile, and agricultural industries (Fortes and de Vries, 2008), and specific occupational chemical exposures are reviewed below.

Those who are employed outdoors may have altered melanoma risk based upon ultraviolet exposure, an independent risk factor for melanoma. In 2005, Gandini *et al.* performed a meta-analysis and found an inverse association of high occupational sun exposure with melanoma (Gandini *et al.*, 2005a), while others have shown that occupational exposure carries an increased risk of melanoma of the head and neck, especially at low latitudes (Chang *et al.*, 2009a). The shift hours associated with one's occupation has also been shown to impact melanoma risk, though the mechanism is not clear. Among 68,336 women in the Nurses' Health Study from 1988–2006, there was a 44% decreased risk of skin cancer among nurses working 10 or more years on rotating night shifts compared to nurses who never worked night shifts, after adjustment for melanoma risk factors (Schernhammer *et al.*, 2011).

### 3.2.2 Ultraviolet exposure

The International Agency for Research on Cancer (IARC) identified solar and ultraviolet radiation as a significant environmental risk factor for cutaneous malignant melanoma (IARC, 1992), and in 2009 an IARC working group classified UV-emitting devices as group 1 carcinogens (El Ghissassi *et al.*, 2009). Ultraviolet radiation reaching the earth's surface is comprised of ultraviolet A and ultraviolet B radiation. Ultraviolet A light generally causes guanosine to thymine transversions, possibly due to oxidation of DNA bases (Pfeifer *et al.*, 2005). Ultraviolet B light characteristically generates mutations at dipyrimidine sequences with cytosine (which occurs in approximately 35% of *p53* gene mutations). Overall, the ultraviolet radiation-induced DNA mutations render DNA repair machinery an important protection against melanoma, which is particularly problematic for patients with defective DNA repair. Some have raised concern that climate change and ozone depletion will lead to increased solar ultraviolet radiation exposure, which may further correlate with increases in skin cancer (Diffey, 2004). Recently, the 10-year follow-up of a prospective study of daily or discretionary sunscreen application showed that daily sunscreen use reduced the rate in total melanomas and significantly reduced the rate of invasive melanomas as well (Green *et al.*, 2011).

Recreational or intermittent sun exposure was associated with increased melanoma risk of the trunk and limbs, but not head and neck, regardless of latitude of residence (Chang *et al.*,

2009a). Intermittent sun exposure is also associated with increased numbers of nevi (a potent melanoma risk factor) and nevi located at intermittently exposed body sites (Newton-Bishop *et al.*, 2010). Solar (actinic) keratoses and reported sun exposure strongly influence melanomas localized to the head and neck, while sporadic intermittent exposures, blistering sunburns, and self-reported sunburns are associated with an overall increased melanoma risk on all major body sites (Olsen *et al.*, 2010; Rigel, 2010).

While intermittent sun exposure and a history of sunburns are associated with up to 65% of malignant melanomas, the cumulative ultraviolet radiation exposure and pattern are also significant considerations. In a systematic review of case-control studies, melanoma risk was positively associated with intermittent sun exposure and sunburn at all ages (adult, adolescence, and childhood), in contrast to a reduced rate of melanoma in individuals with high occupational ultraviolet exposure (Elwood and Jopson, 1997). Ultraviolet exposure pattern can also impart risk for specific melanoma subtypes. The lentigo maligna melanomas were less strongly related to intermittent sun exposure or skin reaction to sun, in contrast to superficial spreading melanomas and nodular melanomas. Of these types, superficial spreading melanomas were most strongly associated with vacation sun exposures (Elwood *et al.*, 1987).

### 3.2.3 Molecular features of mutations

Although UV radiation is strongly associated with risk for development of melanoma, it is striking that signature UV mutations (pyrimidine dimers) are much less frequent within mutated oncogenes of melanomas than in non-melanoma skin cancers. An important terminology is used to discriminate genomic mutations which actively promote oncogenic behavior from those which are biologically silent. "Driver" mutations are functionally important in conferring cancerous phenotypic changes, whereas "passenger" mutations are indicative of carcinogenic exposure, but do not actively contribute to malignant behavior of the cell. A human melanoma was the first malignancy for which complete genomic sequencing was reported, and compared to a matched lymphocyte cell line derived from the same patient (Pleasance *et al.*, 2010). In this study thousands of mutations were observed, including numerous pyrimidine dimers indicative of prior UV exposure. However comparatively few mutations were observed within gene coding regions (vs. intergenic zones of the genome) suggesting relatively efficient transcription-coupled DNA repair. Indeed the patterns of UV signature mutation were more informative about the molecular geneology of the tumor than the nature of its precise oncogenic "drivers."

### 3.2.4 Recreational tanning

A recent study in Denmark examining travel and sun-related behavior from 2007–2009 found that 69% of subjects tanned intentionally, and this was the most important factor in sunburn on vacation (Koster *et al.*, 2011). Prospective data from The Women's Lifestyle and Health Cohort Study including over 100,000 women from Norway and Sweden indicated that sunburns and solarium use (described below), particularly during adolescence and early adulthood (ages 10–39), are associated with increased melanoma risk (Veierod *et al.*, 2003).

Typical 5-minute sunlamp tanning exposures increase melanoma risk by 19% for frequent users (over 10 sessions) and by 3% for occasional users (less than 10 sessions), with primary melanomas most commonly located on sites that are not generally exposed to sunlight

(Fears *et al.,* 2011). Hery *et al.* described a significant increase in melanoma incidence in Iceland between 1954 and 2006, with increased incidence rates in women younger than 50 years (Hery *et al.,* 2010). They had postulated that UV-emitting tanning devices would increase melanoma incidence on the trunk (Boniol *et al.*, 2004) and presented data suggestive of a possible influence of indoor tanning bed use on this increase (Hery *et al.,* 2010). From 1975–2006, SEER data revealed an increase in melanomas arising on the trunk among young women in the United States (Bradford *et al., 2010*). Examination of the Australian Melanoma Family Study data regarding indoor tanning bed use and melanoma risk identified associations of tanning bed use with increased early-onset melanoma, with increased risks for those who use tanning beds more frequently and at an earlier age (Cust *et al., 2010*).
Several studies have indicated clear associations between indoor tanning and elevated melanoma risk. Lazovitch *et al.* observed increased melanoma risk in multiple groups of indoor tanning bed users (Lazovich *et al.*, 2010). The data were in agreement with a prior meta-analysis of the same question published by the The International Agency for Research on Cancer Working Group on artificial ultraviolet (UV) light and skin cancer (*Int J. Cancer,* 2007). This study demonstrated elevated melanoma incidence in users of indoor tanning beds, and formed the basis for the subsequent designation of tanning beds as Class I carcinogens by the World Health Organization. An additional important aspect of indoor tanning is its association with addictive behavioral patterns. Studies by Feldman and colleagues revealed evidence of withdrawal-like symptoms in frequent tanning bed users who volunteered to receive a dose of the opiate antagonist naltrexone (Kaur *et al.*, 2006). Frequent tanners were also able to discriminate UV-emitting tanning beds from "sham" tanning beds in a blinded study (Feldman *et al.*, 2004). A recent questionnaire-based analysis of a cohort of frequent tanners indicated that 39% met DSM IV criteria for addiction to indoor tanning (Mosher and Danoff-Burg, 2010). The precise underlying mechanism(s) of this addiction remain to be determined, but it is plausible that such behaviors may underlie the unremitting increases in melanoma incidence described above.

### 3.2.5 Medications

Medications such as psoralens can artificially increase ultraviolet induced damage, significantly increasing melanoma risk. Patients receiving photochemotherapy with oral methoxsalen and ultraviolet A light have increased melanoma risk with a large number of treatments (at least 250), and the risk increases at 15 years after the first treatment (Stern *et al.*, 1997) and appears to continue to increase with further passing of time (Stern, 2001).
Some data exist for a decreased risk of melanoma with long-term (>5 years) use of cholesterol-lowering drugs in analysis of the Cancer Prevention Study II Nutritional Cohort from 1997–2007 (Jacobs *et al.*, 2011), and higher doses of statin medications were associated with decreased melanoma risk upon analysis of a Vetaran's Administration pharmacy database (Farwell *et al.*, 2008). However, the effect of long-term statin use on melanoma risk was not evident upon analysis of the Kaiser Permanente database (Friedman *et al.*, 2008).
Female sex hormones and oral contraceptive use have been called into question regarding a potential increased risk of melanoma, given the slightly higher risk of breast cancer patients for melanoma (Levi *et al.*, 2003), and the fact that estrogens can increase melanocyte counts and cause cutaneous hyperpigmentation. An examination of Nurses' Health Study and Nurses' Health Study II cohorts revealed a 2-fold increase in melanoma risk among oral contraceptive users, and a further increased risk among premenopausal women who took oral contraceptives for 10 or more years (Feskanich *et al.*, 1999). Since that time, a number of

case reports and small cohort studies have offered conflicting information regarding hormonal therapy and melanoma risk. A Netherlands retrospective study found a cumulative dose-dependent increased risk of melanoma with hormone replacement therapy use (Koomen *et al.*, 2009b), though the same authors found no association of estrogen use with increased anatomic thickness of cutaneous melanoma (Koomen *et al.*, 2009a). Studies in mice demonstrated that the antiestrogen tamoxifen inhibited both development and metastasis in mouse melanoma (Matsuoka *et al.*, 2009), though study of tamoxifen in patients with melanoma showed no improvement in overall response rate, complete response rate, or survival rate when administered with systemic chemotherapy (Lens *et al.*, 2003). Pregnancy had no influence on disease-free survival in patients with a history of stage I cutaneous malignant melanoma (Albersen *et al.*, 2010).

Pooled analysis of case control studies including 5,590 women found a lack of association between melanoma risk and pregnancy, and no relation between melanoma and exogenous hormone use (Lens and Bataille, 2008). Regarding the facts and controversies surrounding a hormonal influence on melanoma risk, at this time, exogenous hormone use is not contraindicated, though counselling should be performed on an individualized basis (Gupta and Driscoll, 2010). While the role of estrogens have not been definitively demonstrated in melanoma, some still suspect melanoma may be a hormone-related neoplasm (de Giorgi *et al.*, 2011).

### 3.2.6 Chemical exposures

A possible association of melanoma exists with ionizing radiation, as well as chemicals and pollutants such as arsenic (Rigel, 2010). Occupational exposures to chemicals such as vinyl chloride, polychlorinated biphenyls, and petrochemicals have been linked to a possible increased risk of melanoma, though the contribution of these exposures to overall melanoma risk has not been consistently demonstrated in clinical studies (Markovic *et al.*, 2007). Fortes and deVries have reviewed the literature for occupation-specific exposures with cutaneous melanoma and summarized the evidence implicating polycyclic aromatic hydrocarbons, benzene, and polychlorinated biphenyls; trichloroethylene solvents, dioxin, and polyvinyl chloride; pesticides; and ionizing and non-ionizing radiation (Fortes and de Vries, 2008). Agricultural pesticides including mancozeb, parathion, and carbaryl were shown to associate significantly with cutaneous melanoma after adjustment for confounding factors (Dennis *et al., 2010*). There is concern that residential pesticide use may also impart increased cutaneous melanoma risk, as data from Italy supports a 2.18 odds ratio for high use of indoor pesticides (four times annually) versus low use (once annually) (Fortes *et al.*, 2007).

### 3.2.7 External factors and melanoma risk modification

Recent prospective data offers a role for daily sunscreen use in the reduction of melanoma frequency and invasion (Green *et al.*, 2011). Whereas prior studies had failed to consistently demonstrate such a benefit, this study incorporated 10-year followup, suggesting a longer latency between UV exposures for melanoma as compared to cutaneous squamous cell carcinoma. Additionally, attempts have been made to demonstrate benefit for supplementation of one's diet with vitamin D or non-steroidal anti-inflammatory drugs, for which conclusive positive effect has not been demonstrated at this time.

There remains controversy regarding the optimal level of serum vitamin D with respect to bone health, cancer, and wellness. A prospective cohort study suggested that vitamin D (serum 25-hydroxy-vitamin D3) levels are associated with lower Breslow thickness of

melanoma at the time of diagnosis, as well as being protective of survival in terms of melanoma relapse and death independent of melanoma thickness (Newton-Bishop *et al.*, 2009). However, at this time, there are no data to indicate that supplementation with vitamin D after diagnosis is protective for melanoma (Hutchinson *et al.*, 2010).
Studies have explored a potential protective effect of non-steroidal anti-inflammatory drugs and acetylsalicylic acids, based on a chemopreventative effect for other cancer types in addition to promising *in vitro* laboratory studies that suggested a potential role in the inhibition of melanoma migration and invasion. A large, Dutch case-control study found that continuous use of low-dose acetylsalicylic acids imparted a significantly reduced incidence of melanoma in women, but not in men (Joosse *et al.*, 2009). A large cohort study of self-reported NSAID use over the previous 10 years found no association between NSAID use and melanoma risk, tumor thickness, invasion, or metastasis, after statistical adjustments for melanoma risk factors and indications for NSAID use (Asgari *et al.*, 2008).

## 4. Melanoma clinical phenotypes

For many years, scientists have noted that there are distinct sets of genetic alterations in melanoma, and some of these are associated with distinct clinical phenotypes. Several of the functionally important signalling pathways in melanoma are depicted in Figure 2. Mutations in either *BRAF* or *NRAS* are found in a significant majority of the most common cutaneous melanoma types, highlighting the importance of the RAS-RAF-MAPK-ERK signaling cascade in disease pathogenesis. A number of genes have emerged as therapeutic targets, but it is not yet known whether they have a particular phenotypic correlation. Conversely, clinical phenotypes such as lentigo maligna melanoma, melanomas arising in chronically sun-exposed skin, aggressive melanomas in the elderly, melanomas of unknown primary site, dysplastic, and amelanotic melanomas do not have a known specific genetic mutation at this time. There is an increasing appreciation of certain clinical phenotypes with genetic associations, and this knowledge may be leveraged for current and future therapeutic approaches.

### 4.1 Intermittent ultraviolet exposures & sunburn-associated melanoma

*BRAF* mutations are identified in over 60% of cutaneous melanomas (Smalley, 2010), with over 80% of these mutations characterized by an amino acid substitution (V600E mutation) (Davies *et al.*, 2002). These melanomas often occur on skin with little histopathologic evidence of chronic sun damage (such as solar elastosis), occur in younger individuals, and are most associated with intense recreational/intermittent sun exposure (Junkins-Hopkins, 2010). Comparison of the characterization of melanomas with and without marked microscopic solar elastosis (associated with chronic sun-induced damage) suggest that *BRAF* mutations were found in patients without chronic actinic damage, and *NRAS* mutations were found only in samples without *BRAF* mutation but were not specific for a melanoma subtype (Curtin *et al.*, 2005). Analysis of Australian patients found that BRAF(V600E) mutation was significantly associated with a younger age at diagnosis of distant metastasis (56 versus 63 years) (Long *et al.*, 2011).

### 4.2 Melanoma in patients with red hair

Individuals with red hair, pale skin, tendency to freckle, and the inability to tan are known to have specific melanocortin-1 receptor (*MC1R*) variant alleles, found in over 80% of

individuals with this pigmentation phenotype (Valverde *et al.*, 1995). In 2000, an Australian study showed that patients with three active *MC1R* alleles (R151C, R160W, and D294H) have a doubled risk of cutaneous malignant melanoma for each active allele they carry. This increased risk persists among medium and dark-skinned individuals who carry one of the three designated *MC1R* variant alleles (Palmer *et al.*, 2000). A meta-analysis on the nine most studied *MC1R* variants suggested that they may play a role in the pathogenesis of melanoma both via pigmentary and non-pigmentary mechanisms (such as generation of reactive oxygen species), as some of the variants were only associated with melanoma and not the pigmentary phenotype (Raimondi *et al.*, 2008).
Based upon their Fitzpatrick skin phototype, red-haired *MC1R* variant allele patients are particularly susceptible to environmental ultraviolet exposure and sunburns, and they should take precautions according to their increased melanoma risk. These patients may lack the phenotype of chronically sun-damaged skin (including microscopic solar elastosis), while acquiring a lifetime of intermittent intense ultraviolet exposure as described above. Accordingly, *MC1R*-melanoma risk has been associated with *BRAF* mutations. In a study of two Caucasian populations with non-chronic solar damage melanomas, *BRAF* mutations were identified in over 80% of patients with two variant *MC1R* alleles and in only approximately 30% of individuals with wild type *MC1R* (Landi *et al.*, 2006). Patients carrying one or two *MC1R* variants in an Italian population were shown to have a 5–15 fold increase risk of *BRAF*-mutant melanomas regardless of actinic damage, and no *BRAF*-negative melanomas were identified among this population (Fargnoli *et al.*, 2008).

### 4.3 Melanomas in specific locations: Uveal, acral, and mucosal melanomas

Melanomas arising in specific locations are associated with specific genetic mutations. Uveal melanoma is characterized by distinct genetic mutations compared to cutaneous melanoma, as 83% of uveal melanomas exhibit somatic activation mutations of *GNAQ* or *GNA11* pathways, and they generally lack mutations in *BRAF, NRAS,* and *KIT* (Van Raamsdonk *et al.*. 2010). Oculodermal melanocytosis or Nevus of Ota is a risk factor for uveal melanoma (Singh *et al.*, 1998), and uveal melanomas often metastasize to the liver (Singh *et al.*, 2005). A large number of blue nevi contain similar genetic mutations (Van Raamsdonk *et al.*, 2010). Acral and mucosal melanomas have been shown to possess more genomic instability and chromosomal aberrations (in terms of DNA losses or gains, changes in amplicons, or changes in total copy-number transitions)(Curtin *et al.*, 2005). The *c-KIT* mutations are seen in up to one-third of acral and mucosal melanomas, in addition to those that arise in chronically actinically damaged skin (Curtin *et al.*, 2006).

### 4.4 Hereditary melanomas

Among newly diagnosed melanoma patients, an estimated 5–10% have an affected primary family member. Familial melanomas account for ~10% of malignant melanomas and about half of these are associated with known genetic lesions. The hereditary melanoma syndrome may involve mutation in the cyclin-dependent kinase inhibitor 2A (*CDKN2A*) gene locus, imparting a loss or inactivation of p16 or its alternative reading frame gene (ARF) (Goldstein *et al.*, 2006). Cell cycle regulator p16 protein mutations are found in 41% of familial cutaneous melanoma cases (Goldstein *et al.*, 2006). The cyclin dependent kinase 4 (*CDK4*) enzyme, which is inhibited by *p16* binding, is also found to be mutated in small sets of cutaneous melanoma families (Zuo *et al.*, 1996). A microsphere-based array assay was recently developed to detect over 30 variants of p16 pathway mutations for genotyping of familial melanoma samples (Lang *et al.,* 2011). Additional familial melanoma genes are being identified using high throughput genomics methodologies.

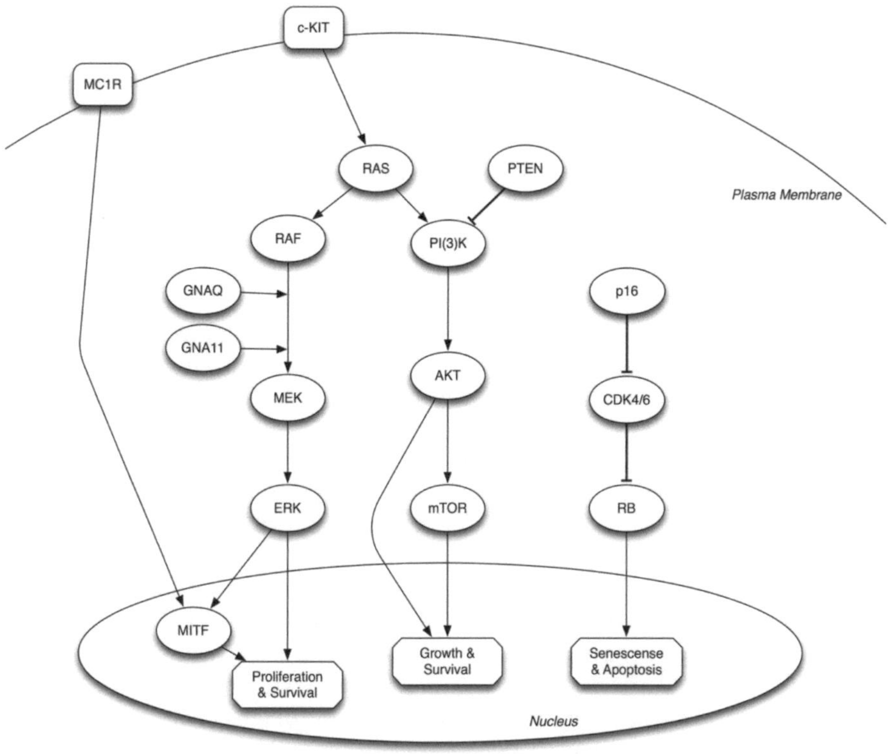


Fig. 2. Cellular Signaling Pathways Relevant to Melanoma Clinical Phenotypes. *BRAF* gene mutations disrupt Ras signaling in patients with intermittent/sunburn ultraviolet exposure, and are also more prominent among red-haired patients carrying *MCR1* variant alleles. Uveal melanomas may carry activating mutations of *GNAQ* or *GNA11,* while mucosal and acral melanomas often have *c*-KIT mutations. Hereditary melanomas with *CDKN2A* mutation have altered p16 pathway signaling. Metastatic melanoma involves transformation of several of these and additional signaling pathways.

### 4.5 Metastatic melanoma

Advances in melanoma genetics have enabled the identification of key oncogenic pathways that promote the transformation of primary to metastatic melanoma. A number of cell cycle regulatory proteins have mutations that contribute to melanoma pathogenesis, such as *AKT* family member activation mutation in up to 43–60% of melanomas (Stahl *et al.,* 2004) and loss of *PTEN* expression in 38% of primary and 58% of metastatic melanomas (Birck *et al.,* 2000). Constitutive activation of several other pathways may contribute to melanoma pathogenesis, including Src, JAK/STAT, Wnt, hedgehog, nuclear factor kappa B, and Notch signaling pathways (Smalley, 2010). A nested case-control study of DNA repair pathway genes in malignant melanoma patients and matched controls found a significant association of a *PARP1* gene variant with melanoma risk (Zhang *et al.,* 2011).

A number of oncogenic pathways have been targeted for therapies for malignant melanoma, including RAS/mitogen-activated protein (MAP) kinase family, RAF family members, MEK, c-KIT, and the P13K/AKT/mTOR pathways, in addition to downstream mediators of pathogenic pathways including apoptosis, anti-angiogenic, and immunological targets (Ko and Fisher, 2011). The MITF transcription factor is a lineage specific master regulator of melanocyte development and is amplified in ~20% of metastatic melanomas (Garraway *et al.*, 2005). It is becoming increasingly apparent that targeting one established mutation (for example, the V600E mutation of *BRAF* or mutant *KIT* in acral/mucosal melanomas) can yield impressive therapeutic responses in some patients (Flaherty *et al.*, 2010; Hodi *et al.*, 2008). Generally, the mutation-specific therapy provides a temporary improvement before disease progression, suggesting the potential for *de novo* mutations, activation of alternative signaling pathways such as NRAS or MAPK signaling, and evolution of melanoma (Johannessen *et al.*, 2010; Nazarian *et al.*, 2010). Clinical trials for combinatorial therapy targeting multiple pathways may provide improved therapeutic outcomes in patients who appear to develop tolerance or resistance to specific genetically-targeted therapeutic approaches (Solit and Sawyers, 2010), and one may consider evaluating the genome of progressing melanoma over time to enable improved personalized medicine, as is currently being pursued for other aggressive carcinomas (Singer, 2011).

## 5. Conclusions

With improved understanding of the risk factors and the relationship between clinical phenotype and genetics of melanoma, there are new opportunities for novel prevention strategies and therapeutic approaches for this devastating disease. Genome sequencing technologies have enabled the analysis and cataloging of somatic mutations from human cancers, and efforts are underway to expand this type of analysis to many additional melanomas in order to discriminate between driver and passenger mutations. Similar high throughput methodologies are being applied to populations at risk for melanoma formation, in order to identify predisposition genes and link them to specific environmental exposures or risks. Simultaneously, unprecedented progress has been made in translating the discovery of melanoma oncogenes into novel therapeutic strategies by exploiting targeted small molecule inhibitors of activated oncogenic kinases. Although the eventual emergence of resistance appears to be common, new research efforts are underway to reveal the mechanism(s) of such resistance and hopefully discover strategies to prevent disease progression. Collectively the past 10 years have produced unprecedented progress in understanding and attacking virtually every aspect of melanoma biology and clinical behavior. The continued characterization of melanoma mutations and risk factors will provide increasing opportunity to understand disease pathophysiology, and hopefully enable us to both meaningfully diminish melanoma risk as well as tailor treatments on the basis of informed molecular targeting.

## 6. Acknowledgments

We gratefully acknowledge Dr. Matthew Hawryluk and Mrs. Kristen Homer for their comments in preparation of this chapter. The authors acknowledge generous support from the Dr. Miriam and Sheldon Adelson Medical Research Foundation, the Melanoma Research Alliance, the Doris Duke Medical Foundation, and the National Institutes of Health.

## 7. References

(1992). IARC monographs on the evaluation of carcinogenic risks to humans. Solar and ultraviolet radiation. IARC Monogr Eval Carcinog Risks Hum *55,* 1-316.

(1999). Cancer risks in BRCA2 mutation carriers. The Breast Cancer Linkage Consortium. J Natl Cancer Inst *91,* 1310-1316.

(2007). The association of use of sunbeds with cutaneous malignant melanoma and other skin cancers: A systematic review. Int J Cancer *120,* 1116-1122.

Albersen, M., Westerling, V.I., and van Leeuwen, P.A. (2010). The influence of pregnancy on the recurrence of cutaneous malignant melanoma in women. Dermatol Res Pract *2010.*

Asgari, M.M., Maruti, S.S., and White, E. (2008). A large cohort study of nonsteroidal anti-inflammatory drug use and melanoma incidence. J Natl Cancer Inst *100,* 967-971.

Baade, P., Meng, X., Youlden, D., Aitken, J., and Youl, P. (2011). Time trends and latitudinal differences in melanoma thickness distribution in Australia, 1990-2006. Int J Cancer.

Balducci, L., and Beghe, C. (2001). Cancer and age in the USA. Crit Rev Oncol Hematol *37,* 137-145.

Bataille, V., and de Vries, E. (2008). Melanoma--Part 1: epidemiology, risk factors, and prevention. BMJ *337,* a2249.

Bates, M.N. (2007). Registry-based case-control study of cancer in California firefighters. Am J Ind Med *50,* 339-344.

Bertoni, J.M., Arlette, J.P., Fernandez, H.H., Fitzer-Attas, C., Frei, K., Hassan, M.N., Isaacson, S.H., Lew, M.F., Molho, E., Ondo, W.G., Phillips, T.J., Singer, C., Sutton, J.P., and Wolf, J.E., Jr. (2010). Increased melanoma risk in Parkinson disease: a prospective clinicopathological study. Arch Neurol *67,* 347-352.

Beswick, S., Affleck, P., Elliott, F., Gerry, E., Boon, A., Bale, L., Nolan, C., Barrett, J.H., Bertram, C., Marsden, J., Bishop, D.T., and Newton-Bishop, J.A. (2008). Environmental risk factors for relapse of melanoma. Eur J Cancer *44,* 1717-1725.

Bilimoria, K.Y., Balch, C.M., Wayne, J.D., Chang, D.C., Palis, B.E., Dy, S.M., and Lange, J.R. (2009). Health care system and socioeconomic factors associated with variance in use of sentinel lymph node biopsy for melanoma in the United States. J Clin Oncol *27,* 1857-1863.

Birck, A., Ahrenkiel, V., Zeuthen, J., Hou-Jensen, K., and Guldberg, P. (2000). Mutation and allelic loss of the PTEN/MMAC1 gene in primary and metastatic melanoma biopsies. J Invest Dermatol *114,* 277-280.

Boniol, M., Autier, P., and Dore, J.F. (2004). Re: A prospective study of pigmentation, sun exposure, and risk of cutaneous malignant melanoma in women. J Natl Cancer Inst *96,* 335-336; author reply 336-338.

Bradford, P.T., Anderson, W.F., Purdue, M.P., Goldstein, A.M., and Tucker, M.A. (2010). Rising melanoma incidence rates of the trunk among younger women in the United States. Cancer Epidemiol Biomarkers Prev *19,* 2401-2406.

Chaillol, I., Boniol, M., Middleton, R., Dore, J.F., Autier, P., and Gavin, A. Seasonality of cutaneous melanoma diagnosis in Northern Ireland with a review. Melanoma Res *21,* 144-151.

Chang, Y.M., Barrett, J.H., Bishop, D.T., Armstrong, B.K., Bataille, V., Bergman, W., Berwick, M., Bracci, P.M., Elwood, J.M., Ernstoff, M.S., Gallagher, R.P., Green, A.C., Gruis, N.A., Holly, E.A., Ingvar, C., Kanetsky, P.A., Karagas, M.R., Lee, T.K., Le

Marchand, L., Mackie, R.M., Olsson, H., Osterlind, A., Rebbeck, T.R., Sasieni, P., Siskind, V., Swerdlow, A.J., Titus-Ernstoff, L., Zens, M.S., and Newton-Bishop, J.A. (2009a). Sun exposure and melanoma risk at different latitudes: a pooled analysis of 5700 cases and 7216 controls. Int J Epidemiol *38*, 814-830.

Chang, Y.M., Newton-Bishop, J.A., Bishop, D.T., Armstrong, B.K., Bataille, V., Bergman, W., Berwick, M., Bracci, P.M., Elwood, J.M., Ernstoff, M.S., Green, A.C., Gruis, N.A., Holly, E.A., Ingvar, C., Kanetsky, P.A., Karagas, M.R., Le Marchand, L., Mackie, R.M., Olsson, H., Osterlind, A., Rebbeck, T.R., Reich, K., Sasieni, P., Siskind, V., Swerdlow, A.J., Titus-Ernstoff, L., Zens, M.S., Ziegler, A., and Barrett, J.H. (2009b). A pooled analysis of melanocytic nevus phenotype and the risk of cutaneous melanoma at different latitudes. Int J Cancer *124*, 420-428.

Curtin, J.A., Busam, K., Pinkel, D., and Bastian, B.C. (2006). Somatic activation of KIT in distinct subtypes of melanoma. J Clin Oncol *24*, 4340-4346.

Curtin, J.A., Fridlyand, J., Kageshita, T., Patel, H.N., Busam, K.J., Kutzner, H., Cho, K.H., Aiba, S., Brocker, E.B., LeBoit, P.E., Pinkel, D., and Bastian, B.C. (2005). Distinct sets of genetic alterations in melanoma. N Engl J Med *353*, 2135-2147.

Cust, A.E., Armstrong, B.K., Goumas, C., Jenkins, M.A., Schmid, H., Hopper, J.L., Kefford, R.F., Giles, G.G., Aitken, J.F., and Mann, G.J. (2010). Sunbed use during adolescence and early adulthood is associated with increased risk of early-onset melanoma. Int J Cancer.

Davies, H., Bignell, G.R., Cox, C., Stephens, P., Edkins, S., Clegg, S., Teague, J., Woffendin, H., Garnett, M.J., Bottomley, W., Davis, N., Dicks, E., Ewing, R., Floyd, Y., Gray, K., Hall, S., Hawes, R., Hughes, J., Kosmidou, V., Menzies, A., Mould, C., Parker, A., Stevens, C., Watt, S., Hooper, S., Wilson, R., Jayatilake, H., Gusterson, B.A., Cooper, C., Shipley, J., Hargrave, D., Pritchard-Jones, K., Maitland, N., Chenevix-Trench, G., Riggins, G.J., Bigner, D.D., Palmieri, G., Cossu, A., Flanagan, A., Nicholson, A., Ho, J.W., Leung, S.Y., Yuen, S.T., Weber, B.L., Seigler, H.F., Darrow, T.L., Paterson, H., Marais, R., Marshall, C.J., Wooster, R., Stratton, M.R., and Futreal, P.A. (2002). Mutations of the BRAF gene in human cancer. Nature *417*, 949-954.

de Giorgi, V., Gori, A., Alfaioli, B., Papi, F., Grazzini, M., Rossari, S., Lotti, T., and Massi, D. (2011). Influence of Sex Hormones on Melanoma. Journal of Clinical Oncology *29*, e94-e95.

Dennis, L.K., Lynch, C.F., Sandler, D.P., and Alavanja, M.C. (2010). Pesticide use and cutaneous melanoma in pesticide applicators in the agricultural heath study. Environ Health Perspect *118*, 812-817.

Diepgen, T.L., and Mahler, V. (2002). The epidemiology of skin cancer. Br J Dermatol *146 Suppl 61*, 1-6.

Diffey, B. (2004). Climate change, ozone depletion and the impact on ultraviolet exposure of human skin. Phys Med Biol *49*, R1-11.

El Ghissassi, F., Baan, R., Straif, K., Grosse, Y., Secretan, B., Bouvard, V., Benbrahim-Tallaa, L., Guha, N., Freeman, C., Galichet, L., and Cogliano, V. (2009). A review of human carcinogens--part D: radiation. Lancet Oncol *10*, 751-752.

Elwood, J.M., Gallagher, R.P., Worth, A.J., Wood, W.S., and Pearson, J.C. (1987). Etiological differences between subtypes of cutaneous malignant melanoma: Western Canada Melanoma Study. J Natl Cancer Inst *78*, 37-44.

Elwood, J.M., and Jopson, J. (1997). Melanoma and sun exposure: an overview of published studies. Int J Cancer *73*, 198-203.

Fargnoli, M.C., Pike, K., Pfeiffer, R.M., Tsang, S., Rozenblum, E., Munroe, D.J., Golubeva, Y., Calista, D., Seidenari, S., Massi, D., Carli, P., Bauer, J., Elder, D.E., Bastian, B.C., Peris, K., and Landi, M.T. (2008). MC1R variants increase risk of melanomas harboring BRAF mutations. J Invest Dermatol *128*, 2485-2490.

Farwell, W.R., Scranton, R.E., Lawler, E.V., Lew, R.A., Brophy, M.T., Fiore, L.D., and Gaziano, J.M. (2008). The association between statins and cancer incidence in a veterans population. J Natl Cancer Inst *100*, 134-139.

Fears, T.R., Sagebiel, R.W., Halpern, A., Elder, D.E., Holly, E.A., Guerry Iv, D., and Tucker, M.A. (2011). Sunbeds and sunlamps: who used them and their risk for melanoma. Pigment Cell Melanoma Res.

Feldman, S.R., Liguori, A., Kucenic, M., Rapp, S.R., Fleischer, A.B., Jr., Lang, W., and Kaur, M. (2004). Ultraviolet exposure is a reinforcing stimulus in frequent indoor tanners. J Am Acad Dermatol *51*, 45-51.

Ferrone, C.R., Ben Porat, L., Panageas, K.S., Berwick, M., Halpern, A.C., Patel, A., and Coit, D.G. (2005). Clinicopathological features of and risk factors for multiple primary melanomas. JAMA *294*, 1647-1654.

Feskanich, D., Hunter, D.J., Willett, W.C., Spiegelman, D., Stampfer, M.J., Speizer, F.E., and Colditz, G.A. (1999). Oral contraceptive use and risk of melanoma in premenopausal women. Br J Cancer *81*, 918-923.

Florez, A., and Cruces, M. (2004). Melanoma epidemic: true or false? Int J Dermatol *43*, 405-407.

Ford, D., Easton, D.F., Bishop, D.T., Narod, S.A., and Goldgar, D.E. (1994). Risks of cancer in BRCA1-mutation carriers. Breast Cancer Linkage Consortium. Lancet *343*, 692-695.

Fortes, C., and de Vries, E. (2008). Nonsolar occupational risk factors for cutaneous melanoma. Int J Dermatol *47*, 319-328.

Fortes, C., Mastroeni, S., Melchi, F., Pilla, M.A., Alotto, M., Antonelli, G., Camaione, D., Bolli, S., Luchetti, E., and Pasquini, P. (2007). The association between residential pesticide use and cutaneous melanoma. Eur J Cancer *43*, 1066-1075.

Friedman, G.D., Flick, E.D., Udaltsova, N., Chan, J., Quesenberry, C.P., Jr., and Habel, L.A. (2008). Screening statins for possible carcinogenic risk: up to 9 years of follow-up of 361,859 recipients. Pharmacoepidemiol Drug Saf *17*, 27-36.

Fusaro, R.M., and Lynch, H.T. (2000). The FAMMM syndrome: epidemiology and surveillance strategies. Cancer Invest *18*, 670-680.

Gandini, S., Sera, F., Cattaruzza, M.S., Pasquini, P., Picconi, O., Boyle, P., and Melchi, C.F. (2005a). Meta-analysis of risk factors for cutaneous melanoma: II. Sun exposure. Eur J Cancer *41*, 45-60.

Gandini, S., Sera, F., Cattaruzza, M.S., Pasquini, P., Zanetti, R., Masini, C., Boyle, P., and Melchi, C.F. (2005b). Meta-analysis of risk factors for cutaneous melanoma: III. Family history, actinic damage and phenotypic factors. Eur J Cancer *41*, 2040-2059.

Gao, X., Simon, K.C., Han, J., Schwarzschild, M.A., and Ascherio, A. (2009). Family history of melanoma and Parkinson disease risk. Neurology *73*, 1286-1291.

Goggins, W.B., and Tsao, H. (2003). A population-based analysis of risk factors for a second primary cutaneous melanoma among melanoma survivors. Cancer *97*, 639-643.

Goldstein, A.M., Chan, M., Harland, M., Gillanders, E.M., Hayward, N.K., Avril, M.F., Azizi, E., Bianchi-Scarra, G., Bishop, D.T., Bressac-de Paillerets, B., Bruno, W., Calista, D., Cannon Albright, L.A., Demenais, F., Elder, D.E., Ghiorzo, P., Gruis, N.A., Hansson, J., Hogg, D., Holland, E.A., Kanetsky, P.A., Kefford, R.F., Landi, M.T., Lang, J., Leachman, S.A., Mackie, R.M., Magnusson, V., Mann, G.J., Niendorf, K., Newton Bishop, J., Palmer, J.M., Puig, S., Puig-Butille, J.A., de Snoo, F.A., Stark, M., Tsao, H., Tucker, M.A., Whitaker, L., and Yakobson, E. (2006). High-risk melanoma susceptibility genes and pancreatic cancer, neural system tumors, and uveal melanoma across GenoMEL. Cancer Res *66*, 9818-9828.

Green, A.C., Williams, G.M., Logan, V., and Strutton, G.M. (2011). Reduced melanoma after regular sunscreen use: randomized trial follow-up. J Clin Oncol *29*, 257-263.

Gupta, A., and Driscoll, M.S. (2010). Do hormones influence melanoma? Facts and controversies. Clin Dermatol *28*, 287-292.

Hardwicke, J., Brunt, A.M., Rylands, G., and Rayatt, S. (2011). Ten-year Audit of Melanoma in a Central England Population*. Acta Derm Venereol.

Hemminki, K., Zhang, H., and Czene, K. (2003). Familial and attributable risks in cutaneous melanoma: effects of proband and age. J Invest Dermatol *120*, 217-223.

Hery, C., Tryggvadottir, L., Sigurdsson, T., Olafsdottir, E., Sigurgeirsson, B., Jonasson, J.G., Olafsson, J.H., Boniol, M., Byrnes, G.B., Dore, J.F., and Autier, P. (2010). A melanoma epidemic in Iceland: possible influence of sunbed use. Am J Epidemiol *172*, 762-767.

Howard, R.A., Dores, G.M., Curtis, R.E., Anderson, W.F., and Travis, L.B. (2006). Merkel cell carcinoma and multiple primary cancers. Cancer Epidemiol Biomarkers Prev *15*, 1545-1549.

Hutchinson, P.E., Osborne, J.E., and Pringle, J.H. (2010). Higher Serum 25-Hydroxy Vitamin D3 Levels at Presentation Are Associated With Improved Survival From Melanoma, But There Is No Evidence That Later Prevailing Levels Are Protective. Journal of Clinical Oncology *28*, e492-e493.

Jacobs, E.J., Newton, C.C., Thun, M.J., and Gapstur, S.M. (2011). Long-term Use of Cholesterol-Lowering Drugs and Cancer Incidence in a Large United States Cohort. Cancer Res *71*, 1763-1771.

Jemal, A., Devesa, S.S., Hartge, P., and Tucker, M.A. (2001). Recent trends in cutaneous melanoma incidence among whites in the United States. J Natl Cancer Inst *93*, 678-683.

Johannessen, C.M., Boehm, J.S., Kim, S.Y., Thomas, S.R., Wardwell, L., Johnson, L.A., Emery, C.M., Stransky, N., Cogdill, A.P., Barretina, J., Caponigro, G., Hieronymus, H., Murray, R.R., Salehi-Ashtiani, K., Hill, D.E., Vidal, M., Zhao, J.J., Yang, X., Alkan, O., Kim, S., Harris, J.L., Wilson, C.J., Myer, V.E., Finan, P.M., Root, D.E., Roberts, T.M., Golub, T., Flaherty, K.T., Dummer, R., Weber, B.L., Sellers, W.R., Schlegel, R., Wargo, J.A., Hahn, W.C., and Garraway, L.A. (2010). COT drives resistance to RAF inhibition through MAP kinase pathway reactivation. Nature *468*, 968-972.

Joosse, A., Koomen, E.R., Casparie, M.K., Herings, R.M., Guchelaar, H.J., and Nijsten, T. (2009). Non-steroidal anti-inflammatory drugs and melanoma risk: large Dutch population-based case-control study. J Invest Dermatol *129*, 2620-2627.

Junkins-Hopkins, J.M. (2010). Malignant melanoma: molecular cytogenetics and their implications in clinical medicine. J Am Acad Dermatol *63*, 329-332.

Kaur, M., Liguori, A., Lang, W., Rapp, S.R., Fleischer, A.B., Jr., and Feldman, S.R. (2006). Induction of withdrawal-like symptoms in a small randomized, controlled trial of opioid blockade in frequent tanners. J Am Acad Dermatol *54*, 709-711.

Ko, J.M., and Fisher, D.E. (2011). A new era: melanoma genetics and therapeutics. J Pathol *223*, 241-250.

Koomen, E.R., Joosse, A., Herings, R.M., Casparie, M.K., Guchelaar, H.J., and Nijsten, T. (2009a). Does use of estrogens decrease the Breslow thickness of melanoma of the skin? Oral contraceptives and hormonal replacement therapy. Melanoma Res *19*, 327-332.

Koomen, E.R., Joosse, A., Herings, R.M., Casparie, M.K., Guchelaar, H.J., and Nijsten, T. (2009b). Estrogens, oral contraceptives and hormonal replacement therapy increase the incidence of cutaneous melanoma: a population-based case-control study. Ann Oncol *20*, 358-364.

Koster, B., Thorgaard, C., Philip, A., and Clemmensen, I.H. (2011). Vacations to sunny destinations, sunburn, and intention to tan: a cross-sectional study in Denmark, 2007-2009. Scand J Public Health *39*, 64-69.

Kraemer, K.H., Lee, M.M., and Scotto, J. (1987). Xeroderma pigmentosum. Cutaneous, ocular, and neurologic abnormalities in 830 published cases. Arch Dermatol *123*, 241-250.

La Vecchia, C., Lucchini, F., Negri, E., and Levi, F. (1999). Recent declines in worldwide mortality from cutaneous melanoma in youth and middle age. Int J Cancer *81*, 62-66.

Lamberg, L. (2002). "Epidemic" of malignant melanoma: true increase or better detection? JAMA *287*, 2201.

Landi, M.T., Bauer, J., Pfeiffer, R.M., Elder, D.E., Hulley, B., Minghetti, P., Calista, D., Kanetsky, P.A., Pinkel, D., and Bastian, B.C. (2006). MC1R germline variants confer risk for BRAF-mutant melanoma. Science *313*, 521-522.

Lang, J.M., Shennan, M., Njauw, J.C., Luo, S., Bishop, J.N., Harland, M., Hayward, N.K., Tucker, M.A., Goldstein, A.M., Landi, M.T., Puig, S., Gruis, N.A., Bergman, W., Bianchi-Scarra, G., Ghiorzo, P., Hogg, D., and Tsao, H. (2011). A flexible multiplex bead-based assay for detecting germline CDKN2A and CDK4 variants in melanoma-prone kindreds. J Invest Dermatol *131*, 480-486.

Lanoy, E., Dores, G.M., Madeleine, M.M., Toro, J.R., Fraumeni, J.F., Jr., and Engels, E.A. (2009). Epidemiology of nonkeratinocytic skin cancers among persons with AIDS in the United States. AIDS *23*, 385-393.

Lasithiotakis, K.G., Leiter, U., Gorkievicz, R., Eigentler, T., Breuninger, H., Metzler, G., Strobel, W., and Garbe, C. (2006). The incidence and mortality of cutaneous melanoma in Southern Germany: trends by anatomic site and pathologic characteristics, 1976 to 2003. Cancer *107*, 1331-1339.

Lazovich, D., Vogel, R.I., Berwick, M., Weinstock, M.A., Anderson, K.E., and Warshaw, E.M. (2010). Indoor tanning and risk of melanoma: a case-control study in a highly exposed population. Cancer Epidemiol Biomarkers Prev *19*, 1557-1568.

Lens, M., and Bataille, V. (2008). Melanoma in relation to reproductive and hormonal factors in women: current review on controversial issues. Cancer Causes Control *19*, 437-442.

Lens, M.B., and Dawes, M. (2004). Global perspectives of contemporary epidemiological trends of cutaneous malignant melanoma. Br J Dermatol *150*, 179-185.

Lens, M.B., Reiman, T., and Husain, A.F. (2003). Use of tamoxifen in the treatment of malignant melanoma. Cancer *98*, 1355-1361.

Levi, F., Randimbison, L., Te, V.C., and La Vecchia, C. (2005). High constant incidence rates of second cutaneous melanomas. Int J Cancer *117*, 877-879.

Levi, F., Te, V.C., Randimbison, L., and La Vecchia, C. (2003). Cancer risk in women with previous breast cancer. Ann Oncol *14*, 71-73.

Linos, E., Swetter, S.M., Cockburn, M.G., Colditz, G.A., and Clarke, C.A. (2009). Increasing burden of melanoma in the United States. J Invest Dermatol *129*, 1666-1674.

Lipsker, D., Engel, F., Cribier, B., Velten, M., and Hedelin, G. (2007). Trends in melanoma epidemiology suggest three different types of melanoma. Br J Dermatol *157*, 338-343.

Long, G.V., Menzies, A.M., Nagrial, A.M., Haydu, L.E., Hamilton, A.L., Mann, G.J., Hughes, T.M., Thompson, J.F., Scolyer, R.A., and Kefford, R.F. (2011). Prognostic and Clinicopathologic Associations of Oncogenic BRAF in Metastatic Melanoma. Journal of Clinical Oncology.

Lynch, H.T., Brand, R.E., Hogg, D., Deters, C.A., Fusaro, R.M., Lynch, J.F., Liu, L., Knezetic, J., Lassam, N.J., Goggins, M., and Kern, S. (2002). Phenotypic variation in eight extended CDKN2A germline mutation familial atypical multiple mole melanoma-pancreatic carcinoma-prone families: the familial atypical mole melanoma-pancreatic carcinoma syndrome. Cancer *94*, 84-96.

Marghoob, A.A., Slade, J., Salopek, T.G., Kopf, A.W., Bart, R.S., and Rigel, D.S. (1995). Basal cell and squamous cell carcinomas are important risk factors for cutaneous malignant melanoma. Screening implications. Cancer *75*, 707-714.

Markovic, S.N., Erickson, L.A., Rao, R.D., Weenig, R.H., Pockaj, B.A., Bardia, A., Vachon, C.M., Schild, S.E., McWilliams, R.R., Hand, J.L., Laman, S.D., Kottschade, L.A., Maples, W.J., Pittelkow, M.R., Pulido, J.S., Cameron, J.D., and Creagan, E.T. (2007). Malignant melanoma in the 21st century, part 1: epidemiology, risk factors, screening, prevention, and diagnosis. Mayo Clin Proc *82*, 364-380.

Matsuoka, H., Tsubaki, M., Yamazoe, Y., Ogaki, M., Satou, T., Itoh, T., Kusunoki, T., and Nishida, S. (2009). Tamoxifen inhibits tumor cell invasion and metastasis in mouse melanoma through suppression of PKC/MEK/ERK and PKC/PI3K/Akt pathways. Exp Cell Res *315*, 2022-2032.

Maubec, E., Chaudru, V., Mohamdi, H., Grange, F., Patard, J.J., Dalle, S., Crickx, B., Paillerets, B.B., Demenais, F., and Avril, M.F. (2011). Characteristics of the coexistence of melanoma and renal cell carcinoma. Cancer *116*, 5716-5724.

McCaul, K.A., Fritschi, L., Baade, P., and Coory, M. (2008). The incidence of second primary invasive melanoma in Queensland, 1982-2003. Cancer Causes Control *19*, 451-458.

McLaughlin, J.M., Fisher, J.L., and Paskett, E.D. (2010). Marital status and stage at diagnosis of cutaneous melanoma: results from the surveillance epidemiology and end results (SEER) program, 1973-2006. Cancer.

Merrill, R.M., Pace, N.D., and Elison, A.N. (2011). Cutaneous malignant melanoma among white Hispanics and non-Hispanics in the United States. Ethn Dis *20*, 353-358.

Moloney, F.J., Comber, H., O'Lorcain, P., O'Kelly, P., Conlon, P.J., and Murphy, G.M. (2006). A population-based study of skin cancer incidence and prevalence in renal transplant recipients. Br J Dermatol *154*, 498-504.

Mosher, C.E., and Danoff-Burg, S. (2010). Addiction to indoor tanning: relation to anxiety, depression, and substance use. Arch Dermatol *146*, 412-417.

Nazarian, R., Shi, H., Wang, Q., Kong, X., Koya, R.C., Lee, H., Chen, Z., Lee, M.K., Attar, N., Sazegar, H., Chodon, T., Nelson, S.F., McArthur, G., Sosman, J.A., Ribas, A., and Lo, R.S. (2010). Melanomas acquire resistance to B-RAF(V600E) inhibition by RTK or N-RAS upregulation. Nature *468*, 973-977.

Negin, B.P., Riedel, E., Oliveria, S.A., Berwick, M., Coit, D.G., and Brady, M.S. (2003). Symptoms and signs of primary melanoma: important indicators of Breslow depth. Cancer *98*, 344-348.

Newton-Bishop, J.A., Beswick, S., Randerson-Moor, J., Chang, Y.M., Affleck, P., Elliott, F., Chan, M., Leake, S., Karpavicius, B., Haynes, S., Kukalizch, K., Whitaker, L., Jackson, S., Gerry, E., Nolan, C., Bertram, C., Marsden, J., Elder, D.E., Barrett, J.H., and Bishop, D.T. (2009). Serum 25-hydroxyvitamin D3 levels are associated with breslow thickness at presentation and survival from melanoma. J Clin Oncol *27*, 5439-5444.

Newton-Bishop, J.A., Chang, Y.M., Iles, M.M., Taylor, J.C., Bakker, B., Chan, M., Leake, S., Karpavicius, B., Haynes, S., Fitzgibbon, E., Elliott, F., Kanetsky, P.A., Harland, M., Barrett, J.H., and Bishop, D.T. (2010). Melanocytic nevi, nevus genes, and melanoma risk in a large case-control study in the United Kingdom. Cancer Epidemiol Biomarkers Prev *19*, 2043-2054.

Nieto, A., Ruiz-Ramos, M., Abdel-Kader, L., Conde, M., and Camacho, F. (2003). Gender differences in rising trends in cutaneous malignant melanoma in Spain, 1975-98. Br J Dermatol *148*, 110-116.

Olsen, C.M., Zens, M.S., Green, A.C., Stukel, T.A., Holman, C.D., Mack, T., Elwood, J.M., Holly, E.A., Sacerdote, C., Gallagher, R., Swerdlow, A.J., Armstrong, B.K., Rosso, S., Kirkpatrick, C., Zanetti, R., Bishop, J.N., Bataille, V., Chang, Y.M., Mackie, R., Osterlind, A., Berwick, M., Karagas, M.R., and Whiteman, D.C. (2010). Biologic markers of sun exposure and melanoma risk in women: Pooled case-control analysis. Int J Cancer.

Palmer, J.S., Duffy, D.L., Box, N.F., Aitken, J.F., O'Gorman, L.E., Green, A.C., Hayward, N.K., Martin, N.G., and Sturm, R.A. (2000). Melanocortin-1 receptor polymorphisms and risk of melanoma: is the association explained solely by pigmentation phenotype? Am J Hum Genet *66*, 176-186.

Penn, I. (1996). Malignant melanoma in organ allograft recipients. Transplantation *61*, 274-278.

Pfeifer, G.P., You, Y.H., and Besaratinia, A. (2005). Mutations induced by ultraviolet light. Mutat Res *571*, 19-31.

Pfutzner, W., and Przybilla, B. (1997). Malignant melanoma and levodopa: is there a relationship? Two new cases and a review of the literature. J Am Acad Dermatol *37*, 332-336.

Pielop, J.A., Brownell, I., and Duvic, M. (2003). Mycosis fungoides associated with malignant melanoma and dysplastic nevus syndrome. Int J Dermatol *42*, 116-122.

Pleasance, E.D., Cheetham, R.K., Stephens, P.J., McBride, D.J., Humphray, S.J., Greenman, C.D., Varela, I., Lin, M.L., Ordonez, G.R., Bignell, G.R., Ye, K., Alipaz, J., Bauer, M.J., Beare, D., Butler, A., Carter, R.J., Chen, L., Cox, A.J., Edkins, S., Kokko-Gonzales, P.I., Gormley, N.A., Grocock, R.J., Haudenschild, C.D., Hims, M.M., James, T., Jia, M., Kingsbury, Z., Leroy, C., Marshall, J., Menzies, A., Mudie, L.J., Ning, Z., Royce, T., Schulz-Trieglaff, O.B., Spiridou, A., Stebbings, L.A., Szajkowski, L., Teague, J., Williamson, D., Chin, L., Ross, M.T., Campbell, P.J., Bentley, D.R., Futreal, P.A., and Stratton, M.R. (2010). A comprehensive catalogue of somatic mutations from a human cancer genome. Nature *463*, 191-196.

Psaty, E.L., Scope, A., Halpern, A.C., and Marghoob, A.A. (2010). Defining the patient at high risk for melanoma. Int J Dermatol *49*, 362-376.

Purdue, M.P., Freeman, L.E., Anderson, W.F., and Tucker, M.A. (2008). Recent trends in incidence of cutaneous melanoma among US Caucasian young adults. J Invest Dermatol *128*, 2905-2908.

Raimondi, S., Sera, F., Gandini, S., Iodice, S., Caini, S., Maisonneuve, P., and Fargnoli, M.C. (2008). MC1R variants, melanoma and red hair color phenotype: a meta-analysis. Int J Cancer *122*, 2753-2760.

Renehan, A.G., Tyson, M., Egger, M., Heller, R.F., and Zwahlen, M. (2008). Body-mass index and incidence of cancer: a systematic review and meta-analysis of prospective observational studies. Lancet *371*, 569-578.

Rigel, D.S. (2010). Epidemiology of melanoma. Semin Cutan Med Surg *29*, 204-209.

Rouhani, P., Pinheiro, P.S., Sherman, R., Arheart, K., Fleming, L.E., Mackinnon, J., and Kirsner, R.S. (2010). Increasing rates of melanoma among nonwhites in Florida compared with the United States. Arch Dermatol *146*, 741-746.

Schernhammer, E.S., Razavi, P., Li, T.Y., Qureshi, A.A., and Han, J. (2011). Rotating Night Shifts and Risk of Skin Cancer in the Nurses' Health Study. J Natl Cancer Inst.

SEER. (website). SEER Stat Fact Sheets: Melanoma of the Skin, accessed 3/19/2011, available from: http://seer.cancer.gov/statfacts/html/melan.html.

Severi, G., Giles, G.G., Robertson, C., Boyle, P., and Autier, P. (2000). Mortality from cutaneous melanoma: evidence for contrasting trends between populations. Br J Cancer *82*, 1887-1891.

Singer, E. (2011). Cancer's Genome. In: Technology Review, Boston, MA: MIT.

Singh, A.D., Bergman, L., and Seregard, S. (2005). Uveal melanoma: epidemiologic aspects. Ophthalmol Clin North Am *18*, 75-84, viii.

Singh, A.D., De Potter, P., Fijal, B.A., Shields, C.L., Shields, J.A., and Elston, R.C. (1998). Lifetime prevalence of uveal melanoma in white patients with oculo(dermal) melanocytosis. Ophthalmology *105*, 195-198.

Siskind, V., Hughes, M.C., Palmer, J.M., Symmons, J.M., Aitken, J.F., Martin, N.G., Hayward, N.K., and Whiteman, D.C. (2011). Nevi, family history, and fair skin increase the risk of second primary melanoma. J Invest Dermatol *131*, 461-467.

Smalley, K.S. (2010). Understanding melanoma signaling networks as the basis for molecular targeted therapy. J Invest Dermatol *130*, 28-37.

Sober, A.J., and Wick, M.M. (1978). Levodopa therapy and malignant melanoma. JAMA *240*, 554-555.

Solit, D., and Sawyers, C.L. Drug discovery: How melanomas bypass new therapy. Nature *468*, 902-903.

Stahl, J.M., Sharma, A., Cheung, M., Zimmerman, M., Cheng, J.Q., Bosenberg, M.W., Kester, M., Sandirasegarane, L., and Robertson, G.P. (2004). Deregulated Akt3 activity promotes development of malignant melanoma. Cancer Res *64*, 7002-7010.

Stam-Posthuma, J.J., van Duinen, C., Scheffer, E., Vink, J., and Bergman, W. (2001). Multiple primary melanomas. J Am Acad Dermatol *44*, 22-27.

Stern, R.S. (2001). The risk of melanoma in association with long-term exposure to PUVA. J Am Acad Dermatol *44*, 755-761.

Stern, R.S., Nichols, K.T., and Vakeva, L.H. (1997). Malignant melanoma in patients treated for psoriasis with methoxsalen (psoralen) and ultraviolet A radiation (PUVA). The PUVA Follow-Up Study. N Engl J Med *336*, 1041-1045.

Swerdlow, A.J., English, J.S., and Qiao, Z. (1995). The risk of melanoma in patients with congenital nevi: a cohort study. J Am Acad Dermatol *32*, 595-599.

Swerlick, R.A., and Chen, S. (1996). The melanoma epidemic. Is increased surveillance the solution or the problem? Arch Dermatol *132*, 881-884.

Swerlick, R.A., and Chen, S. (1997). The melanoma epidemic: more apparent than real? Mayo Clin Proc *72*, 559-564.

Tas, F. (2011). Age-specific Incidence Ratios in Malignant Melanoma in Turkey: Melanoma in Older People is Increasing. Acta Derm Venereol.

Travis, L.B., Curtis, R.E., Boice, J.D., Jr., Hankey, B.F., and Fraumeni, J.F., Jr. (1991). Second cancers following non-Hodgkin's lymphoma. Cancer *67*, 2002-2009.

Travis, L.B., Curtis, R.E., Hankey, B.F., and Fraumeni, J.F., Jr. (1992). Second cancers in patients with chronic lymphocytic leukemia. J Natl Cancer Inst *84*, 1422-1427.

Tucker, M.A., Fraser, M.C., Goldstein, A.M., Elder, D.E., Guerry, D.t., and Organic, S.M. (1993). Risk of melanoma and other cancers in melanoma-prone families. J Invest Dermatol *100*, 350S-355S.

Tucker, M.A., Halpern, A., Holly, E.A., Hartge, P., Elder, D.E., Sagebiel, R.W., Guerry, D.t., and Clark, W.H., Jr. (1997). Clinically recognized dysplastic nevi. A central risk factor for cutaneous melanoma. JAMA *277*, 1439-1444.

Vagero, D., Swerdlow, A.J., and Beral, V. (1990). Occupation and malignant melanoma: a study based on cancer registration data in England and Wales and in Sweden. Br J Ind Med *47*, 317-324.

Valverde, P., Healy, E., Jackson, I., Rees, J.L., and Thody, A.J. (1995). Variants of the melanocyte-stimulating hormone receptor gene are associated with red hair and fair skin in humans. Nat Genet *11*, 328-330.

van der Esch, E.P., Muir, C.S., Nectoux, J., Macfarlane, G., Maisonneuve, P., Bharucha, H., Briggs, J., Cooke, R.A., Dempster, A.G., Essex, W.B., and et al. (1991). Temporal change in diagnostic criteria as a cause of the increase of malignant melanoma over time is unlikely. Int J Cancer *47*, 483-489.

Van Raamsdonk, C.D., Griewank, K.G., Crosby, M.B., Garrido, M.C., Vemula, S., Wiesner, T., Obenauf, A.C., Wackernagel, W., Green, G., Bouvier, N., Sozen, M.M., Baimukanova, G., Roy, R., Heguy, A., Dolgalev, I., Khanin, R., Busam, K., Speicher, M.R., O'Brien, J., and Bastian, B.C. (2010). Mutations in GNA11 in uveal melanoma. N Engl J Med *363*, 2191-2199.

Veierod, M.B., Weiderpass, E., Thorn, M., Hansson, J., Lund, E., Armstrong, B., and Adami, H.O. (2003). A prospective study of pigmentation, sun exposure, and risk of cutaneous malignant melanoma in women. J Natl Cancer Inst *95*, 1530-1538.

Welch, H.G., Woloshin, S., and Schwartz, L.M. (2005). Skin biopsy rates and incidence of melanoma: population based ecological study. BMJ *331*, 481.

WHO. (website). Ultraviolet Radiation and the INTERSUN Programme, vol. 2011: World Health Organization, accessed 3/19/2011, available from: http://www.who.int/uv/faq/skincancer/en/index1.html.

Zell, J.A., Cinar, P., Mobasher, M., Ziogas, A., Meyskens, F.L., Jr., and Anton-Culver, H. (2008). Survival for patients with invasive cutaneous melanoma among ethnic groups: the effects of socioeconomic status and treatment. J Clin Oncol *26*, 66-75.

Zhang, M., Qureshi, A.A., Guo, Q., and Han, J. (2011). Genetic variation in DNA repair pathway genes and melanoma risk. DNA Repair (Amst) *10*, 111-116.

Zuo, L., Weger, J., Yang, Q., Goldstein, A.M., Tucker, M.A., Walker, G.J., Hayward, N., and Dracopoli, N.C. (1996). Germline mutations in the p16INK4a binding domain of CDK4 in familial melanoma. Nat Genet *12*, 97-99.

Zwald, F.O., Christenson, L.J., Billingsley, E.M., Zeitouni, N.C., Ratner, D., Bordeaux, J., Patel, M.J., Brown, M.D., Proby, C.M., Euvrard, S., Otley, C.C., and Stasko, T. (2010). Melanoma in solid organ transplant recipients. Am J Transplant *10*, 1297-1304.

# 2

# Increasing Incidences of Cutaneous Malignant Melanoma by Region Around the World

Dianne E. Godar
*US Food and Drug Administration, Center for Devices and Radiological Health, Silver Spring, USA*

## 1. Introduction

For decades, cutaneous malignant melanoma (CMM) has been steadily increasing among indoor workers in industrialized countries around the world [Godar et al 2009; Godar submitted]. Scientists believe strong, intermittent UVB (290-320 nm) exposures, i.e., sunburn episodes, initiate CMM [Elwood et al 1985], and some believe the UVA (321-400 nm) passing through glass windows in offices and cars promotes it [Godar et al 2009]. In support of those possibilities exists the paradox between indoor and outdoor worker's UV exposures and their incidences of CMM. Although outdoor workers get three to ten times the annual UV doses that indoor workers get [Godar et al 2001; Godar 2005], they have similar or lower incidences of CMM [Gandini et al 2005; Kennedy et al 2003].

To understand what factor(s) may be responsible for the increasing incidence of CMM among indoor workers, we must know the temporal incidence by region around the world, especially by latitude [Godar, In press]. The causative agent of CMM is probably UVB-initiated sunburn episodes [Elwood et al 1985], but the promoting agent is unknown and may be UVA passing through office windows and cars [Godar et al 2009], and earlier (<1988) through UVB-absorbing sunscreens [Gorham et al 2007]. However, there could be a different promoting agent or an additional promoting agent; whatever the promoting agent(s) are, they must have entered and/or left our environment years before the first observed increase in Connecticut, USA in 1935 [EPA 1987; Rousch et al 1988].

We can analyze the CMM incidences of indoor working, industrialized populations over time and by latitudinal regions to get clues to the nature of the promoting agent(s). In this book chapter, we will explore the incidence of CMM all over the world during two decades, 1980 and 2000, by latitudinal regions of each fair-skinned continent: Europe, North America, and Australia (including New Zealand).

## 2. Analysis methods

We can obtain the CMM incidence data for Australia, New Zealand, USA, Canada, and Europe from the International Agency for Research on Cancer (IARC) [Doll et al 1966; Doll et al 1970; Waterhouse et al 1976; Waterhouse et al 1982; Muir et al 1987; Parkin et al 1992; Parkin et el 1997; Parkin et al 2002; Curado et al 2007].

We can average the CMM incidence data of IARC from the following regions for the years 1980 and 2000 to get mean latitudes or latitudinal ranges for each region in a country or continent:

1. Northern Europe (~65°N; range ~60-70°N) – Iceland, Norway, Sweden, and Finland,
2. Middle Europe (~55°N, <20°E; range ~50-60°N) – Ireland, Northern Ireland, Scotland, England, Denmark, the Netherlands, Belgium, and Germany, and either includes or excludes the following countries ≥20°E: Poland, Estonia, Latvia, Lithuania, and Belarus,
3. Southern Europe (~45°N; range 40-50°N) – France, Switzerland, Austria, Czech Republic, Slovakia, and Croatia, and either includes or excludes countries with predominately skin types ≥III: Portugal, Spain and Italy,
4. British Isles data from the year 2000 for the following regions (~53°N, range ~51-56°N): (~54.5°N) Scotland, Northern Ireland, Northern and Yorkshire, (~53.5°N) Ireland, North Western, Merseyside and Cheshire, Trent; (~52.5°N) West Midlands, East Anglia; (~51.5°N) South and Western, Oxford, and Thames,
5. Northernmost Canada and USA (~65°N; ~60-70°N) - Northwest Territories and Alaska,
6. Northern Canada (~55°N; range ~50-60°N) – British Columbia, Alberta, Saskatchewan, Manitoba, and Ontario,
7. Southern Canada (~45°N; range ~40-50°N)- Newfoundland and Quebec; Nova Scotia, New Brunswick, and Prince Edward's Island,
8. Northern USA (~45°N; range ~40-50°N) - Washington, Oregon, Idaho, Montana, Iowa, Wisconsin, Illinois, Indiana, Michigan, Ohio, Pennsylvania, District of Columbia, New Jersey, New York (excludes New York City), Vermont, Rhode Island, Massachusetts, and Maine (2000 yr data was not available for the other states: New Hampshire, Delaware, Maryland, North and South Dakota, Minnesota, Nebraska, Wyoming, and Nevada),
9. Southern USA (~35°N; range ~30-40°N) - California, Arizona, Utah, Colorado, New Mexico, Oklahoma, Texas, Missouri, Louisiana, Kentucky, Alabama, Georgia, South Carolina, Virginia, and Florida (2000 yr data was not available for the other states: Kansas, Arkansas, Mississippi, Tennessee, and North Carolina);
10. Southernmost USA (~20°N) - Hawaii,
11. Southern Hemisphere - Australia - (~19°S) Townsville, Queensland; (range ~20-29°S) Queensland, Western, (32°S) South; (range 30-39°S) New South Wales, Capital Territory, Victoria; (range <39°S) Tasmania and New Zealand
12. New Zealand 1980 regional plots - (~40.5°S; range 34.5-47°S) – (36°S) Northern, (38°S) Midland, (41°S) Central, and (44°S) Southern [regional values are from Bulliard et al 1994],

Figure 1 has averaged IARC data from numbers 1-3 above that either includes (circles) or excludes (squares) Eastern European and Southern European countries. Figure 2 has averaged IARC data from number 4 above. Figure 3 has averaged IARC data from numbers 5-10 above. Figure 4 has averaged IARC data from number 11 above. Figure 5 A and B have data from 12 above [Bulliard et al 1994].

## 3. Results

Figure 1 shows the incidences of CMM in the year 2000 for Europe. The values shown were averaged by latitudinal ranges ~40-50°N (~45°N), ~50-60°N (~55°N) and >60°N (~65°N). The lines with circles in the figure represent all the available European data. The lines with squares represent the European data with excluded Eastern European (≥20°E) countries from latitudes 50°N to 60°N, i.e., Poland, Estonia, Lithuania, Belarus, Lithuania and Latvia, and excluded southern European countries from latitudes ~40°N that have predominately people with skin type III or more, i.e., Spain, Portugal and Italy. Excluding the Eastern European countries and the Southern European countries did not change the trend. The data shows a flat incidence rate of CMM from about 40°N to 55°N and then an increasing incidence with increasing latitude above that.

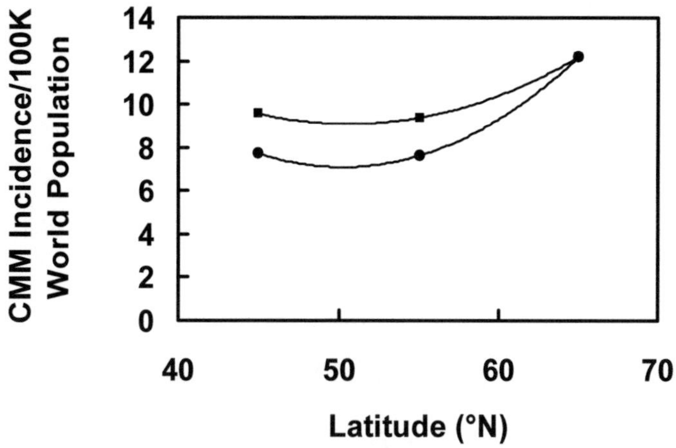


Fig. 1. The CMM incidences in the year 2000 for Europe averaged by latitudinal ranges ~40-50°N (~45°N), ~50-60°N (~55°N) and >60°N (~65°N). The circles include all the data (see the Analysis section), while the squares exclude the Eastern European countries from latitudes 50°N to 60°N, Poland, Estonia, Lithuania, Belarus, Lithuania and Latvia, and the countries with predominately skin types ≥III, i.e., Spain, Portugal and Italy.

Figure 2 shows the CMM incidences in the year 2000 for the British Isles: Ireland, Northern Ireland, Scotland and regions in England. A minimum appears to occur around 53.5°N.

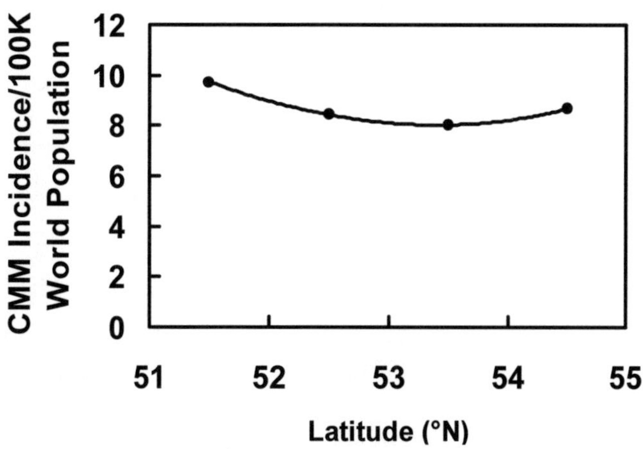


Fig. 2. The CMM incidences in the year 2000 for the British Isles: Ireland, Northern Ireland, Scotland and regions in England.

Figure 3 shows the CMM incidences in the year 2000 for North America: Canada and USA (includes Hawaii and Alaska). The CMM incidence decreases with increasing latitude and are unlike the Western European incidences that increase with increasing latitude above ~50°N.

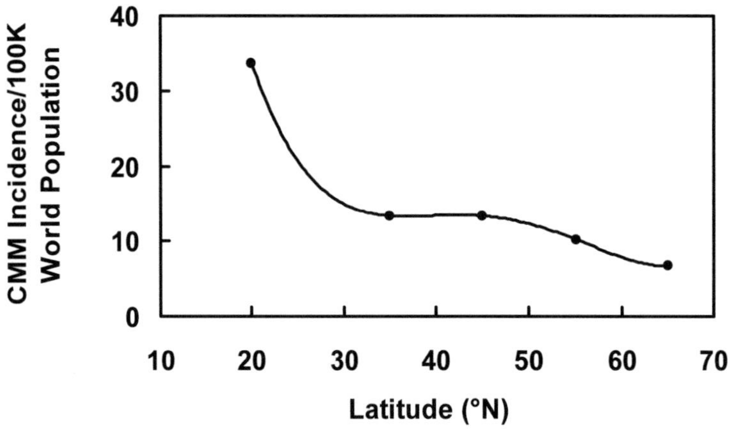


Fig. 3. The CMM incidences in the year 2000 for North America: Canada and USA (includes Hawaii and Alaska).

Figure 4 shows the CMM incidences in the years 1980 and 2000 for Australia by latitude. The CMM incidence decreases with increasing latitude until ~35°S where it appears to increase somewhat with increasing latitude in 2000.

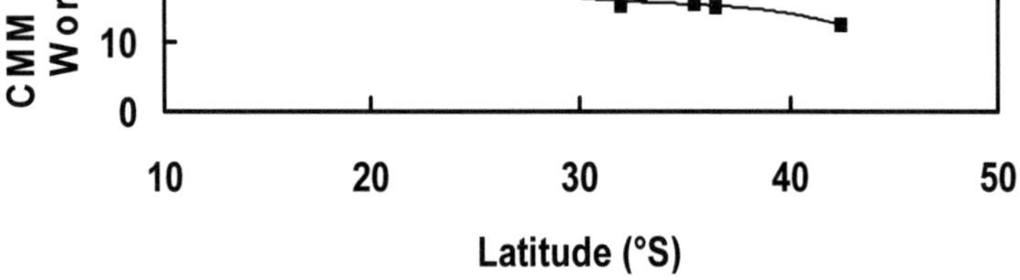


Fig. 4. The CMM incidences in the years 1980 and 2000 for Australia by latitude.

Figure 5A shows an exponential increasing incidence of CMM with latitude in the southern hemisphere. New Zealand by region (1980): Northern (36°S), Midland (38°S), Central (41°S), and Southern (44°N). Figure 5B shows the temporal exponential increase in the incidence of CMM from 1970 to 1985 in the different regions of New Zealand by latitude. There is an exponential increase in the incidence of CMM with increasing latitude and an exponential increase in the incidence of CMM over time as well.

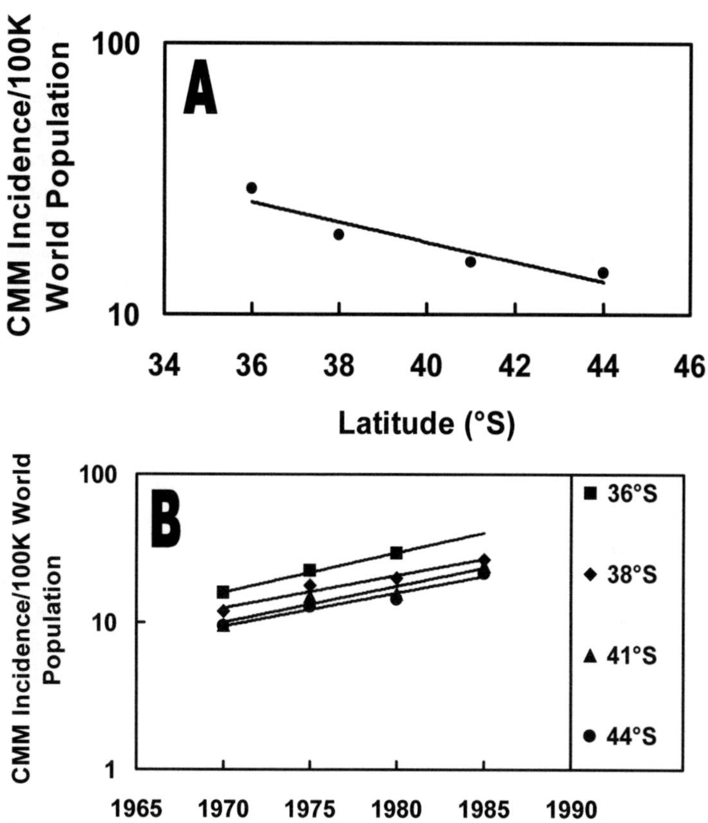


Fig. 5. **A)** Exponential increasing incidence of CMM with latitude in the southern hemisphere. New Zealand (1980) by region: Northern (36°S), Midland (38°S), Central (41°S), and Southern (44°N). **B)** The temporal exponential increase in the incidence of CMM from 1970 to 1985 in different regions of New Zealand by latitude.

## 4. Discussion

The incidences of CMM in fair-skinned, indoor-working people have been steadily increasing in industrialized nations worldwide for decades (Godar et al 2009; Godar submitted). The regions of the world with the lowest CMM incidences are in Southern and Middle Europe ~40-60°N whether or not Eastern and Southern European countries are included or excluded from the analysis (Figure 1). However, regional data for the British Isles begins to show an increasing incidence with increasing latitude around 53.5°N (Figure 2).

That trend is counterintuitive because the amount of UVB present in the terrestrial spectrum decreases with increasing latitude, suggesting something else must be increasing the incidence of CMM with increasing latitude. Separate analysis of the data for the Eastern European countries, Poland, Estonia, Latvia, Lithuania including Saint Petersburg, Russia, gives an incidence of 4.73 (4.82 if Russia is excluded) half the value of Western European countries, which may be due to socio-economic status and/or vacation choices. In North America, there is clearly an increasing incidence of CMM with decreasing latitude (Figure

3); one does not observe the same trend as seen in Europe where an inversion in the incidence of CMM occurs near 53°N. Unlike Europe, the trend in North America continues to decrease with increasing latitude. This may be due to a cultural difference between Northern Europeans and Northern Canadians and Alaskans because we know Northern Europeans tend to take extended vacations at lower latitudes, e.g., Mediterranean. At lower latitudes, they can get sunburned to initiate CMM and then return to their country above 50°N, where there is more UVA relative to UVB, to promote CMM growth the rest of the year. We obtain a clue that vacation choice might be responsible by analyzing the southern Hemisphere data for the years 1980 and 2000 (Figure 4), where during 1980 we see a similar trend as observed in North America in the year 2000, but the trend changes to what we see in Europe in the year 2000. This upward change in the CMM trend for the lower latitudinal regions may be due to increased air travel over the decades leading to more people vacationing closer to the sunny equator. In 1980, New Zealanders displayed an exponential increasing incidence of CMM with increasing latitude (Figure 5A) that increased exponentially over time (Figure 5B). However, the temporal exponential increase with latitude is not only true of New Zealand but is also true for some other countries and regions around the world.

Whether the incidence of CMM is increasing exponentially or not does not change the fact that it is increasing at an alarming rate each year. In order to slow or stop this increasing trend, we must know what is causing it and, if possible, change it. We know whatever started the increasing incidence of CMM either entered or left our environment before 1935, because that is when we have documented data for the first increases in CMM in the USA (Godar et al 2009; Godar In Press). From that data, we know that nothing that came out after the increasing CMM trend began can be responsible for starting it. For example, fluorescent lights (~1938 (http://wweu.wikipedia.org/wiki/Fluorescent_lamp), sunscreens (early 1950's for UVB absorbing and in 1988 for UVA and UVB absorbing; http://en.wikipedia.org/wiki/Sunscreen), and tanning devices (~1978; http://en.wikipedia.org/wiki/Tanning_bed#History) all entered our environment *after* the increasing incidence of CMM was first documented in the USA back in 1935 [EPA, 1987; Rousch et al 1988]. Thus, we should analyze what happened *before* 1935, during the early 20$^{th}$ century, in order to discover what might have affected the incidence of CMM.

During the early 20$^{th}$ century, people in industrialized countries went against evolution by working indoors during the day. That action alone drastically decreased their daily amount of cutaneous vitamin $D_3$ and simultaneously exposed them to only UVA radiation passing through glass windows in offices [Godar et al 2009] and cars [Moehrle et al 2003]. People created an artificial UV barrier with window glass that divides the UVB from the UVA, so that the vitamin D-making UVB wavelengths [MacLaughlin et al, 1982] were excluded while only the vitamin D-breaking [Webb et al 1989] and DNA-mutating UVA wavelengths [Peak and Peak 1991; Jones et al 1987; Halliday et al 2005] were included in our indoor-working environment. Possibly because this unnatural UV environment existed for decades in buildings and later in cars [Moehrle et al 2003], CMM was promoted by UVA, after being initiated by UVB sunburns, and began to steadily increase in the mid-1930's or before.

We also know the ratio of UVA to UVB increases with increasing latitude and that CMM increases with latitude above ~53°N. Evidently, people who live above 50°N go to the beach during the summer and get sunburned at lower latitudes, where they are unfamiliar with the sun's intensity, to initiate CMM, and then they return home to northern latitudes that have primarily UVA for most of the year (inside as well as outside) to promote CMM. The higher latitudes also allows the sun to aim more often at a perpendicular angle to the window glass where more UVA can pass through and directly expose people's skin during their workday[Pope and Godar 2010]. Furthermore, above ~50°N there is little UVB to make cutaneous vitamin $D_3$ most of the year [Webb et al 1988]. Above 37° N, a vitamin $D_3$ "winter" occurs from at least November to February, which extends to October and March at higher latitudes, when the dose-rate of UVB is too low to make any previtamin $D_3$. In contrast, UVB exposure during peak hours occurs to some extent to outdoor workers during their workweek, so that they can maintain adequate levels of vitamin $D_3$ in their skin and blood for most of the year. The blood levels of vitamin D (measured as 25-hydroxyvitamin D in serum) in outdoor workers who get about five times the solar UV dose that indoor workers get is about twice as high as indoor workers [Devgun et al 1981]. Increased cutaneous vitamin D levels, and natural exposure to UVA and UVB together, might explain why outdoor workers have a lower incidence of CMM compared to indoor workers, although they get 3-10 times more UV exposure.

The reason vitamin $D_3$ is important for controlling CMM is because most melanoma cells can directly convert it to the hormone calcitriol [Reichrath et al 2007]. Calcitriol controls the growth rate [Eisman et al 1987; Colston et al 1981; Frampton et al 1983] and apoptotic cell death [Danielson et al 1998] of melanoma cells, while it also affects the immune system [Yang et al 1993a, b] and inhibits tumor promotion [Chida et al 1985]. Increased blood levels of vitamin D might be responsible for increasing the survival of melanoma patients who get regular, moderate sun exposures [Berwick et al 2005; Newton-Bishop et al 2011]. Thus, intermittent, strong UVB-induced sunburns may initiate CMM, while low cutaneous vitamin D levels and UVA-induced DNA damage may promote CMM.

## 5. Conclusions

The incidence of CMM is increasing at an alarming rate around the world in indoor working industrialized populations. In most regions of the world, the CMM incidence decreases with increasing latitude. However, in Europe the incidence appears flat up to ~50°N where it begins to increase with increasing latitude. This may occur because there is more UVA relative to UVB for most of the year at higher latitudes. Windows that allow UVA to enter our vitamin D-deprived indoor-working environments and cars may be partly responsible for the increasing incidence of CMM. If this is true, we can lower the incidence or the rate of increase by simply placing UV filters on our office and car windows to help reduce CMM worldwide.

## 6. References

Berwick M, Armstrong BK, Ben-Porat L, Fine J, Kricker A, Eberle C, Barnhill R. Sun exposure and mortality from melanoma. JNCI 2005;97:195-199.

Bulliard JL, Cox B, Elwood JM. 1994. Latitude gradients in melanoma incidence and mortality in the non-Maori population of New Zealand. Cancer Causes Control. 5:234-240.

Chida K, Hashiba H, Fukushima M, Suda T, Kuroki T. Inhibition of tumor promotion in mouse skin by 1 alpha, 25-dihydroxyvitamin $D_3$. J Cancer Res 1985;45:5426-5430.

Colston K, Colston MJ, Feldman D. 1,25-dihydroxyvitamin $D_3$ and malignant melanoma: the presence of receptors and inhibition of cell growth in culture. Endocrinol 1981;108: 1083-1086.

Curado. M. P., Edwards, B., Shin. H.R., Storm. H., Ferlay. J., Heanue. M. and Boyle. P., eds (2007) Cancer Incidence in Five Continents, Vol. IX IARC Scientific Publications No. 160, Lyon, IARC.

Danielsson C, Fehsel K, Polly P, Carlberg C. Differential apoptotic response of human melanoma cells to 1α,25-dihydroxyvitamin $D_3$ and its analogues. Cell Death Different 1998;5:946-951.

Devgun MS, Paterson CR, Johnson BE, Cohen C. 1981. Vitamin D nutrition in relation to season and occupation. Am J Clin Nutr 34:1501-1504.

Doll, R.,Payne, P.,Waterhouse, J.A.H., eds (1966) Cancer Incidence in Five Continents, Vol. I Union Internationale Contre le Cancer, Geneva

Doll, R.,Muir, C.S.,Waterhouse, J.A.H., eds (1970) Cancer Incidence in Five Continents, Vol. II Union Internationale Contre le Cancer, Geneva

Elwood JM, Gallagher RP, Hill GB, Pearson JCG. Cutaneous melanoma in relation to intermittent and constant sun exposure - The Western Canada Melanoma Study. Br J Cancer 1985;35:427-433.

Eisman JA, Barkla DH, Tutton PJ. Suppression of *in vivo* growth of human cancer solid tumor xenografts by 1,25-dihydroxyvitamin $D_3$. Cancer Res 1987;47:21-25.

Environmental protection agency. Ultraviolet radiation and Melanoma Vol. IV: Appendix A - Assessing the risks of stratospheric ozone depletion. US EPA 400/1-87/001D Dec. 1987. Table 4-1, p. 4-2.

Frampton RJ, Omond SA, Eisman JA. Inhibition of human cancer growth by 1,25-dihydroxyvitamin $D_3$ metabolites. Cancer Res 1983;43:4443-4447.

Gandini S, Sera F, Cattaruza MS, Pasquini P, Picconi O, Boyle P, et al. 2005. Meta-analysis of risk factors for cutaneous melanoma: II. Sun exposure. Eur J Cancer 41:45-60.

Godar DE, Landry RJ, Lucas AD. 2009. Increased UVA exposures and decreased cutaneous Vitamin D(3) levels may be responsible for the increasing incidence of melanoma. Med Hypotheses 72:434-443.

Godar DE, Wengraitis SP, Shreffler J, Sliney DH. 2001. UV doses of Americans. Photochem Photobiol 73:621-629.

Godar DE. 2005. UV Doses Worldwide. Photochem Photobiol 81:736-749.

Godar DE . In press. Worldwide Increasing Incidences of Cutaneous Malignant Melanoma. J. Skin Cancer.

Godar DE. Increasing Incidences of Cutaneous Malignant Melanoma in European Countries: Does UVA Initiate or Promote Melanoma? Submitted to Photochem. Photobiol. Sci.

Gorham ED, Mohr SB, Garland CF, Chaplin G, Garland FC. 2007. Do sunscreens increase risk of melanoma in populations residing at higher latitudes? Ann Epidemiol 17:956-963.

Halliday GM, Agar NS, Barnetson RS, Ananthaswamy HN, Jones AM. UV-A Fingerprint mutations in human skin cancer. Photochem Photobiol 2005;81:3-8.

Jones CA, Huberman E, Cunningham ML, Peak MJ. Mutagenesis and cytotoxicity in human epithelial cells by far- and near-ultraviolet radiations: action spectrum. Radiat Res 1987;110:244-254.

Kennedy C, Bajdik CD, Willemze R, De Gruijl FR, Bouwes Bavinck JN. 2003. The influence of painful sunburns and lifetime sun exposure on the risk of actinic keratoses, seborrheic warts, melanocytic nevi, atypical nevi, and skin cancer. J Invest Dermatol 120:1087-1093.

MacLaughlin J A, Anderson RR, Holick MF. Spectral character of sunlight modulates photosynthesis of previtamin $D_3$ and its photoisomers in human skin. Science 1982;216:1001-1003.

Moehrle M, Soballa M, Korn M. UV exposure in cars. Photodermatol Photoimmunol Photomed 2003;19:175-181.

Muir, C.S.,Waterhouse, J.,Mack, T.,Powell, J.,Whelan, S.L., eds (1987) Cancer Incidence in Five Continents, Vol. V IARC Scientific Publications No. 88, Lyon, IARC

Newton-Bishop JA, Chang YM, Elliott F, Chan M, Leake S, Karpavicius B, Haynes S, Fitzgibbon E, Kukalizch K, Randerson-Moor J, Elder DE, Bishop DT, Barrett JH. 2011. Relationship between sun exposure and melanoma risk for tumours in different body sites in a large case-control study in a temperate climate. Eur J Cancer. 47:732-741.

Parkin, D.M.,Muir, C.S.,Whelan, S.L.,Gao, Y.-T.,Ferlay, J.,Powell, J., eds (1992) Cancer Incidence in Five Continents, Vol. VI IARC Scientific Publications No. 120, Lyon, IARC

Parkin, D.M., Whelan, S.L., Ferlay, J., Raymond, L., and Young, J., eds (1997) Cancer Incidence in Five Continents, Vol. VII IARC Scientific Publications No. 143, Lyon, IARC.

Parkin, D.M., Whelan, S.L., Ferlay, J., Teppo, L., and Thomas, D.B., eds (2002) Cancer Incidence in Five Continents, Vol. VIII IARC Scientific Publications No. 155, Lyon, IARC.

Peak JG, Peak MJ. Comparison of initial yields of DNA-to-protein crosslinks and single-strand breaks induced in cultured human cells by far- and near-ultraviolet light, blue light and X-rays. Mutat Res 1991;246:187-191.

Pope SJ, Godar DE. (2010) Solar UV geometric conversion factors: horizontal plane to cylinder model. Photochem Photobiol. 86:457-466.

Reichrath J, Rech M, Moeini M, Meese E, Tilgen W, Seifert M. 2007. In vitro comparison of the vitamin D endocrine system in 1,25(OH)2D3-responsive and -resistant melanoma cells. Cancer Biol Ther 6:48-55

Roush GC, Schymura MJ, Holford TR. 1988. Patterns of invasive melanoma in the Connecticut Tumor Registry. Is the long-term increase real? Cancer 61: 2586-2595.

Seifert M, Diesel B, Meese E, Tilgen W, Reichrath J. Expression of 25-hydroxyvitamin D-1alpha-hydroxylase in malignant melanoma: implications for growth control via local synthesis of 1,25(OH)D and detection of multiple splice variants. Exp Dermatol 2005;14:153-154.

Waterhouse, J.,Muir, C.S.,Correa, P.,Powell, J., eds (1976) Cancer Incidence in Five Continents, Vol. III IARC Scientific Publications No. 15, Lyon, IARC.

Waterhouse, J.,Muir, C.S.,Shanmugaratnam, K.,Powell, J., eds (1982) Cancer Incidence in Five Continents, Vol. IV IARC Scientific Publications No. 42, Lyon, IARC.

Webb AR, deCosta BR, Holick MF. Sunlight regulates the cutaneous production of vitamin $D_3$ by causing its photodegradation. J Clin Endocrinol Metab 1989;68:882-887.

Webb AR, Kline L, Holick MF. Influence of season and latitude on the cutaneous synthesis of vitamin $D_3$: exposure to winter sunlight in Boston and Edmonton will not promote vitamin $D_3$ synthesis in human skin. J Clin Endocrinol Metab 1988;67:373-378.

Yang S, Smith C, DeLuca HF. 1 α, 25-dihydroxyvitmain $D_3$ and 19-nor-1 α, 25-dihydroxyvitmain $D_3$ suppress immunoglobulin production and thymic lymphocyte proliferation *in vivo*. Biochem Biophys Acta 1993a;1158:279-286.

Yang S, Smith C, Prahl JM, Luo X, DeLuca HF. Vitamin D deficiency suppresses cell-mediated immunity *in vivo*. Arch Biochem Biophys Acta 1993b;303:98-106.

3

# Skin Pigmentation and Melanoma Risk

John A. D'Orazio, Amanda Marsch, James Lagrew and W. Brooke Veith
*University of Kentucky College of Medicine, Markey Cancer Center, Graduate Center for Toxicology and the Departments of Pediatrics and of Molecular and Biomedical Pharmacology, Lexington, KY, USA*

## 1. Introduction

Malignant melanoma of the skin ranks as the number one cause of death from skin cancers. Affecting over 125,000 people worldwide and nearly 70,000 persons annually in the United States alone (Linos et al., 2009), melanoma incidence has been increasing steadily over the last several decades (Erickson and Driscoll, 2010). According to the World Health Organization, approximately 20,000 people worldwide die from melanoma each year. One of the most striking clinical aspects of melanoma is the profound difference in incidence between persons of fair and dark skin complexions (Garbe and Leiter, 2009). Deposition of UV-blocking melanin pigment in the epidermis accounts for much of the protection realized by persons of dark skin complexion, however risk for melanoma does not simply correlate with amount of melanin in the skin. There is now ample evidence that suggests that pheomelanin, the red/blonde sulfated melanin pigment expressed in persons of light complexion may promote UV-mediated oxidative damage to melanocytes and thus contribute to carcinogenesis (Kvam and Tyrrell, 1999; Kadekaro et al., 2006; Abdel-Malek et al., 2008; Smit et al., 2008). In addition, as many as a third of melanomas arise from areas of the skin not generally exposed to UV light, suggesting that UV-induced mutagenesis only partly accounts for melanoma susceptibility. Recent work has shown a link between some of the genes involved in the control of pigmentation and other cancer-relevant processes. In particular, we and others are interested in the melanocortin 1 receptor (MC1R) signaling pathway in melanocytes which determines not only melanoma risk but also the efficiency by which an individual can adaptively tan and repair UV-induced photolesions after UV exposure. Data are now emerging that link this signaling pathway with the DNA repair pathway responsible for clearing UV-induced photodamage from the skin (Kadekaro et al., 2005; Hauser et al., 2006; Robinson et al., 2010). In this chapter, we review the link between melanoma and skin complexion, focusing on the genes that control innate and adaptive skin pigmentation and the mechanisms by which pigmentation differences may account for melanoma risk.

## 2. Melanoma - A growing problem

According to the World Health Organization, about 132,000 people will be diagnosed with malignant melanoma of the skin each year. Mainly a disease of fair-skinned individuals, it is most prevalent in Western nations in which the majority of the population has descended from Northern European ancestry (Tucker, 2009; Rigel, 2010). In the United States, for example, malignant melanoma of the skin currently ranks in the top ten most commonly diagnosed cancers of either men or of women. In 2010, for example, it is estimated that 68,130 individuals (38,870 men and 29,260 women) were diagnosed with the disease and that it claimed the lives of 8,700 people (Croyle, 2011). Melanoma ranks as the second most common cancer in women between the ages of 20 and 35, and represents the leading cause of cancer death in women ages 25 to 30. The melanoma burden is predictably largest in countries with large populations of fair skinned individuals living in sunny climates including the United States, Australia, New Zealand and Europe (Marks, 2000). Worldwide, Australia reports the highest incidences of melanoma (on the order of 40-60 cases per 100,000 individuals) due most likely to their geographic proximity to the equator and the high proportion of their population being fair-skinned immigrants from Europe (Lens and Dawes, 2004).

Race is the primary risk factor for developing melanoma, with fair-skinned races at greater risk than darker-skinned races. For example, fair-skinned Americans are 20 times more likely to develop melanoma than their dark-skinned counterparts (Fig. 1). Ultraviolet radiation in the form of natural sun exposure and, more recently, artificial UV from tanning salons, is also a clear risk factor for melanoma (Linos et al., 2009). The presence of melanin in the skin is thought to explain much of the racial predilection of the disease, with less pigmented individuals having skin of a more UV-permeable nature (Veierod et al., 2010). Because more UV radiation can penetrate the skin, fair-skinned individuals accrue more cancer-causing UV-induced mutations when compared with highly pigmented individuals.

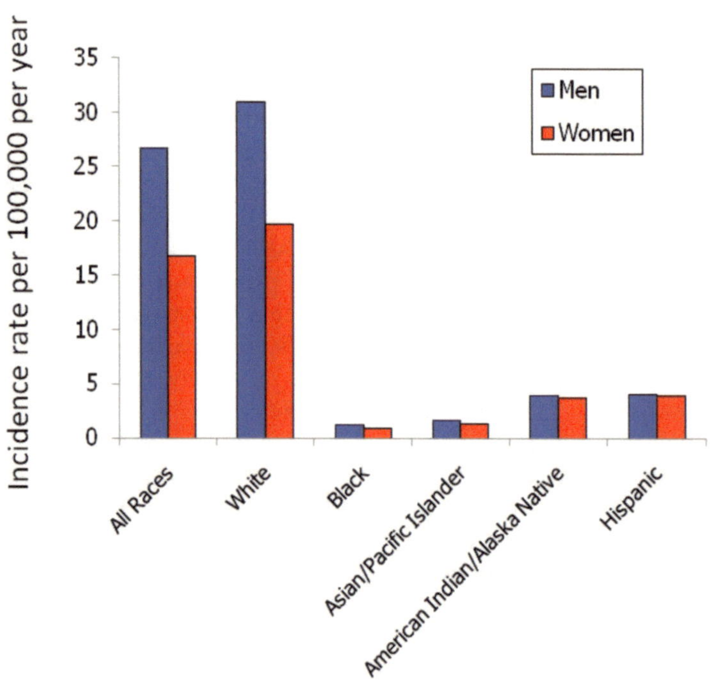


Fig. 1. Incidence of Melanoma by Race in the United States of America, 2004-2008. Note that the disease is much more prevalent among fair-skinned persons (Croyle, 2011).

Nonetheless, melanoma can afflict even the darkest individuals, and there are data to suggest that the disease tends to be diagnosed at a more advanced stage and is therefore associated with a worse prognosis in such persons (Fleming et al., 1975; Halder and Bridgeman-Shah, 1995; Bradford, 2009). Despite advances in many areas of cancer detection and treatment, melanoma incidence and mortality have been rising for the past several decades (Berwick and Wiggins, 2006). The lifetime risk of an American developing melanoma has increased from one in 1500 in 1935 to currently about one in 50 (Fig. 2) (Croyle, 2011). According to the American Cancer Society (ACS), the incidence rate for melanoma has more than doubled since 1973 alone, increasing at annual rate on the order of 3-7% (Fig. 3) (American Cancer Society, 2011). The reason(s) for this alarming increase remain controversial and are likely multifactorial, however, it cannot be argued that melanoma's increasing incidence and high rate of metastatic disease present a legitimate public health problem (Markovic et al., 2007).

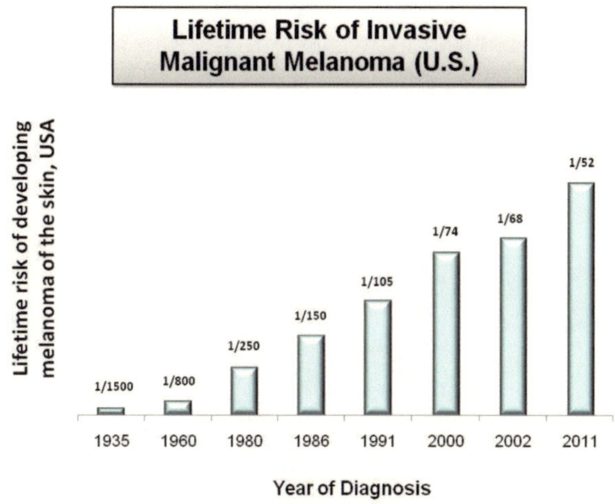


Fig. 2. U.S. Lifetime melanoma risk, 1935 - 2011 (Lens and Dawes, 2004).

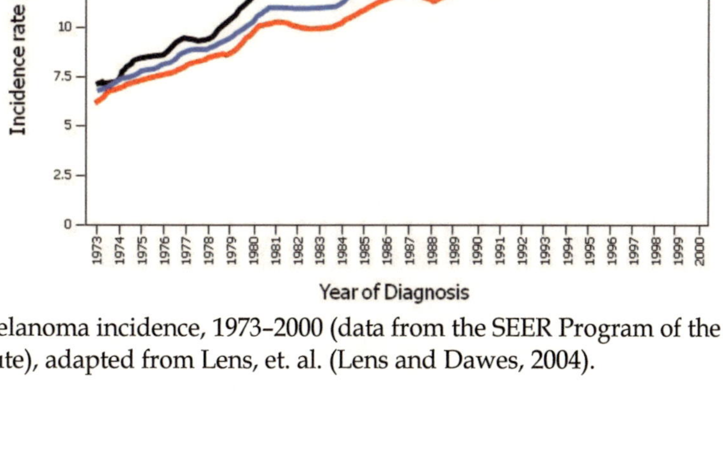


Fig. 3. U.S. Melanoma incidence, 1973–2000 (data from the SEER Program of the National Cancer Institute), adapted from Lens, et. al. (Lens and Dawes, 2004).

## 3. Risk factors

Risk factors for melanoma include both inherited and environmental variables (Cho et al., 2005). Understanding their interaction and relative impact is crucial to optimizing clinical practice and public health efforts.

### 3.1 Age

According to the most recent Surveillance Epidemiology and End Results (SEER) data from the National Cancer Institute (NCI) based on data collected between 2004-2008, the average age at which new patients were diagnosed with melanoma was 60 years (Dennis, 1999; Croyle, 2011). In fact, more than half of all new melanoma diagnoses are made in persons older than 45 years of age (Fig. 4). It should be noted, however, that melanoma can strike persons of any age, and it has been increasingly diagnosed in children and young adults (Cust et al., 2011). The reason(s) why melanoma incidence increases with age are not clearly understood, but may reflect the typical long latency required for accumulation of sufficient mutations caused by environmental factors (in this case UV radiation) to result in carcinogenesis (Liu and Soong, 1996).

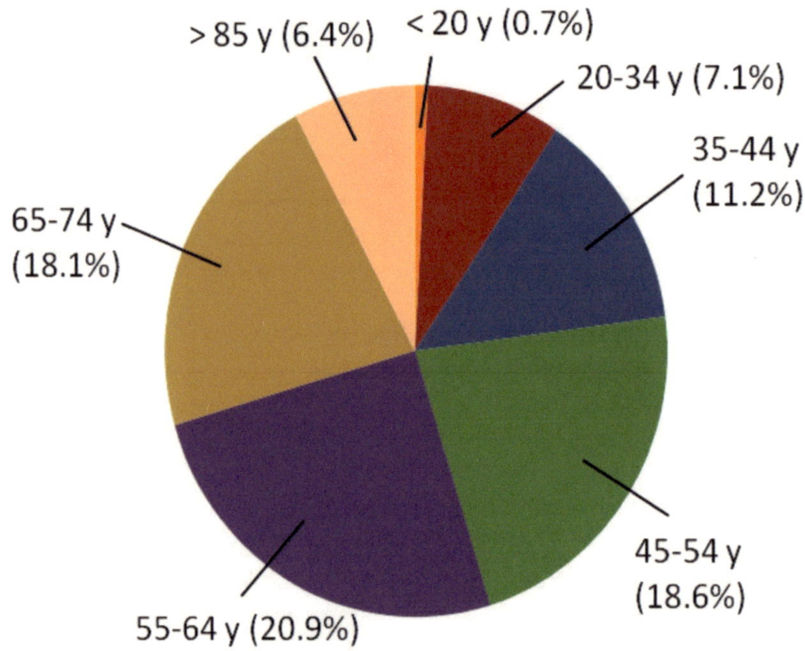


Fig. 4. Age at diagnosis, US Melanoma cases, 2004-2008 (SEER data, NCI).

### 3.2 UV radiation

Though many factors predict melanoma risk (Table 1), UV radiation, in the form of ambient sunlight and artificial UV sources such as tanning beds (Lim et al., 2011) is among the most important. Strong epidemiologic evidence clearly links UV exposure, particularly blistering sunburns early in life, with subsequent melanoma development (MacKie and Aitchison, 1982; Gandini et al., 2005). However, in contrast to squamous cell carcinomas (SCC) and basal cell carcinomas (BCC) which are thought to arise from keratinocytes rather than melanocytes (Leiter and Garbe, 2008), the mechanism of UV-mediated carcinogenesis of melanocytes is not well-characterized. In keratinocyte malignancies, characteristic "UV-signature" transitional mutations between thymidine and cytosine residues are frequently noted in relevant cancer-specific genes such as p53 (Giglia-Mari and Sarasin, 2003); such changes are not typical in melanoma isolates. Nonetheless, most melanomas occur in UV-exposed anatomic locations, and melanoma incidence correlates geographically with doseage of ambient UV. It has been suggested that the mechanism of UV-mediated carcinogenesis in melanocytes may differ fundamentally from that in keratinocytes, possibly mediated by free radicals and oxidative species (Autier et al., 2011), however this has not yet been definitively proven. Because UV is composed of different subtypes (e.g. UV-A, -B and –C) and each are capable of inducing different cellular and DNA damage, the exact wavelengths and mechanisms whereby UVR contributes to the development of melanoma are not clear (Seo and Fisher, 2010). Different exposure patterns appear to predict different cutaneous malignancies (Rass and Reichrath, 2008). Intermittent intense sun exposure such as that received by a fair-skinned vacationer in a sunny environment imparts a significant increase in risk for developing melanoma (Molho-Pessach and Lotem, 2007) whereas chronic sun exposure, typically through occupational or recreational exposure, seems more relevant to keratinocyte malignancies (Gandini et al., 2005). In one study, a history of sunburn at any age, used as a surrogate for periods of intense exposure, conferred a relative risk of melanoma of 2.03 (Tucker, 2009). Serial sunburns across childhood, adolescence, and adulthood result in a dose-dependent increase in risk for melanoma (Dennis et al., 2008).

In 1988, 1% of Americans used a tanning bed. By 2007, that number increased to 27% (Fisher and James, 2010). There are currently roughly 25,000 indoor tanning facilities in the United States alone. The tanning industry represents a multi-billion dollar industry that employs more than 150,00 people and that actively seeks to dispel information linking tanning bed use with skin cancer risk (Fisher and James, 2010). Nonetheless, the UV energy emitted by tanning beds is usually anywhere from two-to ten-fold more intense than direct sunlight, and currently there is no mechanistic way to "get a tan" without assuming the mutagenic risk of UV radiation and the subsequent risk of malignancy. In fact, the profound rise in tanning bed use over the last several years may account for a significant fraction of increased melanoma incidence, particularly among young women. Persons who have ever used a tanning device have a 50% increased risk of BCC and more than a 100% increased risk of SCC (Karagas et al., 2002). Tanning bed use also clearly increases melanoma risk, as determined by at a number of separate clinical studies (Walter et al., 1990; Westerdahl et al., 1994; Chen et al., 1998; Schulman and Fisher, 2009; Lazovich et al., 2010; Mogensen and Jemec, 2010). Together, such meta-analyses suggest that regular use of tanning beds triples or quadruples the risk of developing melanoma, and that first exposure to indoor tanning before 35 years of age raises lifetime risk of melanoma by 75% (Fisher and James, 2010).

Cutaneous UV injury produces both direct and indirect DNA damage, and each can result in accumulation of mutations in skin cells. Direct damage occurs when DNA absorbs UV photons, and undergoes cleavage of the 5-6 double bond of pyrimidines. When two adjacent pyrimidines undergo this 5-6 double bond opening, a covalent ring structure referred to as a cyclobutane pyrimidine dimer (thymine dimer) can be formed.

| | |
|---|---|
| • Age | The incidence of melanoma increases dramatically with age. |
| • Sun exposure | Occupational or recreational UV exposure, living in UV-rich geographies (e.g. equatorial locations), living at altitude. |
| • Tanning bed use | First exposure to indoor tanning before 35 years of age raises lifetime risk of melanoma by 75% |
| • Fair skin complexion | Deficiency of the highly UV-protective eumelanin epidermal pigment allows more UV to penetrate into the skin and promote mutagenesis. |
| • Chronic exposure to heavy metals | Chromium, cobalt and other metals may promote oxidative mutagenesis in melanocytes. |
| • Poor ability to tan | A propensity to burn rather than tan after sun exposure correlates with increased melanoma risk. |
| • History of sunburn | One or more severe blistering sunburns as a child or teenager increases risk |
| • Personal history of melanoma | Once a person has been diagnosed with a melanoma, their risk for others is heightened. Up to 10% of melanoma patients will develop a second melanoma in their lifetime. |
| • Family history of melanoma | Inherited CDKN2A defects (the gene that encodes the p16INK4A and p14ARF tumor suppressors) are associated with familial melanoma |
| • Having a large number of moles (nevi) | Many melanomas appear to arise from pre-existing moles. Benign nevi and melanoma both frequently exhibit gain-of-function mutation in the B-Raf gene. |
| • Immune suppression | Immunosuppressive therapies, for example, as used to prevent rejection of solid organs in transplant recipients, are associated with melanoma. |
| • DNA repair deficiency | Xeroderma pigmentosum (XP) patients who lack one of at least eight enzymes in a common nucleotide excision repair (NER) pathway have a 2,000-fold increased risk of skin cancers, including melanoma. |

Table 1. Melanoma Risk Factors

Alternatively, a pyrimidine 6-4 pyrimidone (6,4)- photoproduct can result when a 5-6 double bond in a pyrimidine opens and reacts with the exocyclic moiety of the adjacent 3' pyrimidine to form a covalent 6-4 linkage (Sarasin, 1999). One day's worth of sun exposure can cause up to 100,000 potentially mutagenic UV-induced photolesions in each skin cell, and UV radiation can also damage cells by free radical formation and oxidative stress (Hoeijmakers, 2009). Oxidative DNA lesions are also mutagenic and form after UV-induced free radical attack (Meyskens et al., 2001). One particularly well-characterized oxidative lesion is 7,8-dihydro-8-oxoguanine (8-oxoguanine; 8-OH-dG), which promotes mutagenesis since this guanine derivative can pair equally well with cytosine (normal pairing) and adenine (abnormal) and consequently cause GC-TA transversion mutations (Schulz et al., 2000). Interestingly, although the cutaneous inflammatory response to solar radiation (sunburn) is clearly caused by the UVB component of solar radiation, it is the UVA component (which actually represents about 95% of ambient sunlight) that penetrates most deeply into the skin. Each has been implicated in skin cancer/melanoma formation. UV energy in the UVA range (roughly 315-400 nm) promotes mainly oxidative damage to DNA (e.g. 8-oxo-guanine formation) although photodimers can result from UVA exposure as well (Cadet et al., 2005). UVB photons (290-320 nm) mainly result in thymine dimer formation but can also cause (6,4)-photoproducts and oxidative adducts to form. Each of the DNA changes caused by UV radiation is potentially mutagenic and actively repaired by cells. Thus, carcinogenesis that results from UV exposure (e.g. melanoma) is influenced not only by the amount of environmental UV exposure but also by the degree to which damage can be repaired.

The mechanism of UV-mediated carcinogenesis for keratinocyte malignancies seems to correlate with direct UV-induced DNA damage (e.g. cyclobutane dimers) because more than half of basal cell and squamous cell carcinomas are found to have signature "UV mutations" in cancer-associated genes like p53 (de Gruijl et al., 2001; Cleaver and Crowley, 2002; Bolshakov et al., 2003). However, in primary human melanoma samples, such C-T transition mutations have not been found with any degree of frequency in known cancer-related genes (Lacour, 2002; Greenman et al., 2007; Rass and Reichrath, 2008). Thus, although UV exposure is clearly linked with melanoma incidence, the actual molecular mechanism of carcinogenesis is unclear. Many groups have hypothesized that UV-induced free radicals and subsequent oxidative damage may be relevant carcinogenic events in melanocytes (Kvam and Tyrrell, 1997; Runger, 1999; Larsson et al., 2005; Runger and Kappes, 2008).

### 3.3 Heavy metal exposure

There is growing interest in the contribution of heavy metals (such as chromium and cobalt) to melanoma risk. Epidemiologic studies of cohorts exposed either occupationally or through joint-replacement (in patients with metal-on-metal hip arthroplasties) to to redox-active heavy metals suggest that such exposure may be a risk factor for melanoma (Meyskens and Berwick, 2008). Through fenton chemistry, heavy metals may contribute independently and in conjunction with UV (particularly UVA) to free radical formation in melanocytes; the interaction between UV and heavy metals is a field of intensive investigation (Meyskens and Yang, 2011). There is also great interest in determining whether heavy metals may influence the ability of melanocytes to recover/repair UV-mediated DNA damage (Beyersmann and Hartwig, 2008; Joseph, 2009; Whiteside et al., 2010).

### 3.4 Large number of moles

Since many melanomas arise from nevi (moles), it is not suprising that having a large number of moles increases an individual's risk for melanoma (Bataille et al., 1996). It is estimated that relative risk for melanoma increases from 1.47 for individuals with 16-40 nevi to 6.89 in people with 101-120 nevi (Tucker, 2009). The moles that seem particularly relevant to melanoma are dysplastic nevi, which are characterized by histologic atypia (Barnhill and Roush, 1990) and may represent a mole in evolution to a less benign state (Hussein, 2005). Still, there is a lack of consensus as to whether melanomas grow from existing benign nevi or whether nevi and melanomas may share one or more genetic factors. Individuals with many nevi are more likely to develop melanomas of the trunk whereas those with lower nevus counts require more sun exposure and typically develop cancer in sun-exposed areas of the body (Whiteman et al., 2003), suggesting that host factors that drive nevus formation may also play a role in carcinogenesis. The role of the BRAF oncogene has been prominently emphasized in recent years, and may represent a critical genetic link between nevi and melanoma. Gain-of-function signaling mutations in the BRAF gene are found in 60-80% of human melanoma isolates (Brose et al., 2002; Davies et al., 2002). Furthermore, about 80% of BRAF-mutated melanomas display a common mutation - the V600E mutation wherein valine is substituted by glutamic acid at position 15- and this very same mutation is found in a large number of benign nevi (Pollock et al., 2003; Yazdi et al., 2003). This mutation leads to increased signaling through the MAP kinase cascade, and is thought to be a contributing factor to melanocyte proliferation.

### 3.5 DNA repair

Nucleotide excision repair (NER) is an evolutionarily-conserved mechanism for repairing bulky DNA lesions, including UV-induced photodimers and (6,4)-photoproducts which, if left unrepaired, underlie characteristic "UV-signature" pyrimidine transition mutations (de Laat et al., 1999; Cleaver et al., 2001). Patients with inherited recessive deficiencies of the NER DNA repair pathway are at much heightened risk of developing melanoma and other skin malignancies (Leibeling et al., 2006). The NER pathway involves the following basic steps: (1) recognition of damage and recruitment of a multiprotein repair complex to the damaged site, (2) nicking the damaged strand several nucleotides away on each side of the damaged base(s) and excision of the damaged region between the two nicks, 3) filling in the resultant gap by a DNA polymerase using the non-damaged strand as a template and (4) ligating the final nick to seal the strand. Xeroderma Pigmentosum (XP) is a rare autosomal recessive condition of defective NER caused by homozygous loss-of-function in any one of eight or more genes central to NER function. XP patients exhibit profound UV hypersensitivity beginning in early childhood, and develop epidermal thinning, telangiectasias, lentigenes and patchy hypo- or hyper-pigmentation by adolescence(Eugene and Joshi, 2006). Furthermore, despite UV-avoidance, most XP patients develop actinic keratosis and frank skin malignancies in the first decade of life (with a median age of 8 years) (Jen et al., 2009). XP patients have at least a 1,000-fold increased risk of skin cancers, and have a median age of onset for non-melanomatous skin cancer roughly fifty years younger than that of the general population. Similarly, XP patients have a markedly higher incidence of cutaneous malignant melanoma, particularly on UV-exposed skin (Van Patter and Drummond, 1953; Lynch et al., 1967; Jung, 1978), highlighting the central relevance of the NER pathway in melanoma prevention. Even though clinical XP has been described in the setting of defects in any one of eight genes (XPA, ERCC3 (XPB), XPC, ERCC2 (XPD), DDB2 (XPE), ERCC4 (XPF), ERCC5 (XPG), and POLH (XP-V)), mutations in XPA or XPC account for at least half of all clinical cases. Though XP is a dramatic phenotype that, fortunately, affects only a small fraction of the population, the mechanistic defects underlying XP may have relevance to the greater population at risk for sporadic melanoma. The contribution of polymorphisms in NER response in the general population's risk of melanoma is an area of active investigation (Li et al., 2006; Millikan et al., 2006; Applebaum et al., 2007).

Resistance to oxidative DNA damage is accomplished on a cellular level by anti-oxidant cellular defenses (e.g. glutathione levels) as well as via repair of oxidative lesions by the base excision repair (BER) pathway, a highly conserved pathway initiated by one of at least eleven damage-specific, monofunctional or bifunctional glycosylases that scan the DNA for specific base alterations (Tudek et al., 2006; Russo et al., 2007). After recognition, altered bases are cleaved from the phosphodiesterase backbone by glycolases and repair is achieved via involvement of an apurinic intermediate which is cleaved out and then replaced (David et al., 2007; Hazra et al., 2007; Klungland and Bjelland, 2007). Each of the distinct types of mutagenic lesions in the DNA of UV-exposed cells (cyclobutane dimers,(6,4)-photoproducts and oxidative lesions such as 8-OH-dG and abasic sites) can promote mutation through aberrant repair and/or incorrect base pairing during replication. Much as is the case with NER, variations in the resistance or repair of UV-induced oxidative lesions may be relevant in determining mutagenesis in the skin and subsequently risk of melanoma (Phillipson et al., 2002; Kadekaro et al., 2006; Runger and Kappes, 2008; Song et al., 2009).

### 3.6 Personal or family history of skin cancer

Either because of inherited predisposition or through environmental factors, individuals who have had melanoma once have as much as an 8% chance of developing a second primary melanoma distinct from their original tumor (Ferrone et al., 2005). Similarly, melanoma risk is higher in people with first-degree relatives affected by melanoma (Gandini et al., 2005). Melanoma-prone family cohorts have been described with mutations in the CDKN2A gene which encodes the p16INK4A and p14ARFtumor suppressors, highlighting the importance of the integrity of this pathway in the ability of melanocytes to resist malignant degeneration (Hussussian et al., 1994; Kamb et al., 1994; Meyle and Guldberg, 2009; Hansson, 2010). Perhaps because of increased surveillance, familial melanoma is characterized by younger age at diagnosis, thinner lesions, better survival, multiple primary lesions, as well as higher incidence of non-melanoma neoplasms (Kopf et al., 1986).

### 3.7 Immunodeficiency

Individuals with defective immunity, particularly T cell immunity, are at increased risk of melanoma. Thus, patients with inherited or acquired immune defects, patients on chronic immunosuppressive therapies such as cyclosporine, tacrolimus or sirolimus (e.g. following solid organ or stem cell transplantation) and cancer patients treated with immunosuppressive chemotherapy all have a higher risk of melanoma than their immunocompetent counterparts (Otley and Pittelkow, 2000; Calista, 2001; Berg and Otley, 2002; Reutter et al., 2007).

### 3.8 Fair skin complexion and defective tanning response

Fair-skinned individuals, especially those who fail to tan after sun exposure, have a much higher lifetime risk of melanoma than individuals with darker complexions (Rees and Healy, 1997). Melanoma occurs about twenty times more frequently in fair-skinned individuals than in their melanized counterparts (Evans et al., 1988; Franceschi and Cristofolini, 1992). Though dark-skinned persons can develop melanoma, the disease is rare in non-white persons and tends to occur in less pigmented sites such as the subungual regions, the palms of the hand and the soles of the feet (Kabigting et al., 2009). Although the incidence of melanoma in non-white patients is lower, the mortality rate is higher, perhaps reflecting the disease's tendency to be diagnosed later at a more advanced stage and thus associated with a poorer prognosis (Bradford, 2009). Many genes have been described that contribute to skin pigmentation , often first identified in animal models with coat color or other pigmentary defects. In our discussion, we will focus on one gene in particular- the melanocortin 1 receptor (MC1R)- because its function seems particularly relevant to melanoma development.

## 4. Skin pigmentation

### 4.1 Melanocytes

Melanocytes are dendritic-type cells derived from the neural crest and are traditionally defined by their ability to produce melanin. Comprising 5-10% of total cells in the epidermal basal layer, there are estimated to be between 1,000 and 2,000 melanocytes in every square millimeter of human skin (Nordlund, 2007). They are found both in dermal hair follicles (where they impart pigment to hair) and in the interfollicular epidermis in the stratum basale where they manufacture pigment that accumulates in the outer layers of the epidermis and that blocks UV penetration into the deeper layers of the skin. Melanocytes cells are the sole manufacturers of melanin in the skin and are thought to be the precursor cell that, upon malignant degeneration, develop into melanoma. Via their dendritic projections, melanocytes in the stratum basale may be in intimate contact with as many as 30-50 maturing keratinocytes. Numerous studies have shown robust contact-dependent as well as paracrine signals between melanocytes and keratinocytes. The "epidermal melanin unit" is a term coined to describe the close association between one melanocyte and numerous keratinocytes in the epidermis (Jimbow et al., 1991). As melanocytes manufacture melanin pigments, they transfer melanin to interdigitating keratinocytes where it accumulates in the epidermis (Seiberg, 2001). Melanin functions as a "natural sunscreen" to protect the skin against harmful effects of UV radiation such as oxidative damage and DNA mutagenesis. The more eumelanin present in the skin, both basally and after UV exposure, the more UV-protected and cancer-resistant is the individual (Vincensi et al., 1998). Persons with albinism have normal numbers of melanocytes in the skin but lack melanin pigments due to loss-of-function of any one of a number of pigment biosynthetic enzymes (Oetting, 1999). Because they lack melanin, albinos are much more UV sensitive than either fair-skinned pheomelanotic or dark-skinned eumelanotic individuals (Oetting, 2000).

### 4.2 Melanin pigments

Skin pigmentation is determined mainly by the type and amount of melanin pigments deposited in the epidermis. Melanin is a large bio-polymer composed of subunits of different melanotic pigment species formed by sequential oxidation and cyclization of the amino acid tyrosine (Riley, 1997) (Fig. 5). Biosynthetic reactions are catalyzed by several pigment enzymes, including tyrosinase, the critical rate-limiting enzyme that catalyzes the first two steps in melanogenesis (conversion of tyrosine into DOPA and then conversion of DOPA into DOPAquinone) (Prota, 1980; Rosei, 2001). Most of the enzymes involved in melanogenesis are exclusively found in melanocytes. The final amount and type of melanin produced in the melanocyte depends upon both inherited and environmental factors (Hearing, 1999).

There are two basic types of melanin: eumelanin and pheomelanin. Eumelanin is a brown-black chemically inert and poorly-soluble pigment polymer that is preferentially expressed in persons of darkest complexion. In contrast, because of incorporation of cysteine into the molecule, pheomelanin is a more red-yellow sulfur-containing compound (Ito et al., 2000). Eumelanin absorbs more UV radiation (is a better "sunscreen") and is much more chemically inert than pheomelanin. The first two reactions of melanin formation are common to both eumelanogenesis and pheomelanogenesis; biosynthetic pathways diverge after the formation of dopaquinone (Fig. 5). Eumelanins are derived from metabolites of dopachrome whereas pheomelanins are produced from sulfhydryl-reduced metabolites including cysteinyldopa (Prota, 2000). UV resistance is mainly determined by the absolute amount of eumelanin in the skin. Thus, while epidermal pheomelanin levels are fairly similar between light-and dark-skinned persons, dark-skinned individuals have much more eumelanin in the skin and are therefore much more UV-resistant (Simon and Peles, 2010). Besides being a poorer blocker of UV energy, pheomelanin may actually contribute to UV-induced cellular and DNA damage. UV radiation of pheomelanin is associated with generation of reactive oxidative species (Hubbard-Smith et al., 1992; Hill et al., 1997) and photosensitized UV-induced DNA damage when added to melanocytes *in vitro* (Wenczl et al., 1998). Moreover, pheomelanin is much more soluble than eumelanin, even being found in the serum and urine of fair-skinned persons(Ito et al., 1983; Ito and Wakamatsu, 1989), raising the possibility that UV-exposed pheomelanin (or its metabolites) could leach out of melanosomes, diffuse into the nucleus, and interact with DNA to promote mutagenesis especially in the context of UV radiation. The contribution of pheomelanin to UV-induced carcinogenesis is an ongoing area of investigation.

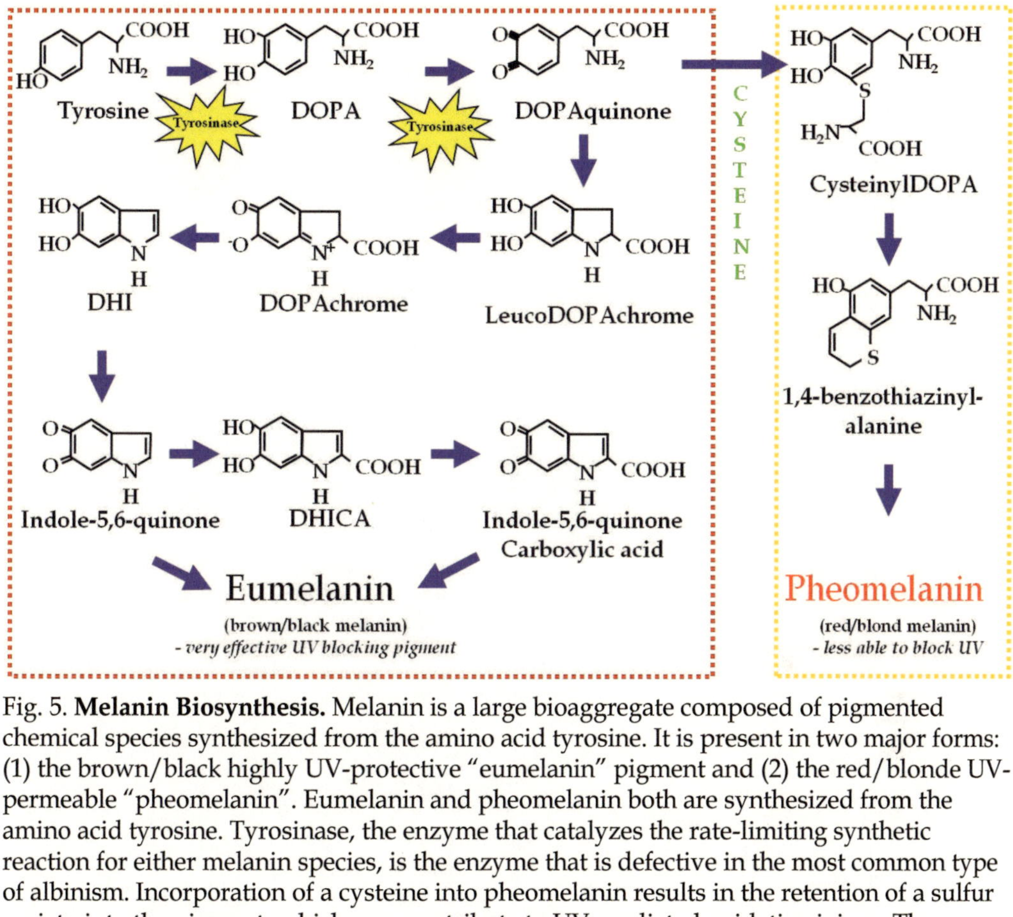


Fig. 5. **Melanin Biosynthesis.** Melanin is a large bioaggregate composed of pigmented chemical species synthesized from the amino acid tyrosine. It is present in two major forms: (1) the brown/black highly UV-protective "eumelanin" pigment and (2) the red/blonde UV-permeable "pheomelanin". Eumelanin and pheomelanin both are synthesized from the amino acid tyrosine. Tyrosinase, the enzyme that catalyzes the rate-limiting synthetic reaction for either melanin species, is the enzyme that is defective in the most common type of albinism. Incorporation of a cysteine into pheomelanin results in the retention of a sulfur moiety into the pigment, which may contribute to UV-mediated oxidative injury. The melanocyte stimulating hormone (MSH) - melanocortin 1 receptor (MC1R) signaling axis is a major determinant of the type and amount of melanin produced by melanocytes in the skin.

### 4.3 Fitzpatrick scale and UV sensitivity

Skin color, mainly determined by the amount of eumelanin in the epidermis, correlates well with UV resistance. Thus, the darker a person's skin, the more eumelanin it contains and the better that person's skin is able to withstand acute (e.g. sunburn) and chronic (e.g. cancer) effects of UV. Dermatologists use the "Fitzpatrick Scale", created in 1975 by a Harvard dermatologist named T.B. Fitzpatrick, to describe skin tone (Andreassi et al., 1999). This scale is comprised of six categories that define individual phototypes by basal skin color and by response to UV radiation (Scherer and Kumar, 2010) (Table 2). Minimal erythematous dose, often abbreviated "MED", is a measure of the skin's response to ultraviolet radiation using erythema (redness, inflammation) as an endpoint. Much more UV radiation is needed to "burn" dark skin, and therefore MED is lowest in fair-skinned persons (Lu et al., 1996; Andreassi et al., 1999; Kawada, 2000). In most cases, phototypes show a strong correlation with MED (Ravnbak, 2010).

| **Fitzpatrick Phototype** | **Phenotype** | **Epidermal eumelanin** | **Cutaneous response to UV** | **MED ($mJ/cm^2$)*** | **Melanoma risk** |
|---|---|---|---|---|---|
| I | Unexposed skin is bright white<br>Blue/green eyes typical<br>Freckling frequent<br>Northern European/British | +/- | Always burns<br>Peels<br>Never tans | 15-30 | ++++ |
| II | Unexposed skin is white<br>Blue, hazel or brown eyes<br>Red, blonde or brown hair<br>European/Scandinavian | + | Burns easily<br>Peels<br>Tans minimally | 25-40 | +++/++++ |
| III | Unexposed skin is fair<br>Brown eyes<br>Dark hair<br>Southern or Central European | ++ | Burns moderately<br>Average tanning ability | 30-50 | +++ |
| IV | Unexposed skin is light brown<br>Dark eyes<br>Dark hair<br>Mediterranean, Asian or Latino | +++ | Burns minimally<br>Tans easily | 40-60 | ++ |
| V | Unexposed skin is brown<br>Dark eyes<br>Dark hair<br>East Indian, Native American, Latino or African | ++++ | Rarely burns<br>Tans easily and substantially | 60-90 | + |
| VI | Unexposed skin is black<br>Dark eyes<br>Dark hair<br>African or Aboriginal ancestry | ++++++ | Almost never burns<br>Tans readily and profusely | 90-150 | +/- |

Minimal erythematous dose (MED) is defined as the least amount of UVB radiation that will result in reddening and inflammation of the skin 24h after exposure (i.e. the lowest UV dose that causes a sunburn). The more UV sensitive an individual is, the lower the MED of their skin.

Table 2. Fitzpatrick Scale of Skin Phototypes

Although innate pigmentation is a major determinant of sun sensitivity, there are other genetic and environmental factors that determine how prone to UV damage an individual will be (Rees, 2003). In particular, UV sensitivity correlates well with the degree to which epidermal melanin can be up-regulated after UV exposure. Adaptive pigmentation, or tanning, is the natural physiologic response of the skin to UV exposure. Adaptive pigmentation involves both an increase in the amount of melanin pigment made by melanocytes as well as epidermal thickening mediated by proliferation of keratinocytes. Both changes serve to increase melanin accumulation in the epidermis so that the skin is better protected against subsequent UV exposures. Individuals with defective adaptive pigmentation are particularly sun-sensitive and melanoma-prone. Thus, individuals with skin phototypes I and II burn easily, have difficulty tanning, and suffer the highest incidence of melanoma whereas persons of higher skin phototypes are much more sun-tolerant and have much lower incidence of melanoma (Ravnbak, 2010).

### 4.4 Genetic determinants of skin color

Several genes are known to be associated with basal pigmentation in humans and natural variation in skin color. Most pigment-determining genes are associated with melanin synthesis or melanosome structure/function (Table 3) (Parra, 2007). Others, such as microphthalmia (MITF) or Kit ligand (KITLG) control melanocyte migration and development (Fleischman et al., 1991; Giebel and Spritz, 1991; Tassabehji et al., 1994}. With the exception of tyrosinase, defects in melanin biosynthetic enzymes generally lead to dilutional pigmentary effects whereas defects that result in defective melanocyte survival or development result in more profound phenotypes such as piebaldism. Many pigmentation genes were identified through detailed study of coat color mutations in mice and other model organisms (Steingrimsson et al., 2006). Tyrosinase deficiency underlies oculocutaneous albinism type I (OCA1) wherein melanocytes are present in normal numbers and distribution in the skin but they fail to make any melanin pigments at all. As a result, individuals with this severe form of albinism are highly UV-sensitive and tend to avoid outdoor activities throughout life. In comparison, SLC45A2, also known as MAPT, encodes a membrane-associated transporter protein (MATP), which when mutated is responsible for the milder OCA4 form of albinism (Newton et al., 2001; Inagaki et al., 2006). Many genes regulate either the ratio or absolute levels of eumelanin or pheomelanin expressed in the skin. For example, solute carrier family 24 member 5 (SLC24A5), purported to encode a cation exchange protein in melanosomes, may account for up to 40% of skin color differences between Europeans and Africans (Lamason et al., 2005) and polymorphisms that result in some decrease in the activity of *TYR, OCA2, MC1R, ASIP* and *IRF4* have been reported to affect skin color in European populations (Sturm, 2009; Edwards et al., 2010; Scherer and Kumar, 2010). Thus, it seems that the protein products of several genes together influence basal skin pigmentation in humans.

### 4.5 Rickets and pigmentation

It would at first seem highly illogical that fair skin would have been evolutionarily selected for over time, as being fair-skinned clearly limits an individual's ability to function in ambient sunlight. However, by considering the native geographical regions from which lightly-pigmented persons originated, we might infer why light skin complexion may have developed in humans over time. Simply put, fair complexion probably evolved so that people living in geographic areas of the world with less intense sun exposure (e.g. celtic populations) would have less risk of rickets. Before widespread supplementation of foods with vitamin D, the major source of this essential vitamin was the natural sunlight-mediated direct chemical conversion of 7-dehydrocholesterol into previtamin D3 that occurs naturally in the epidermis. After synthesis in the skin, previtamin D3 then can be modified sequentially by liver and kidney to form the active hormone cholecalciferol which is intricately involved in a host of homeostatic mechanisms. Deficiency of vitamin D underlies the pathophysiology of rickets, a disease state in which altered calcium metabolism leads to a host of severe health consequences, including osteomalacia and osteoporosis that lead to delayed growth, chronic pain, muscle weakness and disfiguring skeletal abnormalities including bowed legs, scoliosis and abnormal bone structure. Since epidermal eumelanin is a potent blocker of UV penetration and of the direct chemical conversion of 7-dehydrocholesterol into previtamin D3, more UV is needed in dark skin to manufacture sufficient previtamin D3. Therefore, as populations moved away from the equatorial regions in which humans evolved to more polar climates in which the UV energy of sunlight is much weaker, natural selection mechanisms would have favored reduced basal eumelanin in the skin and a lighter skin complexion. Moreover, there would have been much less of a need for photoprotection in such environments, therefore there would have been no evolutionary pressure to maintain a dark phenotype. By gradual lightening of the skin (mediated by reduced melanocytic eumelanin production), sufficient UV-mediated vitamin D production in the skin would still occur in regions with less ambient sunlight so as to prevent rickets (Holick, 1981; Jablonski and Chaplin, 2000). In contrast, in high-UV regions, evolutionary pressure would have favored the photoprotection afforded by eumelanin, as evidenced by the fact that populations native to these regions (e.g. Africans, Australian Aborigines, Indian subcontinent, etc.) typically having much more epidermal melanin than their more-polar counterparts. Thus, it is postulated that the evolution of fair skin may have been a positive adaptation due to the requirement of UV-dependent Vitamin D synthesis (Jablonski and Chaplin, 2000).

### 4.6 The melanocortin 1 receptor (MC1R) and the adaptive tanning response

There are many genes that control human skin pigmentation (Table 3), but we will focus on melanocortin 1 receptor (MC1R), which is a critical locus involved in both pigmentation and the tanning response. More relevant to melanoma, pioneering work done by Jonathan Rees and colleagues in the mid-90's showed that loss-of-function polymorphisms of MC1R correlated directly with melanoma risk. Studies of the interaction between melanocyte stimulating hormone (MSH) and its receptor, the melanocortin 1 receptor (MC1R) have led to some understanding of the molecular basis for differences in inherited and adaptive skin pigmentation. The MC1R is a seven-transmembrane domain G-protein-coupled receptor belonging to the melanocortin receptor subfamily. Ligand-mediated signaling through Mc1r involves G-protein activation and resultant increases in levels of intracellular cAMP. Production of eumelanin is favored with higher intracellular cAMP concentrations, and pheomelanin is preferentially synthesized when cAMP levels are low (Abdel-Malek et al., 2000). Fairness of skin (and melanoma susceptibility) correlates with polymorphisms of the MC1R associated with diminished transmission of MSH signals and a muted cytoplasmic cAMP response (Valverde et al., 1995; Rees and Healy, 1997). Genetic support of this hypothesis is revealed by studies of the C57BL/6 *extension* mutant ($MC1R^{e/e}$) in which red/blonde pigmentation occurs as a result of defective MC1R signaling (Robbins et al., 1993).

| Gene | Pigmentation Disorder | Proposed Function | General Structure |
|---|---|---|---|
| **Tyrosinase (TYR)** | Oculocutaneous albinism type 1 (OCA1) | Rate-limiting enzyme in melanin biosynthesis | Type I transmembrane protein |
| **Tyrosinase-related protein-1 (TRP1)** | Oculocutaneous albinism type 3 (OCA3) | Melanin biosynthesis; tyrosinase stabilization | Type 1 transmembrane protein |
| **Microphthalmia (MITF)** | Waardenburg syndrome type 2 | Myc-like master transcription factor essential for melanocyte differentiation and survival | basic-helix-loop-helix-leucine-zipper transcription factor |
| **Dopachrome tautomerase (TRP2)** | Unknown | Melanin biosynthetic enzyme | Type 1 transmembrane protein |
| **Solute carrier family 24 member 5 (SLC24A5)** | Fair skin | Melanosomal cation exchange | Membrane transporter |
| **stem cell factor/ kit ligand (KITLG)** | Piebaldism | Transmits survival and differentiation signals to melanocytes | Membrane tyrosine kinase |
| **Pmel17 (gp100; ME20)** | Unknown | Striation formation; melanin polymerization | Type 1 transmembrane protein |
| **P/OCA2** | Oculocutaneous albinism type 2 (OCA2) | Melanosome acidification | 12-transmembrane domain-containing protein |
| **OA1 receptor** | Ocular albinism (OA) | Maintenance of melanosome size | G-protein-coupled receptor |
| **Melanocortin 1 receptor (MC1R)** | Red hair, freckling, defective tanning | Binds to melanocyte stimulating hormone and generates cAMP signal | 7 transmembrane Gs-coupled receptor |

Table 3. Partial list of major genes that determine human skin color (Marks and Seabra, 2001).

Inability to tan in response to sunlight is a cardinal feature of fair-skinned, UV-sensitive, melanoma-prone individuals. Normally, melanocytes respond to UV exposure through proliferation and up-regulation of melanin production, the "tanning response". While it is possible that some of this response occurs by direct UV-mediated effects on melanocytes themselves, it is likely that the tanning response depends on signals from other cells. In particular, the melanocyte stimulating hormone (MSH)- melanocortin 1 receptor (MC1R) signaling axis appears to be central to the adaptive tanning response. MSH, the agonistic ligand for MC1R, binds to MC1R on the surface of melanocytes and promotes increases in cytoplasmic cAMP. Basal pigmentation likely results in part from this MSH-MC1R interaction from MSH secreted either central from the pituitary gland or from keratinocytes in the epidermis. There are three common polymorphisms of the MC1R found in UV-sensitive and melanoma-prone individuals: Arg151Cys (R151C), Arg160Trp (R160W) and Asp294His (D294H). These so-called "red hair color" (RHC) mutations correlate with red hair, freckling and tendency to burn rather than tan after UV exposure. Molecularly, the RHC MC1R variants display a muted ability to activate adenylate cyclase after MSH binding, and thus are associated with a blunted cAMP signaling response. Importantly, these loss-of-function polymorphisms of MC1R are also influence susceptibility to melanoma and other skin cancers. Thus, persons with defective MC1R signaling have higher risk of melanoma than their MC1R-intact counterparts.

Using a congenic C57Bl/6 mouse model with humanized skin, we showed that Mc1r signaling is critical to adaptive pigmentation. Thus, animals with intact Mc1r responded to repeated UV exposure by depositing eumelanin in the epidermis, whereas animals that were genetically identical except for loss of Mc1r failed to melanize at all in response to the same UV exposure (Fig. 6). We also found evidence of a cutaneous MSH-MC1R signaling axis in the skin induced by UV and involving MSH production by epidermal keratinocytes. Thus we concluded that adaptive pigmentation is dependent on an effective MSH-MC1R signaling axis in the skin.

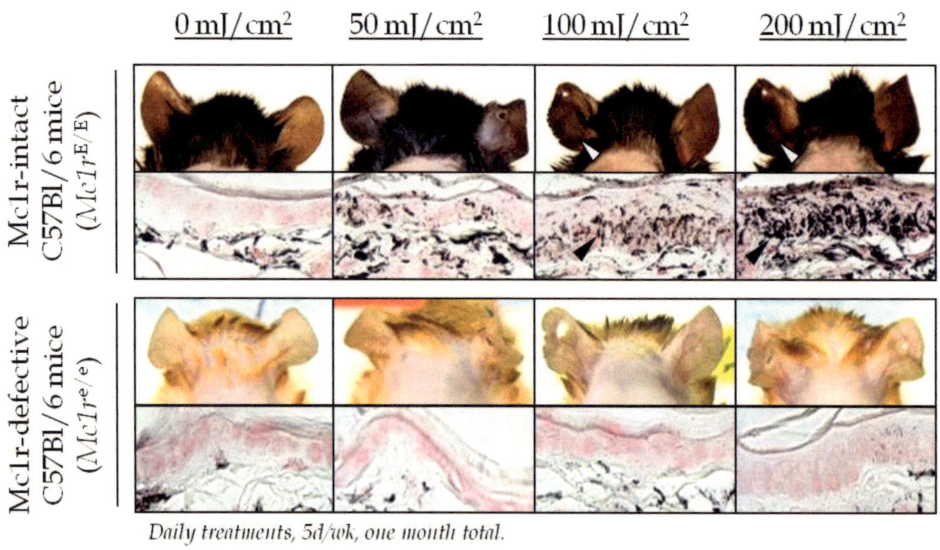


Fig. 6. **Critical role of the melanocortin 1 receptor in the adaptive tanning response.** C57Bl/6 mice genetically identical except for being either wild type (Mc1r$^{E/E}$) or mutant at the MSH receptor (Mc1r$^{e/e}$) were treated with the indicated dose of UV. Top-most rows show UV-induced ear skin darkening, with corresponding skin sections stained for melanin immediately below to show melanin accumulation (black deposits). Note the UV-induced skin darkening (black triangles) and melanin accumulation (white triangles) in Mc1r$^{E/E}$ but not in Mc1r$^{e/e}$ animals (as originally published, D'Orazio, 2006).

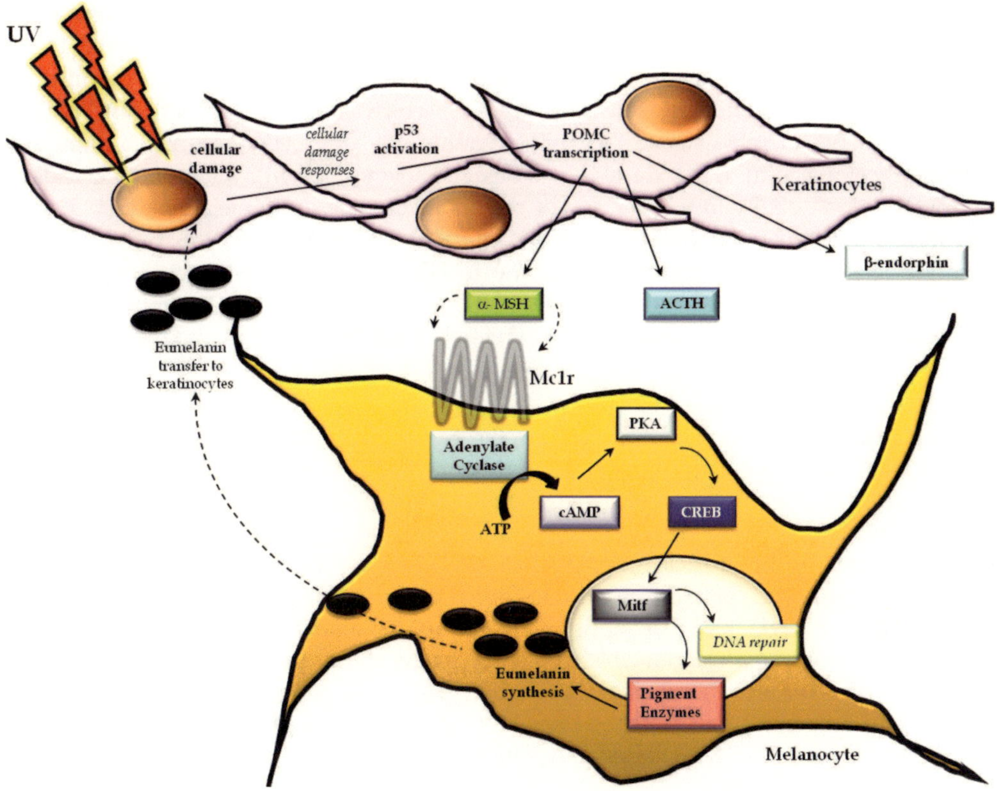


Fig. 7. **The adaptive tanning response.** Epidermal keratinocytes receive the brunt of UV damage because of their proximity to the surface of the body and because they are the most abundant cells in the epidermis. DNA damage in these cells induces activation of the global damage response protein p53, which mediates transcriptional activation of the pro-opiomelanocortin (POMC) gene. The POMC gene encodes a propeptide that is cleaved into three protein products: β-endorphin, adrenocorticotropic hormone (ACTH) and melanocyte stimulating hormone (MSH). MSH is thus produced and secreted from UV-exposed keratinocytes, where it is postulated to interact in a paracrine manner with melanocortin 1 receptors (MC1R) on neighboring melanocytes in the basal epidermis. If MC1R signaling is intact, MSH binding induces generation of the second messenger cAMP via activation of adenylate cyclase. In melanocytes, elevated cAMP levels trigger a number of downstream events including activation of protein kinase A- and subsequent up-regulation of both the cAMP responsive binding element (CREB) and microphthalmia (Mitf) transcription factors. CREB and Mitf mediate up-regulation of melanin production by induction of tyrosinase and other melanin biosynthetic enzymes. Thus, MSH-MC1R signaling leads to enhanced pigment synthesis and subsequent transfer of melanin (in the form of melanosomes) to epidermal keratinocytes. In this manner, the skin is more protected against subsequent UV insults. Recent data suggest that MSH-MC1R signaling may also enhance nucleotide excision repair (NER) in melanocytes, which would favor recovery from potentially mutagenic UV damage.

In subsequent work, David Fisher's group showed that adaptive pigmention was also dependent on p53 function (Cui et al., 2007). Normally thought of in the context as a tumor suppressor, p53 is a central DNA damage response mediator that binds to the POMC promoter and induces its expression. As a result, UV-exposed keratinocytes produce and secrete α-melanocyte stimulating hormone (α-MSH) which may then interact with MC1R on melanocytes and thereby signal the cells to ramp up production of melanin pigment (particularly eumelanin) so that the skin will be more able to cope with subsequent UV insults (Fig. 7). The skin's ability to respond to UV radiation correlates with melanoma risk. Persons with loss-of-function polymorphisms of the MC1R fail to respond to MSH signaling and demonstrate limited melanization in response to UV exposure. These very people with a defective "tanning response" are at very high risk of melanoma; their fair complexion favors accumulation of UV-induced mutation by failing to block UV penetration into the skin.

#### 4.7 MC1R and DNA repair

We and others are now appreciating that the function of Mc1r in melanocytes clearly extends beyond adaptive pigmentation and synthesis of eumelanin. Using genetically heterogeneous human melanocytes transfected with *Mc1r* genes of variable functionality, various groups have reported a reproducible link between nucleotide excision repair (NER), the pathway responsible for clearing UV-induced thymine dimers and [6,4]-photoproducts and Mc1r function and/or cAMP signaling (Bohm et al., 2005; Hauser et al., 2006; Passeron et al., 2008; Smith et al., 2008). Using our congenic animal model divergent only at the Mc1r locus, we also observe a reproducible difference in the ability to recover from UV damage (Fig. 8). Others have also found a correlation between MC1R function and resistance to UV-mediated oxidative and free radical damage (Song et al., 2009). Determining the molecular mechanisms linking MC1R signaling and NER function is an active area of investigation in the melanocyte community.

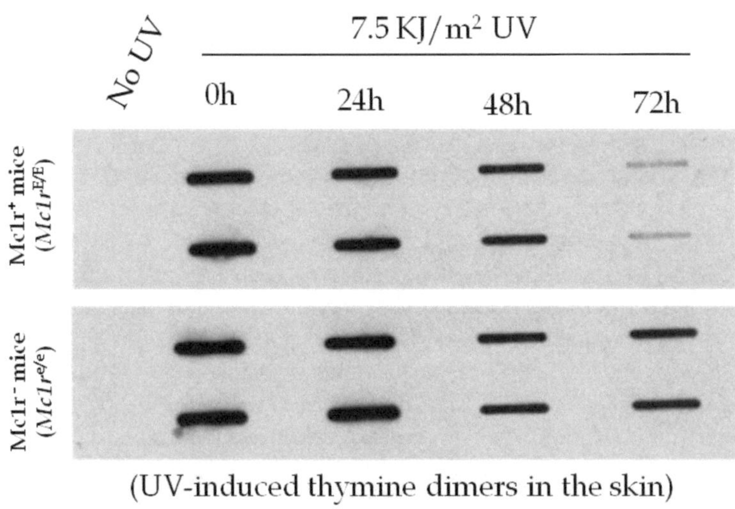


Fig. 8. **Mc1r function influences repair of UV-induced DNA damage.** C57Bl/6 mice differing only at the *Mc1r* locus were irradiated with UV and persistence of thymine dimers in the skin was followed over time. Shown are the results of two animals per group. Note that animals with intact Mc1r cleared thymine dimers more efficiently.

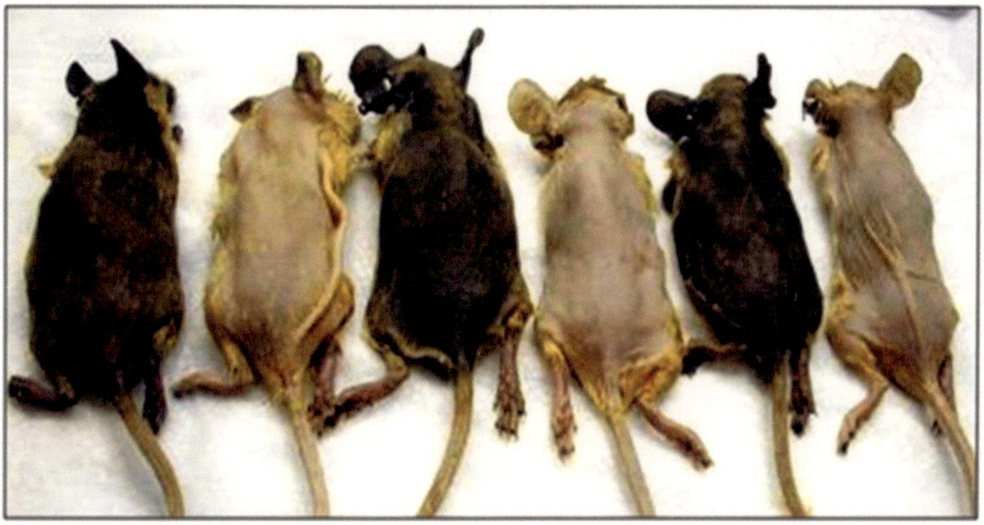


Fig. 9. Pharmacologic induction of melanin in an animal model of the fair-skinned human. C57Bl/6 mice harboring a loss-of-function mutation in the melanocortin 1 receptor ($Mc1r^{e/e}$) were treated daily with topically-applied control (propylene glycol/ethanol) or with forskolin, a drug that directly activates adenylate cyclase and raises cAMP in the skin. Photos of shaved mice were taken after 21 days. Note the robust skin darkening (which proved to be due to accumulation of eumelanin in the epidermis) in the forskolin-treated mice (D'Orazio et al., 2006).

### 4.8 Pharmacologic manipulation of MC1R signaling

Pharmacologic manipulation of melanocytic cAMP levels represents a promising and novel approach to alter UV sensitivity and melanoma risk. Pharmacologic MC1R mimetics include both small peptides that mimic MSH agonist activity (Abdel-Malek et al., 2009) as well as agents that bypass the MC1R to directly manipulate melanocyte cAMP levels. We reported that topical application of the adenylate cylase activating drug forskolin restored melanotic pigmentation in an animal model of the fair-skinned human (Fig. 10) and that this "sunless tanning" was potently protective against UV damage and carcinogenesis of the skin (D'Orazio et al., 2006). More recently, Khaled and coworkers showed that a similar UV-protected phenotype could be induced not by induction of cAMP generation, but rather by pharmacologic interference with clearance of cAMP by topical application of a phosphodiesterase inhibitor (Khaled et al., 2010). Small molecule-based approaches of cAMP manipulation may offer a critical advantage over MSH peptide mimetics in that fair-skinned, UV-sensitive persons most at risk of melanoma are frequently defective in MC1R signaling ability, and thus would not be expected to generate a brisk cAMP response upon MSH peptide binding. Of course, such agents would be expected to have effects in cells other than melanocytes, thus the more melanocyte-targeted approach of the MSH mimetics may offer selective advantages. In any case, rational development of pharmacologic agents capable of safely manipulating cAMP levels in epidermal melanocytes might offer UV- and melanoma protection by a variety of ways. First, by up-regulating melanin in the skin, fair-skinned individuals would be better protected from UV. Second, sunless tanning by small molecules would represent a way to uncouple tanning from UV exposure. Fair-skinned persons seeking tans would no longer need to sunbathe or frequent tanning salons to enjoy the cosmetic and UV-protective benefits of improved skin pigmentation. Lastly, pharmacomimetics of the MC1R pathway hold the promise of enhancing the ability of melanocytes to repair UV-induced damage and would be expected to result in fewer mutations in UV-exposed skin.

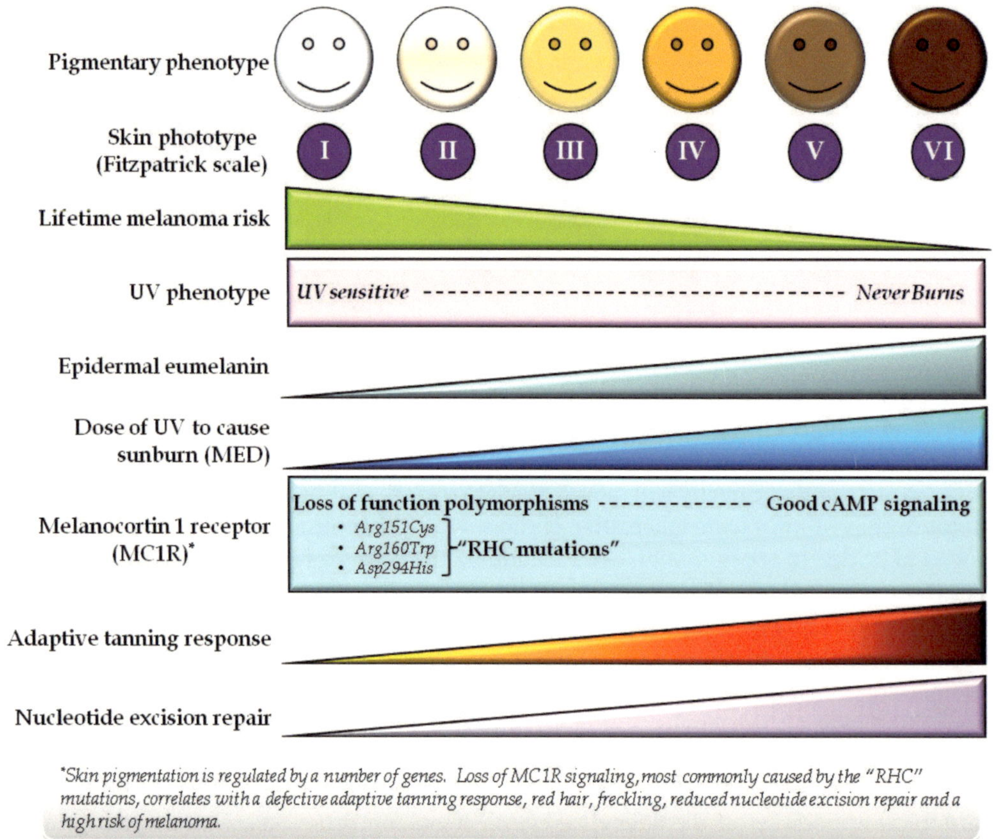


Fig. 10. **Summary of the influence of pigmentation on melanoma risk.** Fair-skinned individuals have a much higher risk of melanoma than their dark-skinned counterparts. Such individuals are much more UV sensitive, tending to burn rather than tan, after UV exposure. Their skin is characterized by much lower levels of epidermal eumelanin and consequently much less UV is needed to induce a sunburn (erythema). Furthermore, fair-skinned persons are more likely to harbor the so-called "red hair color" mutations in their melanocortin 1 receptors. These mutations are associated with a blunted MSH signaling response and reduced ability to tan. Recent data also suggests that MC1R mutations are associated with less efficient nucleotide excision repair. Reduced ability to clear UV-induced DNA photolesions would promote mutagenesis after UV exposure. Thus, MC1R-defective individuals not only suffer a higher realized dose of UV radiation because their skin has insufficient UV-blocking eumelanin but also may accumulate more mutations from UV exposure because of defective DNA repair.

## 5. Conclusions

One of the greatest risk factors for the development of cutaneous melanoma is having a fair skin complexion, which is characterized by comparatively low levels of a UV-blocking dark pigment called eumelanin in the epidermis. Unlike darker-skinned individuals, persons with light complexions suffer much greater skin damage from UV radiation because more UV light penetrates through the superficial epidermis to damage both keratinocytes and melanocytes in the deeper layers of the epidermis. As a result, fair-skinned individuals are exposed to higher "realized" doses of UV radiation in the skin. Thus, UV-induced mutations, which directly contributes to melanoma and other forms of skin cancer, might accumulate preferentially in fair-skinned persons over time. We and others are increasingly interested in the genetic factors that determine melanoma risk to be able to intervene in the carcinogenic process. One of the most important alleles that influences melanoma risk is the melanocortin 1 receptor (MC1R), whose function is central to the adaptive pigmentation (tanning) response in the skin. This protein mediates signals to melanocytes to induce pigment production after UV exposure (the tanning response). Besides regulating adaptive pigmentation (tanning), MC1R seems to have a powerful influence on the ability of melanocytes to repair UV-induced DNA damage by the nucleotide excision repair pathway. Thus, defective MC1R signaling as occurs with the common polymorphisms observed at high frequency in melanoma-prone fair-skinned people may predispose to malignancy by resulting in inadequate pigment deposition (which would favor UV penetration into the skin) and in a sluggish DNA repair response (which would allow UV-induced photodamage to promote mutagenesis). These new insights into the many ways in which MC1R function protects melanocytes from harmful consequences of UV may help explain why people with inherited defects of MC1R signaling suffer a disproportionately high incidence of melanoma (Fig. 10). Our long-term goal is to devise rational MC1R-rescue strategies that would reduce melanoma risk and UV sensitivity in high-risk, melanoma-prone individuals.

## 6. References

Abdel-Malek, Z., M. C. Scott, I. Suzuki, A. Tada, S. Im, et al. (2000). "The melanocortin-1 receptor is a key regulator of human cutaneous pigmentation." Pigment Cell Res 13 Suppl 8: 156-162.

Abdel-Malek, Z. A., J. Knittel, A. L. Kadekaro, V. B. Swope and R. Starner (2008). "The melanocortin 1 receptor and the UV response of human melanocytes--a shift in paradigm." Photochem Photobiol 84(2): 501-508.

Abdel-Malek, Z. A., A. Ruwe, R. Kavanagh-Starner, A. L. Kadekaro, V. Swope, et al. (2009). "alpha-MSH tripeptide analogs activate the melanocortin 1 receptor and reduce UV-induced DNA damage in human melanocytes." Pigment Cell Melanoma Res.

Andreassi, L., M. L. Flori and P. Rubegni (1999). "Sun and skin - Role of phototype and skin colour." Rheumaderm 455: 469-475.

Andreassi, L., M. L. Flori and P. Rubegni (1999). "Sun and skin. Role of phototype and skin colour." Adv Exp Med Biol 455: 469-475.

Applebaum, K. M., M. R. Karagas, D. J. Hunter, P. J. Catalano, S. H. Byler, et al. (2007). "Polymorphisms in nucleotide excision repair genes, arsenic exposure, and non-melanoma skin cancer in New Hampshire." Environ Health Perspect 115(8): 1231-1236.

Autier, P., J. F. Dore, A. M. Eggermont and J. W. Coebergh (2011). "Epidemiological evidence that UVA radiation is involved in the genesis of cutaneous melanoma." Curr Opin Oncol 23(2): 189-196.

Barnhill, R. L. and G. C. Roush (1990). "Histopathologic spectrum of clinically atypical melanocytic nevi. II. Studies of nonfamilial melanoma." Arch Dermatol 126(10): 1315-1318.

Bataille, V., J. A. Bishop, P. Sasieni, A. J. Swerdlow, E. Pinney, et al. (1996). "Risk of cutaneous melanoma in relation to the numbers, types and sites of naevi: a case-control study." Br J Cancer 73(12): 1605-1611.

Berg, D. and C. C. Otley (2002). "Skin cancer in organ transplant recipients: Epidemiology, pathogenesis, and management." J Am Acad Dermatol 47(1): 1-17; quiz 18-20.

Berwick, M. and C. Wiggins (2006). "The current epidemiology of cutaneous malignant melanoma." Front Biosci 11: 1244-1254.

Beyersmann, D. and A. Hartwig (2008). "Carcinogenic metal compounds: recent insight into molecular and cellular mechanisms." Arch Toxicol 82(8): 493-512.

Bohm, M., I. Wolff, T. E. Scholzen, S. J. Robinson, E. Healy, et al. (2005). "alpha-Melanocyte-stimulating hormone protects from ultraviolet radiation-induced apoptosis and DNA damage." J Biol Chem 280(7): 5795-5802.

Bolshakov, S., C. M. Walker, S. S. Strom, M. S. Selvan, G. L. Clayman, et al. (2003). "p53 mutations in human aggressive and nonaggressive basal and squamous cell carcinomas." Clin Cancer Res 9(1): 228-234.

Bradford, P. T. (2009). "Skin cancer in skin of color." Dermatol Nurs 21(4): 170-177, 206; quiz 178.

Brose, M. S., P. Volpe, M. Feldman, M. Kumar, I. Rishi, et al. (2002). "BRAF and RAS mutations in human lung cancer and melanoma." Cancer Res 62(23): 6997-7000.

Cadet, J., E. Sage and T. Douki (2005). "Ultraviolet radiation-mediated damage to cellular DNA." Mutat Res 571(1-2): 3-17.

Calista, D. (2001). "Five cases of melanoma in HIV positive patients." Eur J Dermatol 11(5): 446-449.

Chen, Y. T., R. Dubrow, T. Zheng, R. L. Barnhill, J. Fine, et al. (1998). "Sunlamp use and the risk of cutaneous malignant melanoma: a population-based case-control study in Connecticut, USA." Int J Epidemiol 27(5): 758-765.

Cho, E., B. A. Rosner, D. Feskanich and G. A. Colditz (2005). "Risk factors and individual probabilities of melanoma for whites." J Clin Oncol 23(12): 2669-2675.

Cleaver, J. E. and E. Crowley (2002). "UV damage, DNA repair and skin carcinogenesis." Front Biosci 7: d1024-1043.

Cleaver, J. E., K. Karplus, M. Kashani-Sabet and C. L. Limoli (2001). "Nucleotide excision repair "a legacy of creativity"." Mutat Res 485(1): 23-36.

Croyle, R. T. (2011). "SEER Stat Fact Sheets: Melanoma of the Skin." Cancer Statistics Branch Surveillance Research Program, Division of Cancer Control and Population Sciences, National Cancer Institute, from http://www.seer.cancer.gov/statfacts/html/melan.html#incidence-mortality.

Cui, R., H. R. Widlund, E. Feige, J. Y. Lin, D. L. Wilensky, et al. (2007). "Central Role of p53 in the Suntan Response and Pathologic Hyperpigmentation." Cell 128(5): 853-864.

Cust, A. E., M. A. Jenkins, C. Goumas, B. K. Armstrong, H. Schmid, et al. (2011). "Early-life sun exposure and risk of melanoma before age 40 years." Cancer Causes Control.

D'Orazio, J. A., T. Nobuhisa, R. Cui, M. Arya, M. Spry, et al. (2006). "Topical drug rescue strategy and skin protection based on the role of Mc1r in UV-induced tanning." Nature 443(7109): 340-344.

David, S. S., V. L. O'Shea and S. Kundu (2007). "Base-excision repair of oxidative DNA damage." Nature 447(7147): 941-950.

Davies, H., G. R. Bignell, C. Cox, P. Stephens, S. Edkins, et al. (2002). "Mutations of the BRAF gene in human cancer." Nature 417(6892): 949-954.

de Gruijl, F. R., H. J. van Kranen and L. H. Mullenders (2001). "UV-induced DNA damage, repair, mutations and oncogenic pathways in skin cancer." J Photochem Photobiol B 63(1-3): 19-27.

de Laat, W. L., N. G. Jaspers and J. H. Hoeijmakers (1999). "Molecular mechanism of nucleotide excision repair." Genes Dev 13(7): 768-785.

Dennis, L. K. (1999). "Increasing risk of melanoma with increasing age." JAMA 282(11): 1037-1038.

Dennis, L. K., M. J. Vanbeek, L. E. Beane Freeman, B. J. Smith, D. V. Dawson, et al. (2008). "Sunburns and risk of cutaneous melanoma: does age matter? A comprehensive meta-analysis." Ann Epidemiol 18(8): 614-627.

Edwards, M., A. Bigham, J. Tan, S. Li, A. Gozdzik, et al. (2010). "Association of the OCA2 polymorphism His615Arg with melanin content in east Asian populations: further evidence of convergent evolution of skin pigmentation." PLoS Genet 6(3): e1000867.

Erickson, C. and M. S. Driscoll (2010). "Melanoma epidemic: Facts and controversies." Clin Dermatol 28(3): 281-286.

Eugene, D. W. and K. D. Joshi (2006). "Xeroderma pigmentosa--a disfiguring disease." Kathmandu Univ Med J (KUMJ) 4(1): 78-81.

Evans, R. D., A. W. Kopf, R. A. Lew, D. S. Rigel, R. S. Bart, et al. (1988). "Risk factors for the development of malignant melanoma--I: Review of case-control studies." J Dermatol Surg Oncol 14(4): 393-408.

Ferrone, C. R., L. Ben Porat, K. S. Panageas, M. Berwick, A. C. Halpern, et al. (2005). "Clinicopathological features of and risk factors for multiple primary melanomas." JAMA 294(13): 1647-1654.

Fisher, D. E. and W. D. James (2010). "Indoor tanning--science, behavior, and policy." N Engl J Med 363(10): 901-903.

Fleischman, R. A., D. L. Saltman, V. Stastny and S. Zneimer (1991). "Deletion of the c-kit protooncogene in the human developmental defect piebald trait." Proc Natl Acad Sci U S A 88(23): 10885-10889.

Fleming, I. D., J. R. Barnawell, P. E. Burlison and J. S. Rankin (1975). "Skin cancer in black patients." Cancer 35(3): 600-605.

Franceschi, S. and M. Cristofolini (1992). "Cutaneous malignant melanoma: epidemiological considerations." Semin Surg Oncol 8(6): 345-352.

Gandini, S., F. Sera, M. S. Cattaruzza, P. Pasquini, O. Picconi, et al. (2005). "Meta-analysis of risk factors for cutaneous melanoma: II. Sun exposure." Eur J Cancer 41(1): 45-60.

Gandini, S., F. Sera, M. S. Cattaruzza, P. Pasquini, R. Zanetti, et al. (2005). "Meta-analysis of risk factors for cutaneous melanoma: III. Family history, actinic damage and phenotypic factors." Eur J Cancer 41(14): 2040-2059.

Garbe, C. and U. Leiter (2009). "Melanoma epidemiology and trends." Clin Dermatol 27(1): 3-9.

Giebel, L. B. and R. A. Spritz (1991). "Mutation of the KIT (mast/stem cell growth factor receptor) protooncogene in human piebaldism." Proc Natl Acad Sci U S A 88(19): 8696-8699.

Giglia-Mari, G. and A. Sarasin (2003). "TP53 mutations in human skin cancers." Hum Mutat 21(3): 217-228.

Greenman, C., P. Stephens, R. Smith, G. L. Dalgliesh, C. Hunter, et al. (2007). "Patterns of somatic mutation in human cancer genomes." Nature 446(7132): 153-158.

Halder, R. M. and S. Bridgeman-Shah (1995). "Skin cancer in African Americans." Cancer 75(2 Suppl): 667-673.

Hansson, J. (2010). "Familial cutaneous melanoma." Adv Exp Med Biol 685: 134-145.

Hauser, J. E., A. L. Kadekaro, R. J. Kavanagh, K. Wakamatsu, S. Terzieva, et al. (2006). "Melanin content and MC1R function independently affect UVR-induced DNA damage in cultured human melanocytes." Pigment Cell Res 19(4): 303-314.

Hazra, T. K., A. Das, S. Das, S. Choudhury, Y. W. Kow, et al. (2007). "Oxidative DNA damage repair in mammalian cells: a new perspective." DNA Repair (Amst) 6(4): 470-480.

Hearing, V. J. (1999). "Biochemical control of melanogenesis and melanosomal organization." J Investig Dermatol Symp Proc 4(1): 24-28.

Hill, H. Z., G. J. Hill, K. Cieszka, P. M. Plonka, D. L. Mitchell, et al. (1997). "Comparative action spectrum for ultraviolet light killing of mouse melanocytes from different genetic coat color backgrounds." Photochem Photobiol 65(6): 983-989.

Hoeijmakers, J. H. (2009). "DNA damage, aging, and cancer." N Engl J Med 361(15): 1475-1485.

Holick, M. F. (1981). "The cutaneous photosynthesis of previtamin D3: a unique photoendocrine system." J Invest Dermatol 77(1): 51-58.

Hubbard-Smith, K., H. Z. Hill and G. J. Hill (1992). "Melanin both causes and prevents oxidative base damage in DNA: quantification by anti-thymine glycol antibody." Radiat Res 130(2): 160-165.

Hussein, M. R. (2005). "Melanocytic dysplastic naevi occupy the middle ground between benign melanocytic naevi and cutaneous malignant melanomas: emerging clues." J Clin Pathol 58(5): 453-456.

Hussussian, C. J., J. P. Struewing, A. M. Goldstein, P. A. Higgins, D. S. Ally, et al. (1994). "Germline p16 mutations in familial melanoma." Nat Genet 8(1): 15-21.

Inagaki, K., T. Suzuki, S. Ito, N. Suzuki, K. Adachi, et al. (2006). "Oculocutaneous albinism type 4: six novel mutations in the membrane-associated transporter protein gene and their phenotypes." Pigment Cell Res 19(5): 451-453.

Ito, S., S. Inoue and K. Fujita (1983). "The mechanism of toxicity of 5-S-cysteinyldopa to tumour cells. Hydrogen peroxide as a mediator of cytotoxicity." Biochem Pharmacol 32(13): 2079-2081.

Ito, S. and K. Wakamatsu (1989). "Melanin chemistry and melanin precursors in melanoma." J Invest Dermatol 92(5 Suppl): 261S-265S.

Ito, S., K. Wakamatsu and H. Ozeki (2000). "Chemical analysis of melanins and its application to the study of the regulation of melanogenesis." Pigment Cell Res 13 Suppl 8: 103-109.

Jablonski, N. G. and G. Chaplin (2000). "The evolution of human skin coloration." J Hum Evol 39(1): 57-106.

Jen, M., M. Murphy and J. M. Grant-Kels (2009). "Childhood melanoma." Clin Dermatol 27(6): 529-536.

Jimbow, K., T. G. Salopek, W. T. Dixon, G. E. Searles and K. Yamada (1991). "The epidermal melanin unit in the pathophysiology of malignant melanoma." Am J Dermatopathol 13(2): 179-188.

Joseph, P. (2009). "Mechanisms of cadmium carcinogenesis." Toxicol Appl Pharmacol 238(3): 272-279.

Jung, E. G. (1978). "Xeroderma pigmentosum: heterogeneous syndrome and model for UV carcinogenesis." Bull Cancer 65(3): 315-321.

Kabigting, F. D., F. P. Nelson, C. L. Kauffman, G. Popoveniuc, C. A. Dasanu, et al. (2009). "Malignant melanoma in African-Americans." Dermatol Online J 15(2): 3.

Kadekaro, A. L., R. Kavanagh, H. Kanto, S. Terzieva, J. Hauser, et al. (2005). "alpha-Melanocortin and endothelin-1 activate antiapoptotic pathways and reduce DNA damage in human melanocytes." Cancer Res 65(10): 4292-4299.

Kadekaro, A. L., K. Wakamatsu, S. Ito and Z. A. Abdel-Malek (2006). "Cutaneous photoprotection and melanoma susceptibility: reaching beyond melanin content to the frontiers of DNA repair." Front Biosci 11: 2157-2173.

Kamb, A., D. Shattuck-Eidens, R. Eeles, Q. Liu, N. A. Gruis, et al. (1994). "Analysis of the p16 gene (CDKN2) as a candidate for the chromosome 9p melanoma susceptibility locus." Nat Genet 8(1): 23-26.

Karagas, M. R., V. A. Stannard, L. A. Mott, M. J. Slattery, S. K. Spencer, et al. (2002). "Use of tanning devices and risk of basal cell and squamous cell skin cancers." J Natl Cancer Inst 94(3): 224-226.

Kawada, A. (2000). "Risk and preventive factors for skin phototype." Journal of Dermatological Science 23: S27-S29.

Khaled, M., C. Levy and D. E. Fisher (2010). "Control of melanocyte differentiation by a MITF-PDE4D3 homeostatic circuit." Genes Dev 24(20): 2276-2281.

Klungland, A. and S. Bjelland (2007). "Oxidative damage to purines in DNA: role of mammalian Ogg1." DNA Repair (Amst) 6(4): 481-488.

Kopf, A. W., L. J. Hellman, G. S. Rogers, D. F. Gross, D. S. Rigel, et al. (1986). "Familial malignant melanoma." JAMA 256(14): 1915-1919.

Kvam, E. and R. M. Tyrrell (1997). "Induction of oxidative DNA base damage in human skin cells by UV and near visible radiation." Carcinogenesis 18(12): 2379-2384.

Kvam, E. and R. M. Tyrrell (1999). "The role of melanin in the induction of oxidative DNA base damage by ultraviolet A irradiation of DNA or melanoma cells." J Invest Dermatol 113(2): 209-213.

Lacour, J. P. (2002). "Carcinogenesis of basal cell carcinomas: genetics and molecular mechanisms." Br J Dermatol 146 Suppl 61: 17-19.

Lamason, R. L., M. A. Mohideen, J. R. Mest, A. C. Wong, H. L. Norton, et al. (2005). "SLC24A5, a putative cation exchanger, affects pigmentation in zebrafish and humans." Science 310(5755): 1782-1786.

Larsson, P., E. Andersson, U. Johansson, K. Ollinger and I. Rosdahl (2005). "Ultraviolet A and B affect human melanocytes and keratinocytes differently. A study of oxidative alterations and apoptosis." Exp Dermatol 14(2): 117-123.

Lazovich, D., R. I. Vogel, M. Berwick, M. A. Weinstock, K. E. Anderson, et al. (2010). "Indoor tanning and risk of melanoma: a case-control study in a highly exposed population." Cancer Epidemiol Biomarkers Prev 19(6): 1557-1568.

Leibeling, D., P. Laspe and S. Emmert (2006). "Nucleotide excision repair and cancer." J Mol Histol 37(5-7): 225-238.

Leiter, U. and C. Garbe (2008). "Epidemiology of melanoma and nonmelanoma skin cancer--the role of sunlight." Adv Exp Med Biol 624: 89-103.

Lens, M. B. and M. Dawes (2004). "Global perspectives of contemporary epidemiological trends of cutaneous malignant melanoma." Br J Dermatol 150(2): 179-185.

Li, C., Z. Hu, Z. Liu, L. E. Wang, S. S. Strom, et al. (2006). "Polymorphisms in the DNA repair genes XPC, XPD, and XPG and risk of cutaneous melanoma: a case-control analysis." Cancer Epidemiol Biomarkers Prev 15(12): 2526-2532.

Lim, H. W., W. D. James, D. S. Rigel, M. E. Maloney, J. M. Spencer, et al. (2011). "Adverse effects of ultraviolet radiation from the use of indoor tanning equipment: Time to ban the tan." J Am Acad Dermatol 64(5): 893-902.

Linos, E., S. M. Swetter, M. G. Cockburn, G. A. Colditz and C. A. Clarke (2009). "Increasing burden of melanoma in the United States." J Invest Dermatol 129(7): 1666-1674.

Liu, T. and S. J. Soong (1996). "Epidemiology of malignant melanoma." Surg Clin North Am 76(6): 1205-1222.

Lu, H., C. Edwards, S. Gaskell, A. Pearse and R. Marks (1996). "Melanin content and distribution in the surface corneocyte with skin phototypes." British Journal of Dermatology 135(2): 263-267.

Lynch, H. T., D. E. Anderson, J. L. Smith, Jr., J. B. Howell and A. J. Krush (1967). "Xeroderma pigmentosum, malignant melanoma, and congenital ichthyosis. A family study." Arch Dermatol 96(6): 625-635.

MacKie, R. M. and T. Aitchison (1982). "Severe sunburn and subsequent risk of primary cutaneous malignant melanoma in scotland." Br J Cancer 46(6): 955-960.

Markovic, S. N., L. A. Erickson, R. D. Rao, R. H. Weenig, B. A. Pockaj, et al. (2007). "Malignant melanoma in the 21st century, part 1: epidemiology, risk factors, screening, prevention, and diagnosis." Mayo Clin Proc 82(3): 364-380.

Marks, M. S. and M. C. Seabra (2001). "The melanosome: membrane dynamics in black and white." Nat Rev Mol Cell Biol 2(10): 738-748.

Marks, R. (2000). "Epidemiology of melanoma." Clin Exp Dermatol 25(6): 459-463.

Meyle, K. D. and P. Guldberg (2009). "Genetic risk factors for melanoma." Hum Genet.

Meyskens, F. L., Jr. and M. Berwick (2008). "UV or not UV: metals are the answer." Cancer Epidemiol Biomarkers Prev 17(2): 268-270.

Meyskens, F. L., Jr., P. Farmer and J. P. Fruehauf (2001). "Redox regulation in human melanocytes and melanoma." Pigment Cell Res 14(3): 148-154.

Meyskens, F. L. and S. Yang (2011). "Thinking about the role (largely ignored) of heavy metals in cancer prevention: hexavalent chromium and melanoma as a case in point." Recent Results Cancer Res 188: 65-74.

Millikan, R. C., A. Hummer, C. Begg, J. Player, A. R. de Cotret, et al. (2006). "Polymorphisms in nucleotide excision repair genes and risk of multiple primary melanoma: the Genes Environment and Melanoma Study." Carcinogenesis 27(3): 610-618.

Mogensen, M. and G. B. Jemec (2010). "The potential carcinogenic risk of tanning beds: clinical guidelines and patient safety advice." Cancer Manag Res 2: 277-282.

Molho-Pessach, V. and M. Lotem (2007). "Ultraviolet radiation and cutaneous carcinogenesis." Curr Probl Dermatol 35: 14-27.

Newton, J. M., O. Cohen-Barak, N. Hagiwara, J. M. Gardner, M. T. Davisson, et al. (2001). "Mutations in the human orthologue of the mouse underwhite gene (uw) underlie a new form of oculocutaneous albinism, OCA4." Am J Hum Genet 69(5): 981-988.

Nordlund, J. J. (2007). "The melanocyte and the epidermal melanin unit: an expanded concept." Dermatol Clin 25(3): 271-281, vii.

Oetting, W. S. (1999). "Albinism." Curr Opin Pediatr 11(6): 565-571.

Oetting, W. S. (2000). "The tyrosinase gene and oculocutaneous albinism type 1 (OCA1): A model for understanding the molecular biology of melanin formation." Pigment Cell Res 13(5): 320-325.

Otley, C. C. and M. R. Pittelkow (2000). "Skin cancer in liver transplant recipients." Liver Transpl 6(3): 253-262.

Parra, E. J. (2007). "Human pigmentation variation: evolution, genetic basis, and implications for public health." Am J Phys Anthropol Suppl 45: 85-105.

Passeron, T., T. Namiki, H. J. Passeron, E. Le Pape and V. J. Hearing (2008). "Forskolin Protects Keratinocytes from UVB-Induced Apoptosis and Increases DNA Repair Independent of its Effects on Melanogenesis." J Invest Dermatol 129: 162-166.

Phillipson, R. P., S. E. Tobi, J. A. Morris and T. J. McMillan (2002). "UV-A induces persistent genomic instability in human keratinocytes through an oxidative stress mechanism." Free Radic Biol Med 32(5): 474-480.

Pollock, P. M., U. L. Harper, K. S. Hansen, L. M. Yudt, M. Stark, et al. (2003). "High frequency of BRAF mutations in nevi." Nat Genet 33(1): 19-20.

Prota, G. (1980). "Recent advances in the chemistry of melanogenesis in mammals." J Invest Dermatol 75(1): 122-127.

Prota, G. (2000). "Melanins, melanogenesis and melanocytes: looking at their functional significance from the chemist's viewpoint." Pigment Cell Res 13(4): 283-293.

Rass, K. and J. Reichrath (2008). "UV damage and DNA repair in malignant melanoma and nonmelanoma skin cancer." Adv Exp Med Biol 624: 162-178.

Ravnbak, M. H. (2010). "Objective determination of Fitzpatrick skin type." Dan Med Bull 57(8): B4153.

Rees, J. L. (2003). "Genetics of hair and skin color." Annu Rev Genet 37: 67-90.
Rees, J. L. and E. Healy (1997). "Melanocortin receptors, red hair, and skin cancer." J Investig Dermatol Symp Proc 2(1): 94-98.
Reutter, J. C., E. M. Long, D. S. Morrell, N. E. Thomas and P. A. Groben (2007). "Eruptive post-chemotherapy in situ melanomas and dysplastic nevi." Pediatr Dermatol 24(2): 135-137.
Rigel, D. S. (2010). "Epidemiology of melanoma." Semin Cutan Med Surg 29(4): 204-209.
Riley, P. A. (1997). "Melanin." Int J Biochem Cell Biol 29(11): 1235-1239.
Robbins, L. S., J. H. Nadeau, K. R. Johnson, M. A. Kelly, L. Roselli-Rehfuss, et al. (1993). "Pigmentation phenotypes of variant extension locus alleles result from point mutations that alter MSH receptor function." Cell 72(6): 827-834.
Robinson, S., S. Dixon, S. August, B. Diffey, K. Wakamatsu, et al. (2010). "Protection against UVR involves MC1R-mediated non-pigmentary and pigmentary mechanisms in vivo." J Invest Dermatol 130(7): 1904-1913.
Rosei, M. A. (2001). "Opiomelanins synthesis and properties." Histol Histopathol 16(3): 931-935.
Runger, T. M. (1999). "Role of UVA in the pathogenesis of melanoma and non-melanoma skin cancer. A short review." Photodermatol Photoimmunol Photomed 15(6): 212-216.
Runger, T. M. and U. P. Kappes (2008). "Mechanisms of mutation formation with long-wave ultraviolet light (UVA)." Photodermatol Photoimmunol Photomed 24(1): 2-10.
Russo, M. T., G. De Luca, P. Degan and M. Bignami (2007). "Different DNA repair strategies to combat the threat from 8-oxoguanine." Mutat Res 614(1-2): 69-76.
Sarasin, A. (1999). "The molecular pathways of ultraviolet-induced carcinogenesis." Mutat Res 428(1-2): 5-10.
Scherer, D. and R. Kumar (2010). "Genetics of pigmentation in skin cancer - A review." Mutat Res 705(2): 141-153.
Schulman, J. M. and D. E. Fisher (2009). "Indoor ultraviolet tanning and skin cancer: health risks and opportunities." Curr Opin Oncol 21(2): 144-149.
Schulz, I., H. C. Mahler, S. Boiteux and B. Epe (2000). "Oxidative DNA base damage induced by singlet oxygen and photosensitization: recognition by repair endonucleases and mutagenicity." Mutat Res 461(2): 145-156.
Seiberg, M. (2001). "Keratinocyte-melanocyte interactions during melanosome transfer." Pigment Cell Res 14(4): 236-242.
Seo, S. J. and D. E. Fisher (2010). "Melanocyte photobiology, ultraviolet radiation and melanoma." G Ital Dermatol Venereol 145(5): 603-611.
Simon, J. D. and D. N. Peles (2010). "The red and the black." Acc Chem Res 43(11): 1452-1460.
Smit, N. P., F. A. van Nieuwpoort, L. Marrot, C. Out, B. Poorthuis, et al. (2008). "Increased melanogenesis is a risk factor for oxidative DNA damage--study on cultured melanocytes and atypical nevus cells." Photochem Photobiol 84(3): 550-555.
Smith, A. G., N. Luk, R. A. Newton, D. W. Roberts, R. A. Sturm, et al. (2008). "Melanocortin-1 receptor signaling markedly induces the expression of the NR4A nuclear receptor subgroup in melanocytic cells." J Biol Chem 283(18): 12564-12570.

American Cancer Society (2011). "Melanoma Skin Cancer Overview." from http://www.cancer.org/Cancer/SkinCancer-Melanoma/OverviewGuide/index.

Song, X., N. Mosby, J. Yang, A. Xu, Z. Abdel-Malek, et al. (2009). "alpha-MSH activates immediate defense responses to UV-induced oxidative stress in human melanocytes." Pigment Cell Melanoma Res 22(6): 809-818.

Steingrimsson, E., N. G. Copeland and N. A. Jenkins (2006). "Mouse coat color mutations: from fancy mice to functional genomics." Dev Dyn 235(9): 2401-2411.

Sturm, R. A. (2009). "Molecular genetics of human pigmentation diversity." Hum Mol Genet 18(R1): R9-17.

Tassabehji, M., V. E. Newton and A. P. Read (1994). "Waardenburg syndrome type 2 caused by mutations in the human microphthalmia (MITF) gene." Nat Genet 8(3): 251-255.

Tucker, M. A. (2009). "Melanoma epidemiology." Hematol Oncol Clin North Am 23(3): 383-395, vii.

Tudek, B., M. Swoboda, P. Kowalczyk and R. Olinski (2006). "Modulation of oxidative DNA damage repair by the diet, inflammation and neoplastic transformation." J Physiol Pharmacol 57 Suppl 7: 33-49.

Valverde, P., E. Healy, I. Jackson, J. L. Rees and A. J. Thody (1995). "Variants of the melanocyte-stimulating hormone receptor gene are associated with red hair and fair skin in humans." Nat Genet 11(3): 328-330.

Van Patter, H. T. and J. A. Drummond (1953). "Malignant melanoma occurring in xeroderma pigmentosum; report of a case." Cancer 6(5): 942-947.

Veierod, M. B., H. O. Adami, E. Lund, B. K. Armstrong and E. Weiderpass (2010). "Sun and solarium exposure and melanoma risk: effects of age, pigmentary characteristics, and nevi." Cancer Epidemiol Biomarkers Prev 19(1): 111-120.

Vincensi, M. R., M. d'Ischia, A. Napolitano, E. M. Procaccini, G. Riccio, et al. (1998). "Phaeomelanin versus eumelanin as a chemical indicator of ultraviolet sensitivity in fair-skinned subjects at high risk for melanoma: a pilot study." Melanoma Res 8(1): 53-58.

Walter, S. D., L. D. Marrett, L. From, C. Hertzman, H. S. Shannon, et al. (1990). "The association of cutaneous malignant melanoma with the use of sunbeds and sunlamps." Am J Epidemiol 131(2): 232-243.

Wenczl, E., G. P. Van der Schans, L. Roza, R. M. Kolb, A. J. Timmerman, et al. (1998). "(Pheo)melanin photosensitizes UVA-induced DNA damage in cultured human melanocytes." J Invest Dermatol 111(4): 678-682.

Westerdahl, J., H. Olsson, A. Masback, C. Ingvar, N. Jonsson, et al. (1994). "Use of sunbeds or sunlamps and malignant melanoma in southern Sweden." Am J Epidemiol 140(8): 691-699.

Whiteman, D. C., R. M. Brown, C. Xu, C. L. Paterson, D. Miller, et al. (2003). "A rapid method for determining recent sunscreen use in field studies." J Photochem Photobiol B 69(1): 59-63.

Whiteside, J. R., C. L. Box, T. J. McMillan and S. L. Allinson (2010). "Cadmium and copper inhibit both DNA repair activities of polynucleotide kinase." DNA Repair (Amst) 9(1): 83-89.

Yazdi, A. S., G. Palmedo, M. J. Flaig, U. Puchta, A. Reckwerth, et al. (2003). "Mutations of the BRAF gene in benign and malignant melanocytic lesions." J Invest Dermatol 121(5): 1160-1162.

# Part 2

# Clinical Phenotypes of Melanoma

# 4

# Desmoplastic Melanoma

Lily S. Cheng and April W. Armstrong
*University of California Davis Medical Center*
*United States of America*

## 1. Introduction

Desmoplastic melanoma is a rare variant of spindle cell melanoma that was first described in 1971 by Conley et al. [1] . Between 1988 and 2006, less than 2,000 patients were diagnosed with desmoplastic melanoma in the United States. It accounts for between 1 to 4 percent of all cases of cutaneous melanomas. [2] Early diagnosis of desmoplastic melanoma can often result in favorable outcomes due to the relatively slow-growing nature of the tumor. However, in most patients with desmoplastic melanoma, the diagnosis is usually reached at an advanced stage of the disease due to the significant diagnostic challenges associated with this tumor.

## 2. Epidemiology

An analysis of the National Cancer Insititute's Surveillance, Epidemiology and End Results (SEER) tumor registry database by Wasif et al in 2010 found that the mean age of onset for desmoplastic melanoma to be 66 $\pm$ 4 and a median age of onset of 69. Compared to other cutaneous melanomas, desmoplastic melanoma is more likely to present in an older population with a median age of onset about 10 years older. [3] The study by Wasif et al also identified a 65 percent male predominance. [3] A systematic review of literature on desmoplastic melanoma by Lens et al in 2005 yielded similar epidemiological data with a 63 percent male predominance. While desmoplastic melanoma is most likely to occur in older men, it can affect men or women of any age. [4]

Approximately 51 to 53 percent of desmoplastic melanomas are located in the head and neck; less common locations included the extremities (26 to 30 percent), and the trunk (18 to 20 percent). [3, 4] Although the overall occurrence of desmoplastic melanoma on the extremities is uncommon, compared to the lower extremities, the upper extremities appear to be a more favored location and represent 70 percent of all desmoplastic melanomas occurring on extremities. [4] This distribution for desmoplastic melanoma is similar to the pattern of distribution seen in non-melanoma skin cancers, squamous cell carcinoma and basal cell carcinoma. Overall, desmoplastic melanoma appears to be more likely to be found in chronically sun-exposed areas.

Desmoplastic melanoma is also frequently associated with other types of skin cancers, especially with other cutaneous melanomas that are also associated with sun exposure. [5] Desmoplastic melanoma has been reported to occur in conjunction with atypical lentiginous hyperplasia, lentigo maligna melanoma, and superficial spreading malignant melanoma.

Approximately 30 percent of desmoplastic melanoma occurs in combination with lentigo maligna melanoma, also known as a Hutchinson melanotic freckle, which contributes its presentation as an atypical pigmented lesion in about half of the cases. [5, 6]

## 3. Clinical features

Desmoplastic melanoma is commonly misdiagnosed due to its subtle presentation. It commonly appears as an indurated skin-colored papule, plaque or nodule. These lesions are usually painless. [7, 8] The diagnostic challenge for desmoplastic melanoma is frequently attributed to the observation that more than half of all desmoplastic melanomas are amelanotic, or not possessing pigmentation. Therefore, they are commonly mistaken for benign lesions, such as dermatofibromas or scars. [5] The presence of a new scar without a history of trauma may prompt the clinician to consider the possibility of desmoplastic melanoma among other differential diagnoses, especially if the scar is located on the head and neck region. The differential diagnosis for desmoplastic melanoma also includes basal cell carcinomas and dermal nevi, which can also present as pale, skin-colored lesions in the head and neck region. As previously stated, desmoplastic melanomas that are associated with lentigo melanoma often present with atypical pigmentation patterns that are more reminiscent of other subtypes of melanomas and non-melanoma skin cancers. Desmoplastic melanomas presenting with atypical pigmentation tend to have better prognosis because they are often recognized earlier. Other rare, atypical findings associated with desmoplastic melanoma include macular erythema and alopecia. [4]

## 4. Histological features

As with other skin cancers, a biopsy is required to definitively diagnose desmoplastic melanoma. The pathological presentation of desmoplastic melanoma is characterized by a proliferation of spindle cells, which are non-pigmented spindle-shaped melanocytes. (See Figure 1) Cellular atypia can vary widely from near-normal morphology to moderate atypia. This can lead to significant diagnostic challenge as the cells may display little atypia in many cases. The nuclei of these spindle cells tend to hyperchromatic and may be elongated. The cytoplasm is usually scant an increased nucleus to cytoplasm ratio commonly seen in malignant cells. [5, 8]

These spindle cells of desmoplastic melanoma are found in variable distributions among a background of reactive fibroblasts and collagen bundles. The appearance of collagen bundles is similar to that of a scar; this may account for the scar-like clinical appearance. Islands of lymphoid aggregates may also be seen among the collagenous background. Solar elastosis is routinely found in the dermis, consistent with the association of desmoplastic melanoma with sun exposure. [5, 8]

When desmoplastic melanoma invades surrounding nerves, it is desmoplastic neurotropic melanoma. In desmoplastic neurotropic melanoma, spindle cells may surround and/or invade nerves in the dermis. [9] Spindle cells may also undergo neural transformation to form structures resembling nerves. Typically, this occurs only when the tumor exceeds 1.5 mm in thickness or a Clark stage of greater than IV. [5] Of note, while nerve involvement is not uncommon for large tumors, desmoplastic melanomas tend not to invade the vascular or lymphatic structures with the same frequency.

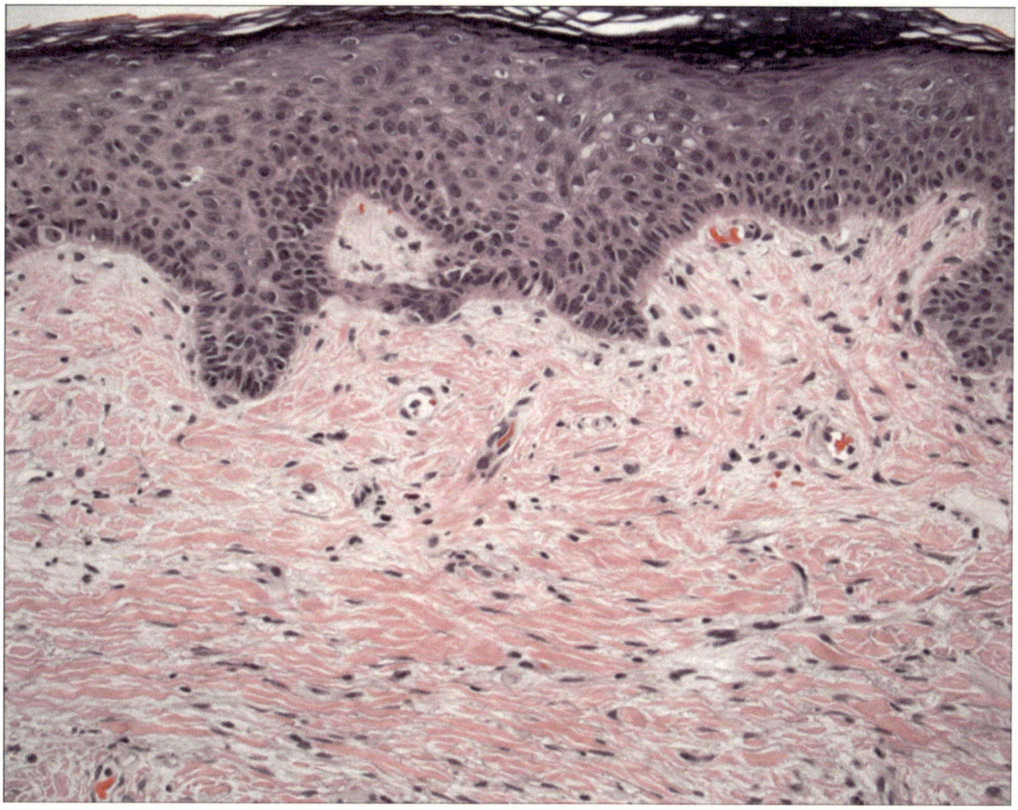

Fig. 1. Histological features of desmoplastic melanoma
(photograph courtesy of Dr. Maxwell Fung)

Immunohistochemistry can a helpful tool to distinguish desmoplastic melanoma from these other forms of cutaneous melanoma and from other benign lesions. Desmoplastic melanomas are typically positive for S100 protein, P75 growth factor, and negative for HMB-45 protein (See Figure 2). [10] Though the S100 marker is currently the most commonly used marker to diagnose desmoplastic melanoma in clinical practice, recently, it has been suggested that the P75 nerve growth factor may be a more sensitive marker. Staining for the P75 nerve growth factor can be used in conjunction with S100 staining for increased sensitivity in diagnosing desmoplastic melanoma. [11]

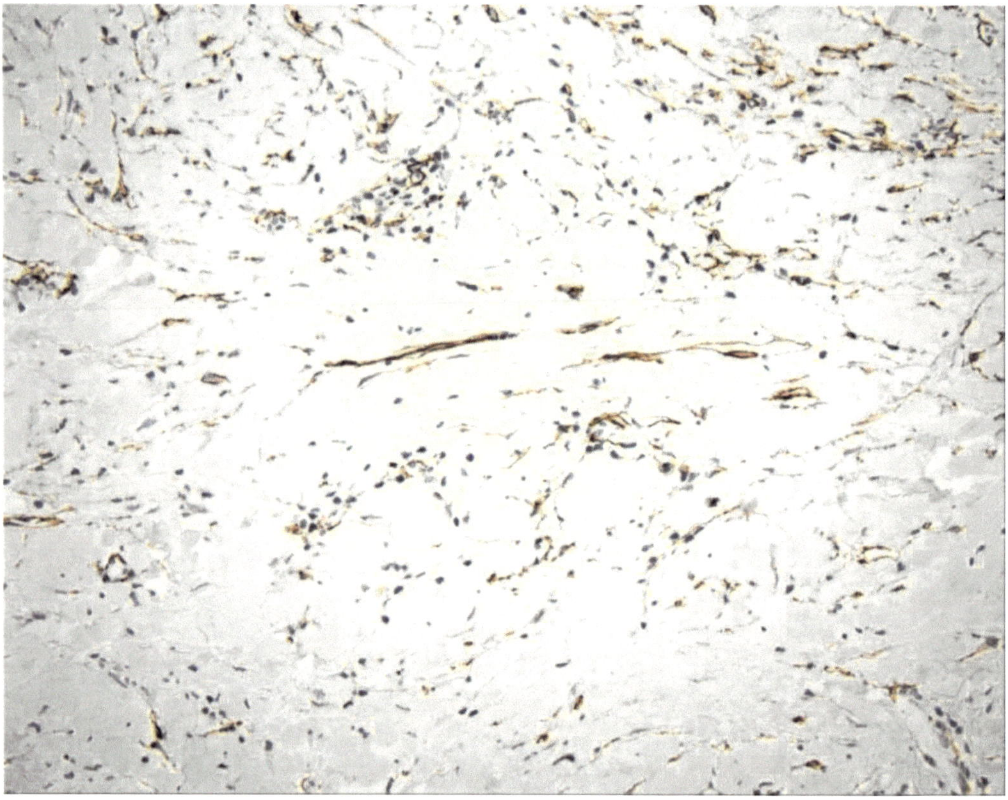

Fig. 2. S100 marker staining for desmoplastic melanoma
(photograph courtesy of Dr. Maxwell Fung)

## 5. Treatment

Desmoplastic melanoma is typically slow-growing but commonly presents in an advanced stage due to its insidious nature. The mean Breslow thickness (measured from the granular layer of the epidermis to the deepest portion of the tumor) at diagnosis ranges from 2.0 mm to 6.5 mm, and most tumors are already Clark stage IV or V at time of diagnosis. Neurotropic involvement ranged from 17 to 78 percent. [4]

As with most skin cancers, surgical excision is the primary treatment modality for desmoplastic melanoma. Wide excision with margins of 1-cm to 2-cm is associated with less risk of recurrence and better prognostic outcomes. [3] It has even been suggested that margins of at least 2-cm are needed for even small lesions. [12]

Despite its tendency to recur locally at the primary site, desmoplastic melanoma is less likely to have nodal metastases than other forms of cutaneous melanoma. In cases where sentinel node biopsies were performed, only 3 percent of these patients were found to have involvement of desmoplastic melanoma cells in the sentinel lymph nodes. Therefore, controversy exists regarding criteria for selecting appropriate patients with desmoplastic melanoma for sentinel lymph node biopsy due to the rare occurrence of nodal invasion. [3, 12] However, the incidence of lymph node involvement is significantly higher when there is nerve involvement, as in DNM. Therefore, sentinel lymph node biopsy is currently recommended for DNM. [9]

The use of post-operative adjuvant radiation for desmoplastic melanoma has been found to be effective in decreasing the rate of recurrence. Adjuvant radiation of the local site is indicated if margins of the tumor are not clearly defined or intense neurotropic invasion is observed. [13] Adjuvant immunotherapy and chemotherapy are not routinely recommended for treatment of desmoplastic melanoma, and the use of these modalities has not been proven to improve outcomes. [4]

## 6. Prognosis

Comparing tumors of the same stage, prognosis of desmoplastic melanoma is more favorable than that of other subtypes of cutaneous melanoma. However, because desmoplastic melanoma is usually diagnosed at a later stage than other cutaneous melanoma, is the overall prognosis for desmoplastic melanoma is poorer. For stage I and II lesions, the 5-year survival rate is approximately 90 percent; however, only 29 percent of cases are diagnosed in stage I. [2] When all stages of the tumor are accounted, the overall 5-year survival rate from desmoplastic melanoma is 72 percent. [2] Of note, survival in desmoplastic melanoma and desmoplastic neurotropic melanoma was found to be comparable despite the wider spread of desmoplastic neurotropic melanoma. This may be due to the success of adjuvant radiation therapy in treatment of more advanced lesions. [2]

Desmoplastic melanomas have a high local recurrence rate that ranges from 7 to 56 percent. [4] The high local recurrence rate of desmoplastic melanoma may be attributed to difficulties in defining surgical margin during resection of the tumor. Local recurrence was more common in desmoplastic neurotropic melanoma than in desmoplastic melanomas without nerve involvement. [2] For desmoplastic melanomas without neural invasion, rates of metastatic disease were generally found to be as low as 7 percent [4] In comparison, desmoplastic neurotropic melanoma metastasize at a higher rate of approximately 15 percent. [9]

## 7. Summary

Desmoplastic melanoma is a rare subtype of cutaneous melanoma that is particular challenging to diagnosis due to its atypical amelanotic appearance. Desmoplastic melanoma is characterized histologically by the proliferation of atypical spindle-shaped melanocytes, and neurotropism is not uncommonly observed with this tumor. While desmoplastic melanoma tends to recur locally at higher frequency compared to other subtypes of melanomas, it is less likely to travel to the nodal basin or metastasize. Treatment of desmoplastic melanoma relies primarily on surgical excision with wide margins and adjuvant radiotherapy for advanced disease. Prognosis tends to be favorable when tumor margins are clearly defined and adequate surgical margin is achieved.

## 8. References

[1] Conley J, Lattes R, Orr W: Desmoplastic malignant melanoma (a rare variant of spindle cell melanoma). Cancer 1971; 28(4): 914-36.
[2] Quinn MJ, Crotty KA, Thompson JF, Coates AS, O'Brien CJ, McCarthy WH: Desmoplastic and desmoplastic neurotropic melanoma: experience with 280 patients. Cancer 1998; 83(6): 1128-35.
[3] Wasif N, Gray RJ, Pockaj BA: Desmoplastic melanoma - the step-child in the melanoma family? J Surg Oncol; 103(2): 158-62.
[4] Lens MB, Newton-Bishop JA, Boon AP: Desmoplastic malignant melanoma: a systematic review. Br J Dermatol 2005; 152(4): 673-8.
[5] McCarthy SW, Scolyer RA, Palmer AA: Desmoplastic melanoma: a diagnostic trap for the unwary. Pathology 2004; 36(5): 445-51.
[6] Anstey A, McKee P, Jones EW: Desmoplastic malignant melanoma: a clinicopathological study of 25 cases. Br J Dermatol 1993; 129(4): 359-71.
[7] Chamberlain A, Ng J: Cutaneous melanoma--atypical variants and presentations. Aust Fam Physician 2009; 38(7): 476-82.
[8] Barnhill RL, Gupta K: Unusual variants of malignant melanoma. Clin Dermatol 2009; 27(6): 564-87.
[9] Chen JY, Hruby G, Scolyer RA, et al.: Desmoplastic neurotropic melanoma: a clinicopathologic analysis of 128 cases. Cancer 2008; 113(10): 2770-8.
[10] Chorny JA, Barr RJ: S100-positive spindle cells in scars: a diagnostic pitfall in the re-excision of desmoplastic melanoma. Am J Dermatopathol 2002; 24(4): 309-12.
[11] Lazova R, Tantcheva-Poor I, Sigal AC: P75 nerve growth factor receptor staining is superior to S100 in identifying spindle cell and desmoplastic melanoma. J Am Acad Dermatol; 63(5): 852-8.
[12] Maurichi A, Miceli R, Camerini T, et al.: Pure desmoplastic melanoma: a melanoma with distinctive clinical behavior. Ann Surg; 252(6): 1052-7.
[13] Vongtama R, Safa A, Gallardo D, Calcaterra T, Juillard G: Efficacy of radiation therapy in the local control of desmoplastic malignant melanoma. Head Neck 2003; 25(6): 423-8.

# 5

# Melanoma During Pregnancy

Lazar Popovic[1], Zorka Grgic[2] and Milica Popovic[2]
[1]*Oncology Institute of Vojvodina, Sremska Kamenica,*
[2]*Clinical Centre of Vojvodina, Novi Sad,*
*Serbia*

## 1. Introduction

Melanoma is the most malignant cutaneous tumor. The incidence of melanoma accounts for the sixth place among malignant diseases, 5% of malignancies among men and 4% of malignancies among women; it stands for 1.4% of deaths caused by malignant disease (Fisher et al., 2008). The incidence of malignant melanoma has constantly been increasing and it has reached 3% per year in the last several years. At the beginning of the 20th century, the population risk for malignant melanoma was in the ratio 1:500 but today 1:73 of women and 1:49 of men are at risk (Fisher et al., 2008). It is anticipated that there will be 68,130 newly diagnose cases of melanoma and approximately 8,700 deaths from the disease in the USA (Jamal et al., 2010). Among the population aged between 20 to 39 years malignant melanoma is on the second place by incidence. Although the disease is more frequent among men, its incidence during the reproductive period is higher among women. In Great Britain, the third of all diagnosed melanomas arise before 50 years of age and about 30% to 35% develop during the reproductive period of women (Anonymus, 2003; Cancer Research UK 2006). The actual incidence of melanoma during pregnancy is unknown. Smith and Randall (Smith RS & Randall, 1969) gave the first reports based on the source documents of a small non-reference Plattsburg Air Force Base Hospital, New York. The incidence of melanoma was 2.8 per 1000 deliveries but studies that are more recent showed that it is between 2.8 and 5 per 100,000 of pregnancies; the registry of German Dermatological Society shows that 1% of female patients affected with melanoma is pregnant (Dillman et al., 1996; Garbe, 1993). A group of Swedish authors analyzed the period from 1973 to 1984 and reported that melanoma is the most common cancer appearing in pregnancy and accounts for 24.5% of cancer cases in pregnant women (Matthiasen & Berg, 1989). From 1958 to 1999, 19,337 women with melanoma were included in the most extensive epidemiology study based on Swedish and regional registries; 0.9% of malignant melanomas were diagnosed during the pregnancy. Of all included patients, 5,533 of women were in reproductive age and 185 (3.3%) of them were diagnosed with melanoma during the pregnancy (Lens et al., 2004.). The prognostic features for melanoma depend on the stage it has been diagnosed. Although the 5-year survival for stage IV melanoma is still less than 5%, overall mortality from melanoma has a decreasing tendency (Rigel et al., 1996). The effect of pregnancy to the course of melanoma has been a researching issue for years. The results of uncontrolled studies conducted from 1950 to 1980 show that pregnancy is an unfavorable prognostic factor in patients' survival (Pack & Scharnagel, 1951; Sutherland et al., 1983; Trapeznikov et al., 1987 ), but the reports of recent controlled studies oppose this finding (Lens et al., 2004; Reintgen et al., 1985; McManamny et al., 1989; Wong et al., 1989; Slingluff et al., 1990; MacKie et al., 1991). The most recent population studies demonstrate equal survival among women with the same melanoma stage regardless they are pregnant or not (Lens et al., 2004; O'Meara et al, 2005). Overall survival rate in both pregnant and nonpregnant patients was 82% (Lens et al., 2004).

## 2. The influence of sex hormones on melanoma

Sun exposure and excessive tanning are the main risk factors for melanoma developing (Katsambas et al., 1996; Lazovich et al., 2010). Because the appearance of malignant melanoma in reproductive period is more often in women than in men (Cancer research UK 2006), the influence of sex hormones, exogenous hormones, and reproductive factors is a broadly investigated topic in the pathogenesis of melanoma ( Osterlind et al., 1988; Smith MA et al., 1998; Karagas et al., 2002; Pfahlberg et al., 1997; Durvasula et al., 2002; Elwood & Coldman, 1978).

### 2.1 The influence of reproductive factors and exogenous hormones

The length of exposure to female sex hormones has no influence on the risk of melanoma development. Osterlind et al. (Osterlind et al., 1988) included in their case-control study 280 patients with melanoma and 536 patients in the control group. They showed that age of menarche, the length of reproductive period, the age of natural menopause appearance, the age of first pregnancy, the number of pregnancies, the number of live newborn infants, and the number of abortions has no influence on melanoma development. In addition, the results of the same study demonstrated that there is no correlation between melanoma appearance and the use of oral contraceptives, their type or time of usage. According to study metioned above, the use of hormone-replacement therapy does not increase the risk of melanoma development. Smith et al. (Smith MA et al., 1998) included in their study 308 women with malignant melanoma and 233 patients in the control group. They investigated the influence of previous pregnancies, the age of the first pregnancy, the use of hormone-replacement therapy, the use of oral contraceptives, and the age when first contraceptive was taken; they found that neither of these parameters had any influence on the increase of the risk of melanoma development. Menopause and body mass index did not have any specific effect to the risk of melanoma development but the incidence of melanoma was three times higher in obese postmenopausal women than in premenopausal women of average weight. This study also reported that multiple pregnancies could partly have protective influence on the development of melanoma. Two meta-analyses of case-control studies found no risk of melanoma development among women who used oral contraceptives. The age when first contraceptive was used, duration of contraceptive use, the length of the period from the first and the last use of contraceptives, and the type of contraceptives did not increase the risk of melanoma development (Karagas et al., 2002; Pfahlberg et al., 1997). The conclusion of Durvasula et al. (Durvasula et al., 2002) study is that there is no need to stop hormone-replacement therapy in patients treated of malignant melanoma because there is no evidence of the negative influence of this therapy to the patients' survival. Although several studies demonstrated the protective effect of multiple pregnancies on melanoma development (Smith MA et al., 1998; Karagas et al., 2006), the results of the last case-control study conducted by Lea et al. (Lea, 2007) are opposite: women with multiple pregnancies are at higher risk for malignant melanoma.

### 2.2 Estrogen receptors

Estrogen effects are expressed by the activation of two estrogen receptors: ERα and ERβ. Up to the discovery of ERβ in 1995, no immunohistochemical analysis pointed to the influence of ER in pathogenesis of malignant melanoma. Contrary to ERα, which is predominant in breast tissue, ERβ is characteristic for skin and other tissues that are not estrogen-dependant, such as prostate, colon, and brain (de Giorgi et al., 2011). ERβ distribution in skin depends on the sex and age of a person. Men have lower ERβ level in skin than women in whom the level of this receptor decreases after menopause because of positive estrogen feedback loosing (Stevenson & Thornton, 2007). Immunohistochemical and real-time polymerase chain reaction (PCR) analyses of ERβ in the tissue of melanoma (de Giorgi et al., 2009; Schmidt et al., 2006) showed that expression of ERβ is reversely proportional to Breslow thickness, which is a significant prognostic factor for survival from melanoma (Rigel et al., 1996). De Giorgi et al. found lower ERβ concentration in thicker and more invasive melanomas and concluded that ERβ had an antiproliferative effect; hence their explanation for the failure of tamoxifen in the treatment of malignant melanoma (Lens et al., 2003). The authors believe that tamoxifen inhibits ERα and ERβ nonselectively and in this way, although it inhibits ERα proliferative effect, it inhibits antiproliferative effect of ERβ (de Giorgi et al., 2011). The influence of estrogen receptors in melanoma pathogenesis is still to be cleared up in future.

### 2.3 The impact of pregnancy

The impact of pregnancies and other reproductive and hormonal factors on melanoma development has been described in previous chapters. Melanomas are relatively often diagnosed during pregnancies; it has led to the speculation that certain hormone effects and immunosuppression in pregnancy may induce malignant transformation (Sadoff et al., 1973; Cochran et al., 1982). However, none of the studies showed that the risk for melanoma occurring is higher during pregnancy. Perhaps, diagnosis of melanoma is more frequent because patients visits the physicians more regular. According to the Connecticut Tumor Registry, the percent of melanoma that are diagnosed among pregnant women equals the one among the general female population (Houghton et al.,1981). In addition, the percent of melanoma arisen by the transformation of existing nevus is from 62% to 68% in pregnant women (Houghton et al.,1981; Colboum et al., 1989), which is similar to 65% found among general female population (George et al., 1960; Friedman et al., 1985).

## 3. Diagnosis

Diagnosis of melanoma in pregnancy does not differ from the diagnosis in other population and it comprises clinical examination, tumor excision or biopsy, and pathological examination. The classic ABCD system for melanoma detection was developed in 1985 by the American Cancer Society and it is the basis of clinical examination (Friedman et al., 1985). ABCD is a simple method for early detection of malignant melanoma and its differentiation from benign nevi and other skin changes. The mnemonic ABCD is formed from the initial letters of the words *Asymmetry*, *Border* irregularity, *Color* variety, and *Diameter* greater than 6 mm (Figure 1).

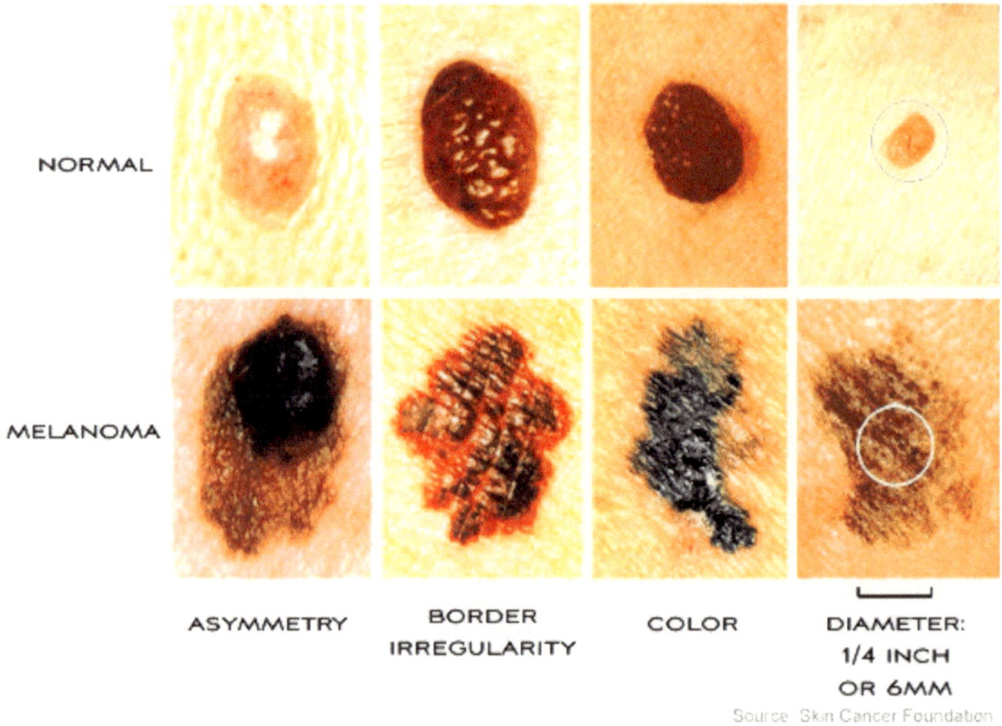


Fig. 1. ABCD diagnostic criteria

The presentation of newly formed or preexisting lesion is of great importance in early detection of melanoma; therefore, the letter E, which stands for *Evolving*, has been added to the ABCD system. The introduction of ABCD criteria has drastically increased the number of melanoma diagnosed in its early, curable stage, without ulceration and with lower Breslow thickness (Rigel et al., 2010). Because of its complexity, Glasgow 7-point checklist (MacKie, 1990) is rarely used, contrary to *Ugly Duckling Sign*. This method is used to mark the nevus that deviate from surrounding lesions and require further examination for suspected malignancy (Scope et al., 2008).

### 3.1 Skin self-examination

The method of skin self-examination should be performed by whole population, especially individuals that are at higher risk for melanoma developing. Melanomas are most often detected by the patients themselves (Rigel et al., 2010). Patients who performed skin self-examination have thinner melanoma than those who did not practice this approach (Pollitt et al., 2009). In addition to the good knowledge of the criteria for melanoma diagnosis by gynecologists and obstetricians, it is of great importance to perform regular skin self-examination during pregnancy.

### 3.2 Problems in pregnancy

Pregnancy triggers a number of physiological changes, skin pigmentation is intensified, and nevi often became darker and bigger (Lens, 2008). These changes complicate the establishment of melanoma diagnosis in pregnancy and physician in charge of a pregnant woman should not assign changed nevus only to physiology mechanisms in pregnancy. Each change of existing or appearance of new nevus should be followed carefully by gynecologist at each patient visit and biopsy should be indicated in case of each suspected lesion. A number of studies report that women diagnosed with melanoma during pregnancy present thicker tumors (Lens et al., 2004, MacKie et al., 1991, Travers et al., 1995.). In Lens study tumor tickness was 1.28 mm in pregnant and 1.07 mm in non-pregnant patients. Same observation was made by Travers et al. (2.28mm vs 1.22 mm). The authors explain this by the impact of hormones and growth factors, and delayed diagnosis compared to general population (Lens et al., 2004). Tumor tickness was independent factor for survival, but once tumor tickness was controlled for survival rate was the same in pregnant and non-pregnant patients.

### 3.3 Excision and pathological examination

Final diagnosis of melanoma is based on excisional biopsy and histopathology analysis. Each lesion suspected for melanoma should be completely removed with free margins. Lidocaine should be used as local anesthetic in pregnant women; epinephrine, usually used for better control hemostasis and prolongation of lidocaine effect, is not recommended because it belongs to group C according to Food and Drug Administration (Lawrence, 1996). A clinician has to provide pathologist with all relevant information about the patient; these information should include: the history of melanoma appearance among the family, the size and the location of excised lesion and its morphological characteristics. Pathological report should include: the type of melanoma, dimesions, status of the margins, disease stage according to Breslow and Clarke, the existence of ulceration, presence of vascular and/or lymphatic invasion, mitotic index, and the growing phase (Lens, 2008).

## 4. Staging

Staging system used for melanoma is based on Union Internationale Contre la Cancer/American Joint Committee on Cancer Staging (UICC.AJCC) guidelines (Balch et al., 2009) (Table 1 and Table 2.). Melanoma staging implies the use of histopathological procedures for measuring the depth of tumor invasion (Breslow thickness), sentinel node, radiology and nuclear medicine procedures. Some of those procedures are contraindicated in pregnancy.

### 4.1 Sentinel node

No locoregional recurrence will occur after local excision without lymphadenectomy in about 80% to 85% of patients with melanomas less than 4 mm thick (Breslow thickness). However, the rest of 15% to 20% of patients will experience locoregional recurrence (Hoekstra, 2008). In order to improve these results a number of authors have tried to routinely perform lymphadenectomy after the excision of primary tumor. Sim et al. (Sim et al., 1986) analyzed the survival of 171 patients with localized malignant melanoma; they preformed an early lymphadenectomy, delayed lymphadenectomy, or no lymphadenectomy at all. No statistically significant difference was found in either metastasis-free survival (MFS) or overall survival (OS). Cacscinelli et al. (Cascinelli et al., 1998) examined 255 patients with melanoma located on the trunk and thicker than 1.5 mm.

They found no statistically significant difference in survival between patients with early lymphadenectomy and patients with lymphadenectomy performed after the diagnosis of lymph node metastases. Balch et al. (Balch et al, 1996) obtained similar results in comparing early lymphadenectomy with only follow-up. However, their extensive study showed certain benefits of lymphadenectomy in case of patients under 60 year of age and those with tumor thickness of 1 mm to 2 mm and no ulceration. Although no statistically significant difference was confirmed, the results of the above-mentioned studies show clearly that there are benefits from early lymphadenectomy for some patients. In 1992, Morton et al. developed the method of sentinel node biopsy (Morton et al., 1992). This technique combine $^{99m}$Tc and blue dye for mapping of affected lymph nodes. When metastases are confirmed by this method, surgeon perform complete lymph node resection in that area. Gershenwald (Gershenwald et al., 1999) and de Vries (de Vries et al., 2005) in their studies have pointed to the importance of sentinel node biopsy in the prognosis of melanoma patients. In addition, Morton (Morton et al., 2006) reports the results of Multicenter Selective Lymphadenectomy Trial I (MSLT I) regarding the sentinel node biopsy in patients with medium thick melanoma of (1.2 mm to 3.5 mm); they show better 5-year survival in patients with early lymphadenectomy than in case of patients with lymphadenectomy after confirmation of metastases development (72.3% vs. 52.4%, p=0.04). Beside, limphoedemas were more frequent in patients with delayed lymphadenectomy ( 20.4 vs 12.4%, p= 0,04) (Faries et al., 2010) After all these results, sentinel node biopsy has become a standard in the treatment of melanoma (Valsecchi et al., 2011; Balch et al., 2009; Dummer et al., 2008).

| **T classification** | | |
|---|---|---|
| T1 | ≤1.0 mm | A: without ulceration |
| T1 | | B: with ulceration or Clarks' level IV or V |
| T2 | 1.01-2.0 mm | A: without ulceration |
| T2 | | B: with ulceration |
| T3 | 2.01-4.0 mm | A: without ulceration |
| T3 | | B: with ulceration |
| T4 | >4.0 mm | A: without ulceration |
| T4 | | B: with ulceration |
| **N classification** | | |
| N1 | One lymph node | A: micrometastasis[a]<br>B: macrometastasis[b] |
| N2 | 2-3 lymph nodes | A: micrometastasis[a]<br>B: macrometastasis[b]<br>C: in-transit met(s)/satellites(s) *without* metastatic lymph nodes |
| N3 | 4 or more metastatic lymph nodes, matted lymph nodes, or combinations of in-transit met(s)/satellite(s), or ulcerated melanoma *and* metastatic lymph node(s) | |
| **M classification** | | |
| M1 | Distant skin, sub-Q, or lymph node mets | Normal LDH |
| M2 | Lung mets | Normal LDH |
| M3 | All other visceral or any distant mets | Normal LDH<br>Elevated LDH with any M |

Table 1. UICC/AJCC TNM staging system

| Clinical Staging[a] | | | |
|---|---|---|---|
| 0 | Tis | N0 | M0 |
| IA | T1a | N0 | M0 |
| IB | T1b | N0 | M0 |
| | T2a | N0 | M0 |
| IIA | T2b | N0 | M0 |
| | T3a | N0 | M0 |
| IIB | T3b | N0 | M0 |
| | T4a | M0 | M0 |
| IIC | T4b | N0 | M0 |
| IIIA | Any T1-4a | N1b | M0 |
| IIIB | Any T1-4a | N2b | M0 |
| IIIC | Any T | N2c | M0 |
| | Any T | N3 | M0 |
| IV | Any T | Any N | Any M |

| Pathologic Staging[b] | | | |
|---|---|---|---|
| 0 | Tis | N0 | M0 |
| IA | T1a | N0 | M0 |
| IB | T1b | N0 | M0 |
| | T2a | N0 | M0 |
| IIA | T2b | N0 | M0 |
| | T3a | N0 | M0 |
| IIB | T3b | N0 | M0 |
| | T4a | N0 | M0 |
| IIC | T4b | N0 | M0 |
| IIIA | T1-4a | N1a | M0 |
| IIIB | T1-4a | N1b | M0 |
| | T1-4a | N2a | |
| IIIC | Any T | N2b,N2c | M0 |
| | Any T | N3 | |
| IV | Any T | Any N | Any M |

Table 2. UICC/AJCC TNM staging system

### 4.1.1 Sentinel node mapping during pregnancy

In spite of being a standard treatment in large healthcare centers sentinel node biopsy has generated a considerably controversy in case of pregnant patients. Because blue dye is contraindicated in pregnant women and $^{99m}Tc$ is a radioactive some surgeons avoid this procedure (Squatrito & Harlow, 2008). The results of at least five studies examined safety of the procedure for fetus in pregnant patients affected with melanoma or breast cancer. Gentilini et al. (Gentilini et al., 2004) have indirectly estimated the possible fetus exposure after application of radiopharmaceutical and its distribution in 26 premenopausal nonpregnant patients. They concluded that fetus exposure would be minimal and therefore the procedure could be safe for application in pregnant patients. Similar study has been performed by Keleher et al (Keleher et al., 2004). Mondi et al. (Mondi et al., 2007) presented the first report on sentinel node biopsy during pregnancy. The procedure has been performed in nine pregnant patients - six patients with melanoma and three with breast cancer. All patients had delivery at term and there were no harms for fetus. A retrospective study conducted in H. Lee Moffitt Cancer Center, Tampa, Florida, USA (Mondi et al., 2007) analyse the results of sentinel node biopsy in 5,563 breast cancer patients. Ten of these patients were pregnant. Median duration of pregnancy was 15.8 weeks. Nine patients delivered a healthy child and one patient had intentional abortion. Another study was performed by Gentilini et al and its results were published last year (Gentilini et al., 2010). The study covered sentinel node biopsy in breast cancer patients applying radiophramaceutical only. Eleven of 12 patients delivered a healthy baby and in case of one baby, ventricular septal defect was operated in the third month of pregnancy. Small number of patients, the fact that most patients had a breast cancer, results from indirect studies, and the studies in which blue dye was not applied refer that sentinel node biopsy has not been proved as a safety procedure yet. Pregnant patients must be warned to both benefits and possible harmfulness of this procedure.

### 4.2 Radiology procedures in melanoma staging

In case of low risk melanoma (tumor thickness less than 1 mm), detailed physical examination is enough and no further radiological procedures are required (Dummer et al., 2008). In patients with locally advanced disease and lymph node involvement, optimal staging is indicated because of the probability for detection of distant metastases (Hoekstra, 2008; Dummer et al., 2008). It is important to identify solitary operable metastases, which increase the chances for cure (Wasif et al., 2011). Ultrasound examination of abdomen and chest X ray are preferable in pregnancy because fetal exposure is minimal (Orecchia et al., 2008). CT scan should be avoided in pregnant patients because of higher radiation doses. If ultrasound and X ray examination reveal suspected metastases that may have effects to further treatment course, CT scan may be used with strict respect of all procedures for fetus protection. Additional imaging examination with contrast medium should be avoided and low-dose protocols and minimal number of slices should be used (Orecchia et al., 2008). Magnetic resonance imaging may replace X-ray based techniques, but it is contraindicate in the first trimester (Campbell FA & Campbell C, 2006).

### 4.3 Nuclear medicine procedures

The use of positron-emission tomography (PET/CT) may change the stage of the disease and thus the change in treatment decision-making (Bastiaannet et al., 2006 a). Standard uptake value is a good prognostic factor of the recurrence in melanoma patients (Bastiaannet et al., 2006 b). On the other hand, PET/CT fails to detect distant metastases within the initial staging of patients with positive sentinel node biopsy (Wagner et al., 2011). Because PET/CT examination is contraindicated during pregnancy, it will not be discussed in this chapter.

## 5. Prognosis

The above chapters deal with the impact of earlier pregnancies and reproductive parameters to the development of malignant melanoma. This chapter presents studies that demonstrate the impact of pregnancy to treatment outcome and occurrence of transplancental metastasis

### 5.1 Impact of pregnancy to melanoma prognosis

From the '50s of the last century to present time, there have been many studies of the impact of pregnancy to melanoma prognosis. Most of these studies and meta-analyses show that malignant melanoma in pregnancy has no influence on patients survival. However, because the conclusions of these studies are inconsistent, it is still unclear whether pregnancy has impact to rapid tumor growth, more rapid occurrence of metastases, and poorer survival of patients (Sampson et al., 1998; Karagas et al., 2002). From the first report on this issue, which was published in 1951 (Pack & Scharnagel , 1983), up to the '80s of the last century almost all studies demonstrate poorer survival rate from melanoma diagnose during pregnancy (Pack et al., 1951; Sutherland et al., 1983; Trapeznikov et al., 1987; Reintgen et al.,

1085; McManamny et al., 1989; Wong et al., 1989; Slingluff et al., 1990; MacKie et al., 1991; O'Meara et al., 2005; Katsambas et al., 1996; Lazovich et al., 2010; Osterlind et al., 1988; Smith MA et al., 1998; Shiu et al., 1976; Houghton et al., 1981). These findings were mostly the consequence of diagnosing tumors in their higher stages during the pregnancy than in case of tumor diagnosis in nonpregnant women of the same age (Shiu et al., 1976; Houghton et al., 1981; Landthaler & Braun-Falco, 1985), and frequent appearance of trunk melanoma (Houghton et al., 1981). The first study that demonstrated no difference inthe overall survival rate was the one published by Wong et al. in 1989 (Wong et al., 1989). The authors compared the survival of 66 pregnant patients in stage I melanoma with 619 nonpregnant patients of the same age and found no difference in the 5-year survival. In the study of Slingluff et al. (Slingluff et al., 1990) there was no difference in the survival time, but pregnant patients were presented with a larger number of involved lymph nodes (39% versus 26%, p=0.053) at diagnosis, lymph node metastases appeared in shorter interval after the diagnosis of stage I disease (p=0.021), and shorter disease free survival (DFS). The results of following studies have not reported difference in survival among pregnant patients (MacKie et al., 1991; Stein et al., 1990; Driscoll et al., 1993; Travers et al., 1995; Grin et al., 1996; Daryanani et al., 2003), but in some a caution has been stressed to the diagnosis of thicker melanoma in pregnancy (MacKie et al., 1991; Travers et al., 1995). In already mentioned Lens et al. study (Lens et al., 2004) (Figure 2.), the results of investigate cohort of 5,533 women (185 of them were pregnant) showed no difference in survival time between pregnant patients and general population with melanoma diagnosis.

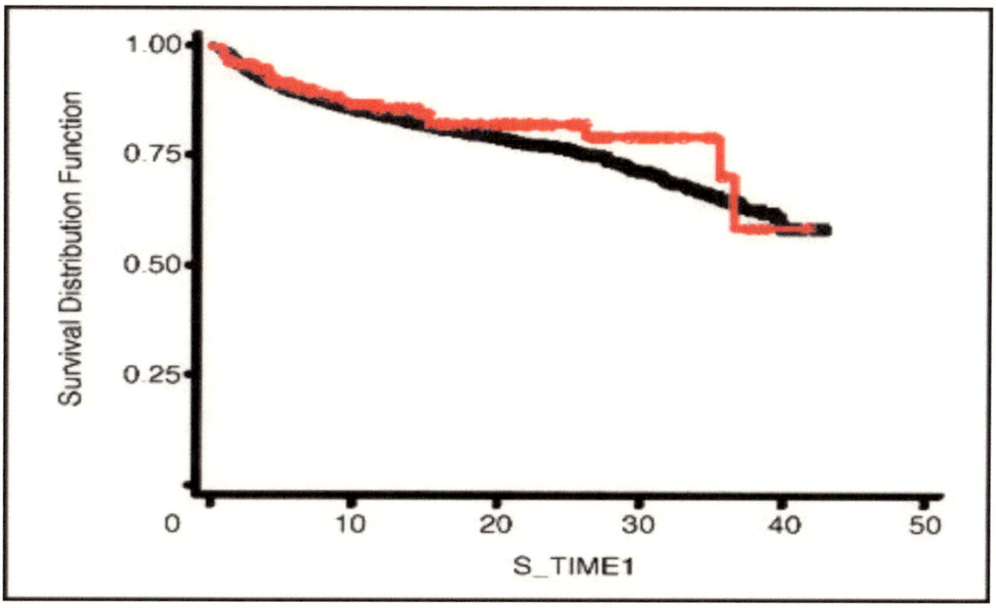


Fig. 2. Kaplan-Meier curve of the survival in pregnant patients with melanoma compared women in generative period (Lens et al., 2004)

Another influential study is a meta-analysis by Karagas et al. (Karagas et al., 2006), which include results obtained in ten case-control studies. Their analysis also did not give evidence for the survival difference between pregnant and nonpregnant melanoma patients. After this study, the general opinion is that there is no difference in the survival between these two patient groups. Yet, the last study that was conducted with a smaller group of patients gave opposite results (Miller et al., 2010) and points out that not all issues in this sphere has been cleared up.

### 5.2 Transplancental metastases and risk for fetus

The occurrence of transplancental metastases in fetus is rare and when it occurs, the most common neoplasm is melanoma. Sporadic case reports can be found in current literature. The study, which particularly dealt with this phenomenon in melanoma, was conducted by Alexander et al. They analyzed MEDLINE database for the period 1966-2002 and found 87 patients with placental metastases. Twenty-seven (31%) of these patients were diagnosed with metastatic melanoma and the rest of cases were breast and lung cancer, leukemia, and lymphoma. The involvement of fetus was found in six of 27 patients with placental metastases from melanoma. Five of six newborn infants died. Because occurrence of melanoma in newborn infant is rare, no diagnostic standards exist. Some recommendations regarding the follow-up include complete skin examination, abdominal ultrasound, and screening for melanocytic proteins in urine (Alexander et al., 2003).

### 5.3 Pregnancy after treatment of melanoma

Contrary to the studies, that analyzed the impact of pregnancy to the treatment outcome of melanoma, the results of the studies that analyse the safety of pregnancy after melanoma diagnosis and treatment are more consistent. The results of all studies show that pregnancy after the treatment of melanoma is safe (Lens et al., 2004; Sutherland et al., 1983; Reintgen et al., 1985; Wong et al., 1989; MacKie et al., 1991; 71 28, Driscoll et al., 1993; o'Meara et al., 2005; Driscoll & Grant-Kels, 2008). The risk of disease recurrence is mainly associated with the stage of the disease before the diagnosis and thus the opinion that the patient's decision regarding the pregnancy should be based on the level of that risk (MacKie et al., 1991). There are authors that advice patients to avoid pregnancy during first two or three years after the treatment of melanoma (Lens st al., 2004, McManamny et al., 1989). Also, there is a report of successful pregnancy with no disease recurrence after the treatment of metastatic melanoma (Nikolin et al., 2005).

## 6. Treatment

Treatment of melanoma in pregnancy does not greatly differ from the treatment of melanoma in general population. However, certain problems such as somewhat more difficult inguinal lymphadenectomy in late pregnancy, as well as the application of some teratogenic medications, complicate the optimal treatment of pregnant women.

### 6.1 Surgical treatment

#### 6.1.1 Excision of primary lesion

More than hundred years ago, it was observed that the skin tumors spread in a star-like shape and that malignant cells exist even a few centimeters away from the visible tumor margins. However, many years later, it was proved that the probability of the surrounding spread depends on the size of the primary tumor. Initially, for all melanomas, regardless the tumor size, a technique that included 5 cm width of healthy tissue around the tumor was applied. With this kind of surgery, skin grafts were transplanted for most of the operations (Brady et al., 2009). After that, a large number of studies were performed, which proved that for tumors of smaller size, it is not necessary for the margin to be so wide. Today's recommendation of the sufficient margin for in situ melanomas is 0.5 cm, for those with the Breslow thickness less than 2 mm, it is 1 cm, while larger melanomas require the margin of more than 2 cm. In an early stage of the disease, there are no specificities related to pregnancy. If it is not possible to achieve a sufficiently wide excision, it is possible to use a skin graft, while the transfers of any deeper tissues are not recommendable because they postpone diagnosis of a local relapse (Hoekstra, 2008). Sentinel node biopsy is described earlier in this chapter.

### 6.1.2 Regional lymphadenectomy

Patients with, clinically observed, enlarged regional lymph nodes without any evidence of distant metastases, should be treated with regional lymphadenectomy. In some specific cases of enlarged lymph nodes, prior to this procedure, a fine needle aspiration should be performed (FNA) (Brady et al., 2009). In patients where lymph nodes are not enlarged, the performance of lymphadenectomy depends on the results of sentinel node biopsy, which is today a standard in melanoma staging (Valsecchi et al., 2011; Balch et al., 2009; Dummer et al., 2008). After a positive sentinel node biopsy, a regional lymphadenectomy is performed (Brady et al., 2009). This procedure may be more difficult due to pregnancy if it is a group of deep groin and loin lymph nodes. In case of late pregnancy, it is allowed to postpone lymphadenectomy after the childbirth (Hoekstra, 2008).

### 6.1.3 Ocular melanoma

Ocular melanoma mostly occurs in choroidea, although it may occur in the iris or cilliary body as well. When less than 3 mm, it usually does not have any symptoms, although, as the tumor grows, the patient notices a brown or a yellow spot in his visual field. In certain number of cases, melanoma causes an increase of intraocular pressure, and sometimes pain (Grgic et al., 2009). As an eye does not have any lymphatic vessels, melanoma does not have lymphogenous metastases, surgical postulates for cutaneous melanomas could not be applied. Some small and peripheral lesions can be excised with minimal loss of vision. Such melanomas can also be treated with the laser photocoagulation, transpupillary thermotherapy, and radiotherapy. However, the radiotherapy possibilities in pregnancy are limited. In the largest number of cases, it is necessary to perform enucleation, and sometimes the exenteration of the orbit. Besides that, the COMSG randomized study showed that implantation of the radioactive gold plaque behind the tumor, gives survival results similar to enucleation, with eye preservation, but again, there are no experiences with this method during the pregnancy (Brady et al., 2009; Grgic et al., 2009).

### 6.1.4 Surgery of locoregional recurrences

Locoregional metastases (satellite metastases, in-transit metastases) represent the recurrence of melanoma in the area between the primary lesion and the local lymph nodes. They are the consequence of intralymphatic spread outside the excision area (Heenan & Ghaznawie, 1999). It is necessary to treat them like thick primary melanoma, because in this way the patient could be cured. Nevertheless, such treatment is not always possible and it depends on the number, location, and size of the lesions. The treatment is directed towards excision with healthy margins, while the amputation of the extremity is not indicated, because it does not increase survival. Besides, it is possible to treat small lesions with laser ablation (Testori et al., 2009). Certain studies proved successful the treatment with isolated extremity perfusion by melphalan and tumor necrosis factor α (TNFα) (Lienard et al., 1992; Grunhagen et al., 2004). However, as there is no experience in this procedure during pregnancy, some authors consider it contraindicated for the time being (Hoekstra, 2008), while others consider that in specific situations it can be applied due to minimal systemic absorption (Dummer et al., 2008).

#### 6.1.5 Surgery in stage IV disease

Some studies showed that resection of single metastasis is related to the prolonged survival (Sarnaik et al., 2007; McLoughlin et al., 2008). However, there are no studies that compared surgical and conservative treatment of single metastasis. Most of authors advise metastasis resection in such a case (Testori et al., 2009). This recommendation is surely the safest and the most efficient in pregnant patients.

### 6.2 Radiotherapy

Because surgical treatment of cutaneous melanoma achieves good results, the use radiotherapy in the treatment of primary melanoma does not have its place (Testori et al., 2009). Vontgama et al. showed certain efficacy of radiotherapy in desmoplastic melanoma, when the clean margins after surgery could not be achieved (Vongtama et al., 2003). On the other hand, radiotherapy of the primary melanoma of the nasal cavity and the paranasal sinuses is successfully applied because melanoma of this region has tendency of more often local than systemic relapse and it is sometimes very difficult to access this region for complete surgery (Testori et al., 2009). Furthermore, seems like postoperative therapy gives better results than surgery alone in melanoma of this region (Stevens & mcKay, 2006; Kirova et al., 1999). However, there are no randomized studies, which could support this. Depending on the number, size and localization of the lymph nodes, local relapse after lymphadenectomy is found in 20%-50% of cases (Calabro et al., 1989). Since such relapse is very difficult for treatment, there were attempts to obtain better results with postoperative radiotherapy. Although some phase II studies showed certain efficacy (Testori et al., 2009), the only randomized study did not show any difference, neither in DFS, nor in OS (Creagan et al., 1978). Radiotherapy in metastatic melanoma is especially significant for symptoms palliation, primarely of pain due to bone metastases (Testori et al., 2009). In pregnancy, such treatment would be theoretically possible if the metastases are not located in the area of lower thoraces and lumbar vertebrae, which shall be discussed later. The greatest significance of radiotherapy in metastatic melanoma is the treatment of brain metastases. CNS metastases occur in 10%-40% of melanoma patients (Douglas & Margolin, 2002). A median survival without treatment is about 1 month. A whole brain radiotherapy treatment (WBRT) in 60%-70% of patients reduces the symptoms, improves neurological status, and prolongs survival up to 6 months (Patchell, 2003). Furthermore, in solitary metastases, WBRT after surgery prolongs survival when compared to surgery alone (Tarhini & Agarwala, 2004). In addition, stereotactic radiosurgery (e.g. gamma knife), irradiation by linear accelerator (Linac) and surgery, have equal results in treatment of one operable metastasis (Grob et la., 1998).

#### 6.2.1 Radiotherapy of melanoma in pregnancy

Due to risk of death or heavy malformation of the fetus, radiotherapy in pregnancy was the subject of controversies due to the necessary balance between the benefits for the mother and the harmful effect to the fetus (Kal & Struikmans, 2005). Some authors postpone irradiation therapy of breast carcinoma during the pregnancy (Pavlidis, 2002; Gwyn 2000), while the others recommend the termination of pregnancy if the doses received by the fetus are larger than 0.05-0.1 Gy (Greer et al., 1997). There is no doubt that high X-ray doses are extremely harmful for the fetus, but more current approaches show that irradiation therapy can be safely applied in most of the cases (Kal & Struikmans, 2005). During the earliest pregnancy, doses above 0.1-0.2 Gy lead to the death of the embryo; in weeks 2 to 8 of organogenesis they may cause heavy anomalies, while in the later period of CNS development hinder development of intelligence and cause consequential mental retardation consequentially. The occurrence of neoplasms in children is more frequent to some extent (Kal & Struikmans, 2005). Regardless these data, the greatest number of irradiation therapies outside the pelvis can be safely applied. The first prerequisite for this is a careful planning, a properly functioning device that does not dissipate irradiation and an adequate protection of abdomen and pelvis of a pregnant woman. Van der Giesen et al. calculated the doses for breast cancer irradiation, which are received by the fetus during the standard therapy of 50 Gy (Van der Giessen 1997). Namely, the dosage was 0.03 Gy in week 8, 0.2 Gy in week 24, and 1.43 Gy in week 36 because the fetus is larger and thus closer to the irradiation source. Several cases of births of healthy children after the irradiation therapy of breast carcinoma are reported. A large number of series of irradiation therapy of supradiaphragmally localized Hodgkin lymphoma in pregnant women, who gave birth to healthy children, is also presented in literature (Zucali et al., 1981; Mazonakis et al., 2003; Lishner et al., 1992). Fetal dose in brain irradiation with 54 Gy at Varian accelerator is about 0.22 Gy, and even without any shielding, the fetus dosage almost never exceeds 0.1 Gy (Haba et al., 2004; Mazonakis et al., 1999). There was one case of a pregnant patient who underwent a gamma-knife treatment due to melanoma metastases without any consequences upon her child (Yu et al., 2003). A case of a pregnant patient irradiated with 66 Gy for head and neck tumor was also presented (Podgorsak et al., 1999). In melanoma treatment during pregnancy, the benefits and the harmfulness of the radiotherapeutic treatment should be properly balanced. A possible irradiation of some distant regions postoperatively, due to positive margins, could be taken into consideration. Sinusal melanoma irradiation was proved useful and it is safe for the fetus. Adjuvant irradiation after lymphadenectomy proved no benefit in a randomized study (Creagan et al., 1978), so it should be avoided in pregnancy. A specific question is when to irradiate a pregnant patient with metastatic melanoma. In our opinion, palliative irradiation of the lower thoracic and lumbar vertebrae should be avoided. In the case of brain metastases, the fetus receives a minimal dosage of irradiation, which sometimes could be useful for patient's prolongation of life and ending of pregnancy in a due term. Indications for pregnancy termination in irradiated patients, who were not aware of being pregnant at the moment of irradiation, are the doses over 0.5 Gy upon the fetus, because that would almost certainly lead to fetus malformation, while the doses of 0.2 Gy bear the risk of mental retardation of a child (Kal & Struikmans, 2005).

### 6.3 Systemic treatment

#### 6.3.1 Adjuvant therapy

Adjuvant treatment, for stage II/III melanoma is a subject of controversy. The reason is a large number of studies, which tested various agents, chemotherapy, immunomodulators, and therapeutic vaccines with more or less success (Eggermont et al., 2009). Although Wheatley et al. (Wheatley et al., 2007) and Mocellina et al. (Mocellina et al., 2010), demonstrated a prolonged DFS and OS in meta-analyses of interferon α (IFNα) studies, such therapy did not become a standard because neither the optimal dose of IFNα nor the optimal duration of treatment is still known. It is considered that the control arm, used in clinical trials, should be just follow up after the complete surgery (Wheatley et al., 2007). The EORTC 18991 study, in which high doses of a pegylated IFNα were used, demonstrated a prolonged DFS (p=0.01), but without any effect either to distant-metastasis-free survival (DMFS), or to OS. The greatest benefit was observed in patients with micrometastases detected by the sentinel node biopsy, while the patients with palpable lymph nodes did not have any benefits (Eggermont et al., 2008). Several studies with small doses of IFNα showed the effect to DFS (Grob et al., 1998; Pehamberger et al., 1998; Cameron et al., 2001; Kirkwood et al., 2000; Hancock et al., 2004), of which, only one showed significant importance for OS (Grob et al., 1998). On the other hand, the WHO-16 study, which tested low doses of IFNα in duration of 3 years in patients in stadiums IIIB and IIIC, did not show any significant effect to DFS or OS (Cascinelli et al., 2001). Some other drugs were tested in combination with IFNα, although dacarbazine (Garbe et al., 2008), Melacine (Mitchell et al., 2007), IL-2 (Hauschild et al., 2003), or isotretinoin (Richtig et al., 2005) did not show any difference in comparison to IFNα alone. As the results of various studies are very different, there is a question if an adjuvant therapy should be applied, especially in the case of a pregnant patient. On the one side toxicity and a possible teratogenicity of drugs that would be used are opposed to higher aggressiveness of melanoma in pregnancy, observed in several studies (Shiu et al., 1976; 73 36; Landthaler & Braun-Falco, 1985). There are no sufficient data on IFNα safety during pregnancy. One study of a smaller scope did not observe any defects in the fetuses after their birth although the patients were treated with IFNα (Egberts et al., 2006). However, IFNα was used during pregnancy in some other indications. In 14 patients with immune thrombocytopenia, 2 of which were in their first trimester, there were no observed changes in the fetus (Vantroyen & Vanstraelen, 2002). However, in the study where the patients were treated from a chronic hepatitis or myeloproliferative syndrome (6 were in the first trimester), there were 4 cases of a premature childbirth and 6 cases of intrauterine growth retardation (Hiratsuka et al., 2002).

### 6.3.2 Metastatic disease

Median 5-year survival of the melanoma patients in stage IV is less than 5% (Rigel et al., 1996). Until two years ago, there was no drug that prolongs survival in patients with distant melanoma metastases. For the purpose of palliation, the most frequently used drug was dacarbazine with small RR and the median survival, not longer than the natural survival duration in melanoma patients. A large number of different drugs, alone or in combination with dacarbazine did not show any difference in relation to RR, DFS, or OS (Brady et al., 2009). Thus, a major question rises, whether to administer dacarbazine to pregnant patients with a metastatic disease, having in mind the risk, which it carries for the fetus and its minimal benefit for the patient. However, some patients demand treatment and some physicians think that it would be unethical if they do not try a cytotoxic therapy. There are certain experiences in administration of dacarbazine-based therapy in pregnancy. Thirty-six patients were administered dacarbazine during pregnancy, 8 of them during their first and 28 of them during their second and third trimesters. Malformations were observed in two fetuses exposed to chemotherapy during the first trimester. In one fetus, a micorophthalmus with secondary heavy hypermetropia was observed, while the other experienced floating thumb malformation. In administration of chemotherapy after the first trimester, one fetus died in utero, while in the other one a syndactyly was observed. Other fetuses were born without any malformations and after a short follow up of 14 months, they were still healthy. In the last two cases, a polychemotherapy was used (Pages et al., 2010). Intensive research in metastatic melanoma treatment achieved significant results in the past few years. Several new drugs proved to be better than standard dacarbazine therapy. Immunotherapy based treatment has been tested for decades and is used in melanoma treatment. Ipilimumab and tremelimumab are monoclonal antibodies, which bind to cytotoxic T-lymphocyte-associated antigen (CTLA4). Under natural conditions, this receptor binds to receptor B7 at the antigen presenting cells and thus, prevents connecting of molecule CD28 that binds to this receptor and conditions the T-cells activation. Under normal conditions, this reaction induces self-tolerance. By blockage of CTLA4 receptors, an undisturbed connecting of CD28 and B7 occurs, and induction of antitumor effect of T-cells to melanoma cells (Schadendorf et al., 2009). In the largest study published until now, median overall survival was 10.1 months (Hodi et al., 2010). Some other immunomodular drugs were tested in metastatic melanoma: human anti-CD137 antibody, anti-integrin antibodies volociximab and etaracizumab, as well as various vaccines: MAGE-3, dendritic, peptide vaccines, etc. (Schadendorf et al., 2009). These agents are mostly in phase I or II of clinical trials and the results are expected in the following period. Cell signal transition inhibitors take very important role in oncology in the last decade. RAF/RAS/MEK signaling pathway is very important in melanoma because it participates in proliferation induction and apoptosis inhibition. A large number of inhibitors of this signaling pathway are in different phase of clinical trials: sorafenib, AZD6244, tipifarnib, (Hersey et al., 2009). A most remarkable result in treatment was achieved with direct B-Raf inhibitor PLX4032 (Flaherty et al., 2010). In the phase I/II study 32 patients with V600 BRAF mutation, 24 partial and two complete remissions were achieved, with DFS of over 7 months. Besides that, the inhibitors of some other signaling pathways are also intensively tested. They include various inhibitors like tyrosine kinase, PI3K, Akt, mTOR, Stat3 inhibitors, and many other agents (Hersey et al., 2009). Since these drugs are mostly present in clinical trials, and in most of the trials, pregnancy is an exclusion criteria, there is no experience in treatment of childbearing women. A drug, which would most likely be the first to enter regular clinical practice, ipilimumab, causes autoimmunity (Schadendorf et al., 2009), which may be expressed through a syndrome, similar to lupus or antiphospholipid syndrome, which may be fatal both for the fetus and the mother. Experience with imatinib in chronic myeloid leukemia in pregnant patients shows that imatinib is teratogenous (Apperley, 2009). Nevertheless, there was a case where the patient was treated with dasatinib and two cases of treatment with nilotinib where healthy children were born (Conchon et al., 2010; Conchon et al., 2009).

## 7. Future remarks

Since etiology and the connection between the hormones, pregnancy and melanoma is not entirely clarified, and the results of metastatic melanoma treatment are poor, there are still many unanswered questions related to the etiology, but also to the treatment of melanoma. Huu et al. (Huu et al., 2009) tested the presence of fetal cells in human melanomas, diagnosed during pregnancy. They found that the fetal cells were present in 63% of melanoma, 12% of nevus during pregnancy and 0% in healthy skin. Since fetal cells are capable of developing in various tissues and since they precipitate angiogenesis, it remains to be seen, whether they have any, and what their role in melanoma development during pregnancy is. Estrogen receptors, their relationship, and the possibility of the hormone therapy in melanoma shall also be the subject of further research. Namely, relationship between ERα and ERβ is probably of the key significance for the response to the hormone therapy (de Giorgi et al., 2011). Efficacy and safety of the new drugs' administration in pregnancy is still to be seen.

## 8. References


Abbasi NR, Shaw HM, Rigel DS, et al. (2004) Early diagnosis of cutaneous melanoma: revisiting the ABCD criteria. *JAMA*. 2004; 292:2771-2776

Alexander A, Samlowski WE, Grossman D, et al. (2003) Metastatic melanoma in pregnancy: risk of transplacental metastases in the infant. *J Clin Oncol* 2003; 21(11): 2179–2186

Anonymous (2003) Stat bite: incidence of and mortality from melanoma of the skin, 1975–2000. *J Natl Cancer Inst* 2003; 95(13): 933

Antypas C, Sandilos P, Kouvaris J, et al. (1998) Fetal dose evaluation during breast cancer radiotherapy. *Int J Radiat Oncol Biol Phys* 1998; 40: 995–99.

Apperley J. (2009) Issues of imatinib and pregnancy outcome *J Natl Compr Canc Netw* 2009; 7(10): 1050-8

Balch CM, Gershenwald JE, Soong SJ, et al. (2009) Final version of 2009 AJCC melanoma staging and classification. *J Clin Oncol.* 2009 Dec 20;27(36):6199-206

Balch CM, Morton DL, Gershenwald JE, et al.(2009) Sentinel node biopsy and standard of care for melanoma.*J Am Acad Dermatol.* 2009 May;60(5):872-5

Balch CM, Soong SJ, Bartolucci AA, et al.(1996) Efficacy of an elective regional lymph node dissection of 1 to 4 mm thick melanomas for patients 60 years of age and younger. *Ann Surg* 1996; 224: 255–263

Bastiaannet E, Hoekstra OS, Oyen WJ, et al. (2006). Level of fluorodeoxyglucose uptake predicts risk for recurrence in melanoma patients presenting with lymph node metastases.*Ann Surg Oncol.* 2006 Jul;13(7):919-26

Bastiaannet E, Oyen WJ, Meijer S, Hoekstra OS,et al. (2006). Impact of [18F]fluorodeoxyglucose positron emission tomography on surgical management of melanoma patients. *Br J Surg.* 2006 Feb;93(2):243-9

Brady M, Kaushal A, Ko C. et al. (2009) Melanoma and other skin cancers In: *CancerManagement: A Multidiciplinary Approach 12th Edition,* Pazdur M, Wagman L, Camphausen K et al. CMP Healthcare Media LLC

Calabro A, Singletary SE, Balch CM. (1989) Patterns of relapse in 1001 consecutive patients with melanoma nodal metastases. *Arch Surg* 1989; 124: 1051–1055.

Cameron DA, Cornbleet MC, Mackie RM et al. (2001) Adjuvant interferon alpha 2b in high risk melanoma—the Scottish study. *Br J Cancer* 2001; 84: 1146–1149.

Campbell FA, Campbell C. Magnetic resonance imaging for stage IV melanoma during pregnancy. (2006) *Arch Dermatol* 2006;142:393

Cancer Research UK Malignant melanoma factsheet May 2006. Available at: www.info.cancerresearchuk.org. Accessed November 9, 2006

Cascinelli N, Belli F, MacKie RM et al. (2001) Effect of long-term adjuvant therapy with interferon alpha-2a in patients with regional node metastases from cutaneous melanoma: a randomised trial. *Lancet* 2001; 358: 866–869.

Cascinelli N, Morabito A, Santinami M, et al. (1998) Immediate or delayed dissection of regional nodes in patients with melanoma of the trunk: a randomized trial. WHO Melanoma Programme. *Lancet* 1998; 351: 793–796

Cochran AJ, Todd G, Hart DM, et al. (1982) Reaction of the leukocytes of melanoma patients and control donors, including pregnant women, with melanoma and fetus-derived materials. *Cancer Immunol Immunother* 1982; 14:78-81

Colboum DS, Nathanson L, Belilos E (1989) Pregnancy and malignant melanoma. *Semin Oncol* 1989; 16:377-387

Conchon M, Sanabani SS, Bendit I, et al. (2009) Two successful pregnancies in a woman with chronic myeloid leukemia exposed to nilotinib during the first trimester od her second pregnancy: case study *J Hematol Oncol* 2009 Oct;2:42

Conchon M, Sanabani SS, Serpa M, et al. (2010) Suucessful pregnancy and delivery in a patient with chronic myeloid leukemia while on dasatinib therapy *Adv Hematol* 2010 Epub Mar 7

Creagan ET, Cupps RE, Ivins JC et al. (1978) Adjuvant radiation therapy for regional nodal metastases from malignant melanoma: a randomized, prospective study. *Cancer* 1978; 42: 2206–2210.

Daryanani D, Plukker JT, De Hullu JA,et al. (2003). Pregnancy and early-stage melanoma. *Cancer* 2003 May 1;97(9):2248-53

de Giorgi V, Mavilia C, Massi D, et al (2009) Estrogen receptor expression in cutaneous melanoma: A real-time reverse transcriptase-polymerase chain reaction and immunohistochemical study. *Arch Dermatol* 2009;145:30-36

de Giorgi V, Gori A, Alfaioli B,et al. (2011) .Influence of sex hormones on melanoma. *J Clin Oncol.* 2011 Feb 1;29(4):e94-5

de Vries M, Jager PL, Suurmeijer AJ, et al. (2005) .Sentinel lymph node biopsy for melanoma: prognostic value and disadvantages in 300 patients *Ned Tijdschr Geneeskd.* 2005 Aug 13;149(33):1845-51

Dillman RO, Vandermolen LA, Barth NM, et al. (1996) Malignant melanoma and pregnancy. *West J Med* 1996;164: 156–161

Douglas JG, Margolin K. (2002) The treatment of brain metastases from malignant melanoma. *Semin Oncol* 2002; 29: 518–524.

Driscoll MS, Grant-Kels JM. (2008) Melanoma and pregnancy. *G Ital Dermatol Venereol.* 2008 Aug;143(4):251-7

Driscoll MS, Grin-Jorgensen CM, Grant-Kels JM. (1993) Does pregnancy influence the prognosis of malignant melanoma? *J Am Acad Dermatol.* 1993 Oct;29(4):619-30.

Dummer R, Hauschild A, Jost L; (2008) ESMO Guidelines Working Group Cutaneous malignant melanoma: ESMO clinical recommendations for diagnosis, treatment and follow-up. *Ann Oncol.* 2008 May;19 Suppl 2:ii86-8.

Durvasula R, Ahmed SM, Vashisht A, et al. (2002) Hormone replacement therapy and malignant melanoma: to prescribe or not to prescribe? *Climacteric* 2002; 5(2): 197–200

Egberts F, Lischner S, Russo P, et al. (2006) Diagnostic and therapeutic procedures for management of melanoma during pregnancy: risks for the fetus? *J Dtsch Dermatol Ges.* 2006 Sep;4(9):717-20

Eggermont AM, Suciu S, Santinami M et al. (2008) Adjuvant therapy with pegylated interferon alpha-2b versus observation alone in resected stage III melanoma: final results of EORTC 18991, a randomised phase III trial. *Lancet* 2008; 372: 117–126.

Eggermont AM, Testori A, Marsden J, et al. (2009) Utility of adjuvant systemic therapy in melanoma.*Ann Oncol.* 2009 Aug;20 Suppl 6:vi30-4.

Elwood JM, Coldman AJ (1978) Previous pregnancy and melanoma prognosis. *Lancet* 1978; 2(8097): 1000–1001

Faries MB, Thompson JF, Cochran A, et al. (2010) The impact on morbidity and length of stay of early versus delayed complete lymphadenectomy in melanoma: results of the

Multicenter Selective Lymphadenectomy Trial (I) *Ann Surg Oncol.* 2010 Dec;17(12):3324-9

Fisher D, Kwong L, Chin L (2008) Molecular Biology of Cutaneous Melanoma In De Vita, Hellman, Rosberg *Cancer: Principle and Practice of Oncology* LWW 2008: 1889-1897

Flaherty K, Puzanov I, Kim K, et al. (2010) Inhibition of Mutated, Activated BRAF in Metastatic Melanoma *N Engl J Med* 2010; 363:809-819

Friedman RJ, Rigel DS, Kopf AW (1985) Early detection of malignant melanoma: the role of physician examination and self-examination of the skin. *CA Cancer J Clin* 1985; 35: 130–151

Garbe C (1993) Pregnancy, hormone preparations and malignant melanoma *Hautarzt* 1993;44: 347–352

Garbe C, Radny P, Linse R et al. (2008) Adjuvant low-dose interferon {alpha}2a with or without dacarbazine compared with surgery alone: a prospective-randomized phase III DeCOG trial in melanoma patients with regional lymph node metastasis. *Ann Oncol* 2008; 19: 1195–1201.

Gentilini O, Cremonesi M, Toesca A, et al. (2010) Sentinel lymph node biopsy in pregnant patients with breast cancer.*Eur J Nucl Med Mol Imaging.* 2010 Jan;37(1):78-83

Gentilini O, Cremonesi M, Trifirò G, et al. (2004) Safety of sentinel node biopsy in pregnant patients with breast cancer.*Ann Oncol.* 2004 Sep;15(9):1348-51

George PA, Fortner JG, Pack GT (1960) Melanoma with pregnancy. *Cancer* 1960; 13:854-859

Gershenwald JE, Thompson W, Mansfield PF, et al. (1999) Multi-institutional melanoma lymphatic mapping experience: the prognostic value of sentinel lymph node status in 612 stage I or II melanoma patients *J Clin Oncol* 1999 Mar;17(3):976-83

Greer BE, Goff BA, Koh W. (1997) Cancer in the pregnant patient. In Hoskins WJ, Perez CA, Young RC, eds. *Principles and practice of gynecologic oncology, 2nd edn.* New York: Lippincott Raven, 1997: 463–70.

Grgic Z, Oros A, Rasic D, Popovic L, Popovic M (2009) Ocular malignant melanoma in pregnancy: Is a happy ending possible? *Arch Oncol* 2009; 17: 83-85

Grin CM, Driscoll MS, Grant-Kels JM (1996) Pregnancy and the prognosis of malignant melanoma *Semin Oncol.* 1996 Dec;23(6):734-6.

Grob JJ, Dreno B. de la Salmonie` re P et al.(1998) Randomised trial of interferon alpha- 2a as adjuvant therapy in resected primary melanoma thicker than 1.5 mm without clinically detectable node metastases. *Lancet* 1998; 351: 1905–1910.

Grob JJ, Regis J, Laurans R et al. (1998) Radiosurgery without whole brain radiotherapy in melanoma brain metastases. Club de Cancerologie Cutanee. *Eur J Cancer* 1998; 34: 1187–1192.

Grunhagen DJ, Brunstein F, Graveland WJ et al. (2004) One hundred consecutive isolated limb perfusions with TNF-alpha and melphalan in melanoma patients with multiple in-transit metastases. *Ann Surg* 2004; 240: 939–948.

Gwyn KM, Theriault RL.(2000) Breast cancer during pregnancy. *Curr Treat Options Oncol* 2000; 1: 239–43.

Haba Y, Twyman N, Thomas SJ, et al. (2004) Radiotherapy for glioma during pregnancy: fetal dose estimates, risk assessment and clinical management. *Clin Oncol (R Coll Radiol)* 2004; 16: 210–14.

Hancock BW, Wheatley K, Harris S et al. (2004) Adjuvant interferon in high-risk melanoma: the AIM HIGH Study–United Kingdom Coordinating Committee on Cancer Research randomized study of adjuvant low-dose extended-duration interferon alfa-2a in high-risk resected malignant melanoma. *J Clin Oncol* 2004; 22: 53–61.

Hauschild A, Weichenthal M, Balda BR et al. (2003) Prospective randomized trial of interferon alfa-2b and interleukin-2 as adjuvant treatment for resected intermediate- and high-risk primary melanoma without clinically detectable node metastasis. *J Clin Oncol* 2003; 21: 2883–2888.

Heenan PJ, Ghaznawie M. (1999) The pathogenesis of local recurrence of melanoma at the primary excision site. *Br J Plast Surg* 1999; 52: 209–213.

Hersey P, Bastholt L, Charion-Sileni V, et al. (2009) Small molecules and targeted therpies in distant metastatic disease *Ann Oncol* 2009 Aug;20 Suppl 6: vi35-vi40

Hiratsuka M, Minakami H, Koshizuka S, et al. (2002) Administration of interferon-alpha during pregnancy: effects on fetus. *J Perinat Med* 2002; 28: 372–376

Hodi S, O'Day S, McDermott D, et al. (2010) Improved Survival with Ipilimumab in Patients with Metastatic Melanoma *N Engl J Med* 2010; 363:711-723

Hoekstra HJ Melanoma during pregnancy: Therapeutic Management and Outcome In Surbone A., Peccatori F, Pavlidis N *Cancer and Pregnancy* Recent Results in Cancer Research vol. 178; Springer 2008: 175-181

Houghton AN, Flannery J, Viola MV (1981) Malignant melanoma of the skin occurring during pregnancy. *Cancer* 1981; 48:407-410

Huu SN, Oster M, Avril MF, et al. (2009) Fetal microchimeric calls participate in tumour angiogenesis in melanomas occuring during pregnanvy *Am J Pathol* 2009; 174 (2): 630-7

Jemal A, Siegel R, Xu J, et al. (2010) Cancer Statistics, 2010 *CA Cancer J Clin* 2010; 60:277-300

Karagas MR, Stukel TA, Dykes J, et al. (2002) A pooled analysis of 10 case-control studies of melanoma and oral contraceptive use. *Br J Cancer* 2002; 86(7):1085–1092

Karagas MR, Zens MS, Stukel TA, et al. (2006) Pregnancy history and incidence of melanoma in women: a pooled analysis. *Cancer Causes Control* 2006; 17(1): 11–1929.

Kal H, Struikmans H (2005) Radiotherapy during pregnancy: fact and fiction *Lancet Oncol* 2005;6:328-33

Katsambas A, Nicolaidou E (1996) Cutaneous malignant melanoma and sun exposure. Recent developments in epidemiology. *Arch Dermatol.* 1996 Apr;132(4):444-50

Lawrence C. (1996) Drug management in skin surgery. *Drugs* 1996;52:805-17.

Keleher A, Wendt R, Delpassand E, et al. (2004) The safety of lymphatic mapping in pregnant breast cancer patients using Tc-99m sulfur colloid. *Breast J* 2004;10:492-5

Landthaler M, Braun-Falco O. (1985) Malignant melanomas in pregnancy. *Dtsch Med Wochenschr.* 1985 Aug 30;110(35):1319-23

Khera SY, Kiluk JV, Hasson DM, et al. (2008) Pregnancy-associated breast cancer patient can safely undergo lymphatic mapping *Breast J* 2008; 14(3):250-4

Kirkwood JM, Ibrahim JG, Sondak VK et al. (2000) High- and low-dose interferon alfa-2b in high-risk melanoma: first analysis of intergroup trial E1690/S9111/C9190. *J Clin Oncol* 2000; 18: 2444–2458.

Kirova YM, Chen J, Rabarijaona LI et al. (1999) Radiotherapy as palliative treatment for metastatic melanoma. *Melanoma Res* 1999; 9: 611–613.

Lazovich D, Vogel RI, Berwick M, et al (2010) Indoor tanning and risk of melanoma: A case-control study in a highly exposed population. *Cancer Epidemiol Biomarkers Prev* 2010; 19:1557-1568

Lea CS, Holly EA, Hartge P et al. (2007) Reproductive risk factors for cutaneous melanoma in woman: a case-control study *Am J Epidemiol* 2007; 165(5): 505-513

Lens MB, Melanoma during pregnancy: epidemiology, diagnosis, staging, clinical picture In Surbone A., Peccatori F, Pavlidis N *Cancer and Pregnancy* Recent Results in Cancer Research vol. 178; Springer 2008:165-174

Lens MB, Reiman T, Husain AF (2003) Use of tamoxifen in the treatment of malignant melanoma. *Cancer* 2003; 98:1355-1361

Lens MB, Rosdahl I, Ahlbom A, et al. Effect of pregnancy on survival in women with cutaneous malignant melanoma. *J Clin Oncol* 2004; 22(21): 4369–4375

Lienard D, Ewalenko P, Delmotte JJ et al. (1992) High-dose recombinant tumor necrosis factor alpha in combination with interferon gamma and melphalan in isolation perfusion of the limbs for melanoma and sarcoma. *J Clin Oncol* 1992; 10: 52–60.

Lishner M, Zemlickis D, Degendorfer P, et al. (1992) Maternal and foetal outcome following Hodgkin's disease in pregnancy. *Br J Cancer* 1992; 65: 114–17

MacKie RM. (1990) Clinical recognition of early invasive malignant melanoma. *BMJ.* 1990;301:1005-1006

MacKie RM, Bufalino R, Morabito A, et al. (1991) Lack of effect of pregnancy on outcome of melanoma—The World Health Organisation Melanoma Programme. *Lancet* 1991; 337:653–655

Matthiasen L, Berg G (1989) Malignant melanoma, the most common cancer type, first appearing during pregnancy. *L臾artidningen* 1989;86:2845–2848

Mazonakis M, Damilakis J, Theoharopoulos N, et al. (1999) Brain radiotherapy during pregnancy: an analysis of conceptus dose using anthropomorphic phantoms. *Br J Radiol* 1999; 72: 274–78.

Mazonakis M, Varveris H, Fasoulaki M, et al. (2003) Radiotherapy of Hodgkin's disease in early pregnancy: embryo dose measurements. *Radiother Oncol* 2003; 66: 333–39.

McLoughlin JM, Zager JS, Sondak VK, et al. (2008) Treatment options for limited or symptomatic metastatic melanoma. *Cancer Control* 2008; 15: 239–247.

McManamny DS, Moss ALH, Pocock PV, et al. (1989) Melanoma and pregnancy: a long-term follow-up. *Br J Obstet Gynaecol* 1989; 96: 1419–1423

Miller E, Barnea Y, Gur E, et al. (2010) Malignant melanoma and pregnancy: second thoughts. *J Plast Reconstr Aesthet Surg.* 2010 Jul;63(7):1163-8.

Mitchell MS, Abrams J, Thompson JA et al. (2007) Randomized trial of an allogeneic melanoma lysate vaccine with low-dose interferon alfa-2b compared with highdose interferon alfa-2b for resected stage III cutaneous melanoma. *J Clin Oncol* 2007; 25: 2078–2085.

Mocellin S, Pasquali S, Rossi D, et al. (2010) Interferon alpha adjuvant therapy in patients with high-risk melanoma: a systematic review and meta-analysis *J Natl Cancer Inst* 2010; 102: 493-501120.

Mondi MM, Cuenca RE, Ollila DW, et al. (2007) Sentinel lymph node biopsy during pregnancy: initial clinical experience. *Ann Surg Oncol* 2007;14 (1):218-21

Morton DL, Thompson JF, Cochran AJ, et al. (2006) Sentinel-node biopsy or nodal observation in melanoma. *N Engl J Med* 2006; 355: 1307–1317

Morton DL, Wen DR, Wong JH, et al. (1992) Technical details of intraoperative lymphatic mapping for early stage melanoma. *Arch Surg* 1992; 127: 392–399

Ngu SL, Duval P, Collins C. (1992) Foetal radiation dose in radiotherapy for breast cancer. *Australas Radiol* 1992; 36: 321–22.

Nikolin B, Sveljo O. (2005) Metastatic melanoma in pregnancy *Arch Oncol* 2005;13(1):31-4

O'Meara AT, Cress R, Xing G, et al. (2005) Malignant melanoma in pregnancy. A population-based evaluation. *Cancer* 2005; 103(6):1217–1226

Orecchia R, Lucignani G, Tosi G Prenatal iradiation and pregnancy: the effects of diagnsotic imaging and radiation therapy In Surbone A., Peccatori F, Pavlidis N *Cancer and Pregnancy* Recent Results in Cancer Research vol. 178; Springer 2008: 3-20

Osterlind A, Tucker MA, Stone BJ, et al. (1998) The Danish case-control study of cutaneous malignant melanoma. III. Hormonal and reproductive factors in women. *Int J Cancer* 1988; 42(6): 821–824

Pack GT, Scharnagel IM (1951) Prognosis of malignant melanoma in pregnant women. *Cancer* 1951; 4:324–334

Pages C, Robert C, Thomas L, et al. (2010) Management and outcome of metastatic melanoma during pregnancy *Br J Dermatol* 2010; 162: 274-81

Patchell RA. (2003) The management of brain metastases. *Cancer Treat Rev* 2003; 29: 533–540.

Pavlidis NA. (2002) Coexistence of pregnancy and malignancy. *Oncologist* 2002; 7: 279–87.

Pehamberger H, Soyer HP, Steiner A et al. (1998) Adjuvant interferon alfa-2a treatment in resected primary stage II cutaneous melanoma. Austrian Malignant Melanoma Cooperative Group. *J Clin Oncol* 1998; 16: 1425–1429.

Pfahlberg A, Hassan K, Wille L, et al. (1997) Systematic review of case-control studies: oral contraceptives show no effect on melanoma risk. *Publ Health Rev* 1997; 25: 309–315

Podgorsak MB, Meiler RJ, Kowal H, et al. (1999) Technical management of a pregnant patient undergoing radiation therapy to the head and neck. *Med Dosim* 1999; 24: 121–28.

Pollitt RA, Geller AC, Brooks DR, et al. (2009) Efficacy of skin self-examination practices for early melanoma detection. *Cancer Epidemiol Biomarkers Prev.* 2009;18:3018-3023

Reintgen DS, McCarty KS Jr, Vollmer R, et al. (1985) Malignant melanoma and pregnancy. *Cancer* 1985; 55: 1340–1344

Richtig E, Soyer HP, Posch M et al. (2005) Prospective, randomized, multicenter, double-blind placebo-controlled trial comparing adjuvant interferon alfa and isotretinoin with interferon alfa alone in stage IIA and IIB melanoma: European Cooperative Adjuvant Melanoma Treatment Study Group. *J Clin Oncol* 2005; 23:8655–8663.

Rigel DS, Friedman RJ, Kopf AW et al. (1996) The incidence of malignant melanoma in the United States: Issues as we approach the 21st century. *J Am Acad Dermatol* 1996; 34: 839–847

Rigel DS, Russak J, Friedman R (2010) The evolution of melanoma diagnosis: 25 years beyond the ABCDs.*CA Cancer J Clin.* 2010 Sep-Oct;60(5):301-16

Sadoff L, Winkley J, Tyson S (1998) Is malignant melanoma an endocrinedependent tumor? *Oncology* 1973; 27:244-257

Sampson JH, Carter JH Jr, Friedman AH, et al. (1998) Demographics, prognosis, and therapy in 702 patients with brain metastases from malignant melanoma. *J Neurosurg* 1998; 88: 11–20.

Sarnaik AA, Zager JS, Sondak VK. (2007) Multidisciplinary management of special melanoma situations: oligometastatic disease and bulky nodal sites. *Curr Oncol Rep* 2007; 9: 417–427.

Schadendorf D, Algarra SM, Bastholt L, et al. (2009) Immunotherapy of distant metastatic disease *Ann Oncol* 2009 Aug;20 Suppl 6: vi41-vi50

Schmidt AN, Nanney LB, Boyd AS, et al (2006)Oestrogen receptor-beta expression in melanocytic lesions. *Exp Dermatol* 2006;15:971-980

Scope A, Dusza SW, Halpern AC, et al. (2008) The "ugly duckling" sign: agreement between observers. *Arch Dermatol.* 2008;144:58-64

Shiu MH, Schottenfeld D, Maclean B, et al. (1976) Adverse effect of pregnancy on melanoma: a reappraisal *Cancer.* 1976 Jan;37(1):181-7.

Sim FH, Taylor WF, Pritchard DJ, et al. (1986) Lymphadenectomy in the management of stage I malignant melanoma: a prospective randomized study. 1986; *Mayo Clin Proc* 61: 697–705

Slingluff CL Jr, Reintgen DS, Volmer RT, et al. (1990) Malignant melanoma arising during pregnancy—a study of 100 patients. *Ann Surg* 1990; 211: 552–559

Smith MA, Fine JA, Barnhill RL, et al. (1998) Hormonal and reproductive influences and risk of melanoma in women. *Int J Epidemiol* 1998; 27(5): 751–757

Smith RS, Randall P (1969) Melanoma during pregnancy. *Obstet Gynecol* 1969;34: 825–829

Squatrito RC, Harlow SP. (1998) Melanoma complicating pregnancy. *Obstet Gynecol Clin North Am* 1998;25:407-16

Stein M, Fried G, Borovik R, et al. (1990). Malignant melanoma occurring during pregnancy: a report of the Northern Israel Oncology Center (1968-1988). *J Surg Oncol.* 1990 Oct;45(2):117-20

Stevens G, McKay MJ. (2006) Dispelling the myths surrounding radiotherapy for treatment of cutaneous melanoma. *Lancet Oncol* 2006; 7: 575–583.

Stevenson S, Thornton J (2007) Effect of estrogens on skin aging and the potential role of SERMs. *Clin Interv Aging* 2007;2:283-297

Sutherland CM, Loutfi A, Mather FJ, et al. (1983) Effect of pregnancy upon malignant melanoma. *Surg Gynecol* Obstet 1983; 157:443–446

Tarhini AA, Agarwala SS. (2004) Management of brain metastases in patients with melanoma. *Curr Opin Oncol* 2004; 16: 161–166.

Testori A, Rutkowski P, Marsden J, et al. (2009) Surgery and radiotherapy in the treatment of cutaneous melanoma. *Ann Oncol.* 2009 Aug;20 Suppl 6:vi22-9.

Trapeznikov NN, Khasanov SR, Iavorskii VV (1987) Melanoma of the skin and pregnancy. *Voproxy Onkologii* 1987;33: 40–46

Travers RL, Sober AJ, Berwick M, et al. (1995) Increased thickness of pregnancy-associated melanoma *Br J Dermatol.* 1995 Jun;132(6):876-83.

Valsecchi ME, Silbermins D, de Rosa N, et al. (2011). Lymphatic Mapping and Sentinel Lymph Node Biopsy in Patients With Melanoma: A Meta-Analysis. *J Clin Oncol.* 2011 Mar 7. [Epub ahead of print]

Van der Giessen PH. (1997) Measurement of the peripheral dose for the tangential breast treatment technique with Co-60 gamma radiation and high energy X-rays. *Radiother Oncol* 1997; 42: 257–64.

Vantroyen B, Vanstraelen D (2002) Management of essential thrombocythemia during pregnancy with aspirin, interferon alpha-2a and no treatment. A comparative analysis of literature. *Acta Haematol* 2002; 107: 158–169

Vongtama R, Safa A, Gallardo D et al. (2003) Efficacy of radiation therapy in the local control of desmoplastic malignant melanoma. *Head Neck* 2003; 25: 423–428.

Wagner T, Meyer N, Zerdoud S, et al. (2011) FDG PET fails to detect distant metastases at initial staging of melanoma patients with metastatic involvement of sentinel lymph node. *Br J Dermatol.* 2011 Feb 17.. [Epub ahead of print]

Wasif N, Bagaria SP, Ray P, et al. (2011) Does metastasectomy improve survival in patients with stage IV melanoma? a cancer registry analysis of outcomes. *J Surg Oncol.* 2011 Mar 4. [Epub ahead of print]

Wheatley K, Ives N, Eggermont AM et al. (2007) Interferon-a as adjuvant therapy for melanoma: An individual patient data meta-analysis of randomised trials. 2007 ASCO Annual Meeting Proceedings Part I. *J Clin Oncol* 2007: 25 Abstr 8526.

Wong JH, Sterns EE, Kopald KH, et al. (1989) Prognostic significance of pregnancy in stage I melanoma. *Arch Surg* 1989; 124: 1227–1231

Yu C, Jozsef G, Apuzzo ML, et al. (2003) Fetal radiation doses for model C gamma knife radiosurgery. *Neurosurgery* 2003; 52: 687–93.

Zucali R, Marchesini R, De Palo G.(1981) Abdominal dosimetry for supradiaphragmatic irradiation of Hodgkin's disease in pregnancy: experimental data and clinical considerations. *Tumori* 1981; 67: 203–08.

# 6

# Familial Melanoma in Italy: A Review

Gloria Funari[1], Chiara Menin[2], Lisa Elefanti[1],
Emma D'Andrea[1,2] and Maria Chiara Scaini[1]
[1]*Section of Oncology, Department of Oncology and Surgical Sciences, University of Padua,*
[2]*Immunology and Molecular Oncology Unit, Istituto Oncologico Veneto, IRCCS, Padua, Italy*

## 1. Introduction

Looking back to history, the first accredited description of melanoma appeared in the writings of Hippocrates (5th century, BC) as a "fatal black disease"; over the centuries, several other physicians have described pigmented malignant skin lesions, but only during the 1800s significant gains were obtained in the comprehension and treatment of melanoma. In 1820 William Norris suggested for the first time a genetic basis for the disease, reporting the development of a skin neoplasm in a father and his son, and in 1838 Carswell used the medical term "melanoma" to describe pigmented lesions.
Cutaneous melanoma represents a malignant skin cancer, which arises from the neoplastic transformation of specialized pigment-producing cells, the melanocytes. Its aggressive features, in terms of tendency to develop metastasis and strong resistance to therapy, make melanoma one of the deadliest forms of cancer.

### 1.1 Origin and pathogenesis

During embryogenesis, cellular precursors emerge from the neural crest and migrate to various sites, as uveal tracts, meninges, ectodermal mucosa and skin, where they finally establish to the epidermal-dermal junction, where they differentiate into melanocytes (Bennett, 1993), making dendridic contacts with the basal keratinocytes and thus forming the so called "epidermal melanin unit". The melanin produced by the melanocytes is transferred to keratinocytes for the adsorption and scattering of light radiation. The quantity of pigment dictates skin pigmentation and protection degree from UV-induced damage.

#### 1.1.1 Melanoma stages

As reported in Figure 1, the pathogenesis of melanoma is characterized by a series of histological and molecular alterations; in particular, five distinct stages have been proposed for melanoma development (Chin, 2003): (I) acquired and/or congenital nevi represent benign forms of melanocytic proliferation, different from (II) dysplastic nevi with some degree of structural atypia and a deeper disorder in the melanin unit organization; both benign and dysplastic nevi may evolve to (III) radial growth phase melanoma, characterized by a lateral growth, that remains mostly limited to the epidermis, due to the dependence of melanocyte proliferation from growth factors released by keratinocytes (*in situ* melanoma). Subsequently, melanoma can shift to (IV) vertical, mitogens- and anchorage-independent, growth phase, with dermis and subcutaneous tissue invasion, that, further on, may give rise to a (V) fully metastatic melanoma. These stages, describing melanoma natural history, have corresponding molecular counterparts, providing a biochemical basis for the main cellular events responsible for melanomagenesis. Accordingly, mutations in genes, normally regulating proliferation, differentiation and cell death, are involved in all of the main steps of melanoma progression, as briefly summarized in Figure 1.

### 1.1.2 Clinical forms

The vast majority of melanomas arise from cutaneous sites and different clinical forms have been described so far. Superficial spreading melanoma, most common in 30-50 year-old patients, spreads horizontally with an early flat appearance, and irregular pigmentation and margins; lentigo maligna melanoma is typically located on sun-exposed sites (head, neck and arms) and presents large (3-4 cm in diameter) and irregular lesions with a very slow growth over 5-20 years; nodular malignant melanoma develops from dark and uniformly coloured lesions, which may ulcerate and bleed, it lacks the radial growth phase and can result in a rapid invasion of the dermis. These three types account together for approximately 85% of all melanoma cases. Other less frequent forms include desmoplastic melanoma, with a highly variable clinical appearance, mucosal lentiginous melanoma and acral lentiginous melanoma, the most common type in dark-skinned populations (Africans and Hispanics).

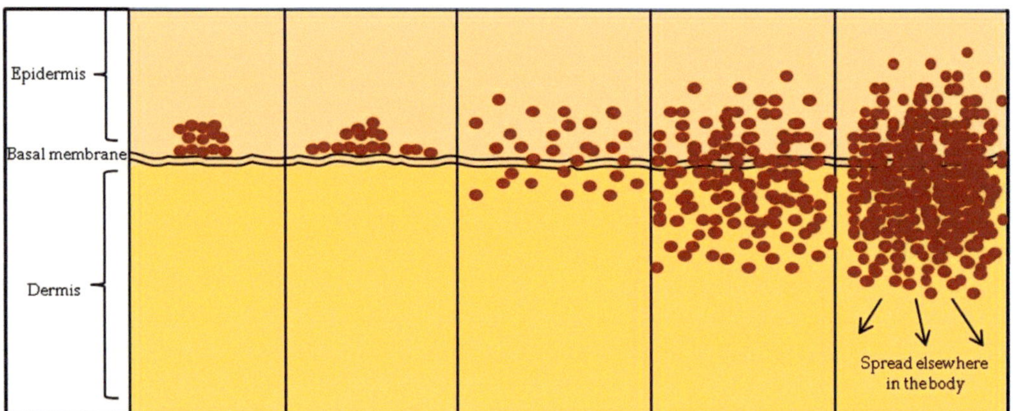


| Histological stage | Congenital and/or acquired nevus (I) | Atypical/dysplastic nevus (II) | Radial growth phase (III) | Vertical growth phase (IV) | Metastatic melanoma (V) |
|---|---|---|---|---|---|
| Molecular alterations | Mutations in:<br>BRAF<br>NRAS<br><br>MC1R alleles | Loss of CDKN2A<br>PTEN<br><br>CDK4 mutations | Decreased:<br>SILV<br>MLANA<br>TRPM1<br><br>E-caderin expression | Expression of:<br>N-caderin<br>αVβ3 integrin<br>MMP2<br><br>E-caderin loss | Additional events |

Fig. 1. Melanoma natural history.

Five proposed stages for melanoma development and corresponding molecular events involved in malignant melanoma pathogenesis. (MC1R: *M*elano*C*ortin *1* *R*eceptor; CDKN2A: *C*yclin-*D*ependent *K*inase i*N*hibitor *2A*; PTEN: *P*hosphate and *TEN*sin homolog; CDK4: *C*yclin *D*ependent *K*inase 4; MLANA: *MeLAN*in-*A*; TRPM1: *T*ransient *R*eceptor *P*otential cation channel sub-family *M* member 1; MMP2: *M*atrix *M*etallo*P*roteinase 2).

### 1.2 Melanoma epidemiology and etiology

It was reported that melanoma incidence rose during the last century worldwide. In recent decades, the annual increase in incidence rate was reported to be in the order of 3-7% for fair skinned Caucasians (Armstrong & Kricker, 1994) and to vary among populations with age, gender (Jemal et al., 2001) and geographical area. Melanoma is the third more frequent cancer in 30-45 years age group, with a higher occurrence in female and in fair-skinned populations living in sunny areas. Some dermatologists questioned whether this rising in melanoma incidence could reflect a real increase of disease occurrence or if it could be ascribed to a more intensive surveillance. Undoubtedly, implementation of screening programs has allowed the early detection of a larger number of pigmented and potentially suspect skin lesions (Dennis, 1999), with a corresponding larger number of new cases per year, that could, at least in part, justify the overall incidence increase. Moreover, some initially unsuspected lesions can be correctly diagnosed as true malignant melanomas (the so called "incidental melanomas") later on by histo-pathological analysis, because of persisting diagnostic limitations for very early lesions (Swerlick & Chen, 1997). Importantly, despite a higher incidence, melanoma mortality remains stable over the years.

Italy is considered a low melanoma incidence country, with geographical variations according to a decreasing North-South gradient, as reported by the Italian Cancer Registries. Melanoma incidence rates in Italy were reported to be of 8.5 cases per 100,000 in male and 10.2 case per 100,000 in female (Boi et al., 2003).

#### 1.2.1 Risk factors

Melanoma epidemiology involves not only incidence and mortality rates, but also possible causal factors. Melanoma is characterized by a complex etiology, concerning both constitutional and environmental factors, that mostly in combination determine the likelihood of developing the disease. There is no question that sun exposure is the major environmental risk factor (Oliveria et al., 2006). Several data from epidemiological analysis on migration and geographical residence showed an increased risk in sunny areas, especially for individuals exposed during childhood and adolescence, both crucial ages for subsequent melanoma development (Autier et al., 1997; Robsahm & Tretli, 2001). Conflicting evidence, however, were reported to this end, since several studies did not confirm the role of childhood/adolescence as "critical time periods" (Kaskel et al., 2001; Pfahlberg et al., 2001). Intermittent sun exposure and sunburns, in particular, appear to be relevant factors as well (Gandini et al., 2005a).

To date, limited data are available on melanoma risk factors in Mediterranean populations, one of the largest Italian collaborative case-control study investigated the role of different potential risk factors, comprising modalities of sun reaction and history of sunburns (Naldi et al., 2000). Moreover, an Italian research group recently reported a protective effect of the so-called Mediterranean diet on cutaneous melanoma onset (Fortes et al., 2008).

On the other hand, several constitutional risk factors were shown to be involved in melanomagenesis. Phenotypic traits, including skin phototype and pigmentation (fair complexion and sensitivity to sunburns), presence of freckles and light-coloured eyes are additional examples of host-related risk factors (Gandini et al., 2005b). Several evidence suggested that while the number of melanocytic nevi can represent a proper melanoma predictor, the presence of atypical nevi may assume an independent role (Bataille et al., 1998; Tucker et al., 1997). Thus, melanoma risk raises with nevus number and clinical atypia degree, with the highest risk for individuals presenting multiple atypical nevi (MacKie et al., 1993).

### 1.2.2 Familial melanoma

Probably, the most important and well documented host-related risk factor is familial history of melanoma, defined by the presence of two or more relatives affected by melanoma within a family branch. Familial melanoma accounts for approximately 5-10% of all melanoma cases and segregation analysis revealed an autosomal dominant mode of transmission. Moreover, likewise other inheritable cancer syndromes, familial melanoma is characterized by peculiar features (Kopf et al., 1986) including early age of onset, multiple primary melanomas and association with other cancers, namely pancreatic carcinoma in the so-called "Familial Melanoma/Pancreatic Cancer Syndrome" (Lynch et al., 2002). On the other hand, as for histological and clinical aspects, familial melanoma is indistinguishable from sporadic cases. Even though exposure to common environmental risk factors cannot be excluded, familial aggregation can be prevalently attributed to shared genetic factors and several melanoma-predisposing genes were identified so far. A crucial aspect of familial melanoma, as well as any cancer syndromes, is that what is inherited is a genetic predisposition, i.e. a greater risk, rather than the disease itself. The reason is that a mutated allele of a specific cancer-predisposing gene is constitutively present in every cell of the body (Knudson's "first-hit"). Thus, individuals belonging to melanoma-prone families, once carriers of genetic predisposition, have a markedly higher risk to develop melanoma during their lifetime, compared to the general population.

Aim of the present review is the description of the genetic basis of familial melanoma, the role of genetic counseling in its early diagnosis, the laboratory assessment of pathogenic gene mutations and an overview of the main studies and research investigations performed on familial melanoma in Italy.

## 2. Genetic basis of familial melanoma

During oncogenesis, both inherited and/or acquired genetic alterations take part in a multistep process that finally results in an invasive and metastatic neoplastic growth. Hereditary cancer syndromes, in particular, represent a model for the analysis of how germline mutations of specific genes can modulate cancer risk and hence influence the development of disease.

Several genes involved in familial melanoma susceptibility were reported and recent advances in molecular genetics, including genome-wide association studies (GWAS), may identify additional melanoma-predisposing alleles in the future.

### 2.1 High risk genes

The identified melanoma susceptibility genes include rare high risk and more common, moderate/low risk genes. It is important to point out that there is not an absolute distinction, in terms of conferred risk, between these two categories, but most likely a continuous gradient of gene effects, leading to a variable (from strong to weak) melanoma risk.

### 2.1.1 CDKN2A

The first real clues about the existence of a major melanoma susceptibility gene came from molecular cytogenetic evidence. Melanoma cell lines were found to have frequent deletions of the 9p21-p22 chromosome region and linkage with markers at 9p13-p22 was subsequently reported in several melanoma families. Some years later, a combination of tumour deletion and recombination mapping studies in melanoma families was used to further limit the position of a candidate gene that was then cloned, sequenced and recognized to be identical to a previously characterized cell cycle regulatory gene. This gene was variably called INK4A, CDK4I or MTS1, but designed by now as CDKN2A (for Cyclin-*D*ependent *K*inase i*N*hibitor *2A*) by the Human Genome Organization Nomenclature Committee.

CDKN2A is the most common high risk susceptibility gene identified to date in familial malignant melanoma. The CDKN2A locus possesses a rather unique genomic organization: it consists of two upstream exons, 1α and 1β, driven by different promoters, that are combined to the common exons 2 and 3 to produce two distinct proteins. The transcript for p16INK4A is initiated from the proximal promoter of exon 1α that is joined to exons 2 and 3, while p14ARF transcript starts from the upstream promoter and is made of exon 1β plus exons 2 and 3 read with a different frame (ARF stands for *A*lternative *R*eading *F*rame). Thus, the CDKN2A particular genome arrangement (Figure 2), likely arisen by gene duplication (Gil & Peters, 2006), and its alternative exon splicing allow to produce two totally distinct proteins from a shared coding sequence (Sherr, 2001).

#### 2.1.1.1 p16INK4A/p14ARF structure and function

More in detail, p16INK4A (p16 for simplicity) belongs to the INK4 protein family, of four members with the capacity to inhibit cell cycle progression; p16 consists of 156 amino acidic residues, spatially organized into four ankirin repeats, which are structural motifs involved in a large number of protein-protein interactions. A single ankyrin repeat is composed by approximately 33 residues that fold into anti-parallel helix-loop-helix structures, linked by β-hairpins (Zhang & Peng, 2000). All these four ankirin repeats are needed for the interaction of p16 with its target: p16 binds to CDK4/6 (Cyclin-*D*ependent *K*inases) and inhibits the catalytic activity of cyclin D-CDK4/6 complexes, hence maintaining the oncosuppressor pRb in its hypo-phosphorilated state (Lukas et al., 1995), thus preventing G1/S transition.

The p14ARF protein (p14 for simplicity), instead, is made up by 132 residues and there are no recognizable protein motifs in its structure. It can limit aberrant cell proliferation by binding to and blocking MDM2 and, thus, stabilizing p53 (Stott et al., 1998); increased intracellular levels of p53, in turn, mediate cell cycle arrest and apoptosis. Recent evidence, however, support additional roles of p14 in mediating p53-independent responses (Eymin et al., 2003). Although p16 and p14 act on distinct molecular pathways, it is important to point out that both are involved in tumour suppression, despite of species- and cell type-specific differences between the two; moreover, their functions show some overlap, due to functional interconnections between p53 and pRb pathways (Bates et al., 1998; Sherr & McCormick, 2002).

Due to the wide role of CDKN2A in tumour suppression and together with the ubiquitous expression of both p16 and p14 oncosuppressors, one wonders why there is such a specific predisposition to melanoma, and not to other malignancies. This type of "tissue specificity of gene defects" is commonly found in the majority of hereditary tumour syndromes and a possible explanation relies on how the same gene might possess entirely distinct functions, depending on its cell type specific expression. In the case of p16, in particular, the role of this protein in activating replicative senescence, an irreversible G1 arrest of still metabolically active cells (Campisi, 1997), has been well established. In human melanocytes, p16 is the master regulator of cell senescence (Sviderskaya et al., 2002) that has no other redundant or compensatory pathways in this particular cell type; this might explain why individuals and families with a germline CDKN2A mutation are prone to melanoma development, due to the specific impairment of melanocyte senescence, a crucial barrier against tumorigenesis.

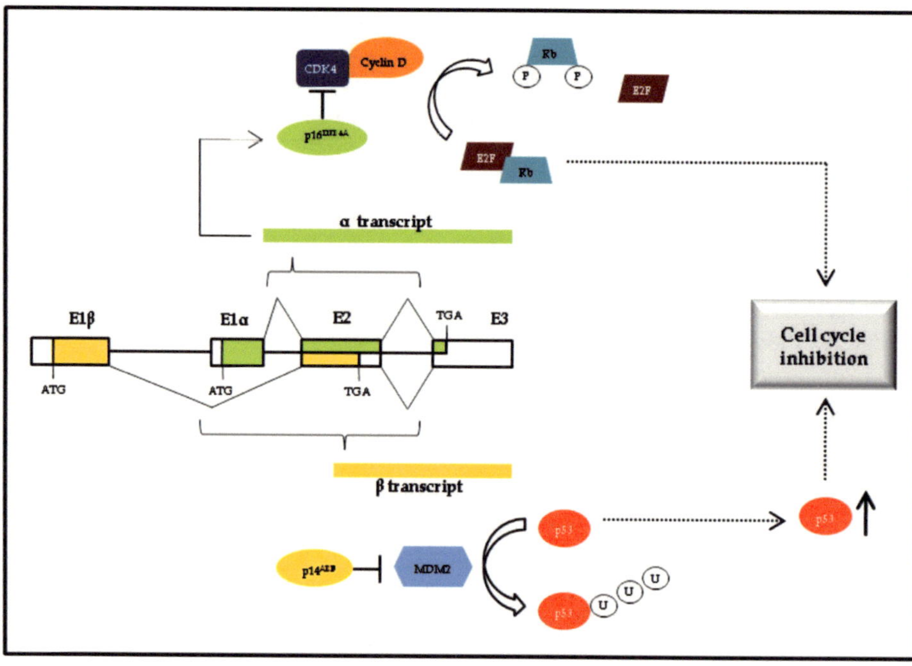


Fig. 2. Genomic organization of CDKN2A locus.

Exons 1α, 2 and 3 code for p16INK4A, able to bind CDK4 and block its activity, thus maintaining the pRb in a hypo-phosphorilated state and, hence, E2F transcriptional factors inactive. Exons 1β, 2 and 3 are joined into the β transcript, coding p14ARF, that inhibits the ubiquitin-ligase activity of MDM2, with a following p53 accumulation. Both, the pRb and the p53 pathways, finally result in G1 cell cycle arrest.

### 2.1.1.2 CDKN2A and melanoma predisposition

A variety of CDKN2A germline mutations have been identified to date in melanoma-prone families, while they are reported to be rare in the general population. The relative risk of melanoma development conferred by CDKN2A mutations in the general population was estimated by an international case-control study (Berwick et al., 2006). This study determined an overall relative risk of melanoma associated with CDKN2A mutations of 4.3, with considerable variations of this value, depending on the particular type of mutation.

In order to better characterize mutations in this high-risk melanoma susceptibility gene, the International Melanoma Genetics Consortium (GenoMEL), comprising most familial melanoma research groups from North America, Europe, Australia and Middle East, performed a large study on 446 families with at least three malignant melanoma patients, for a total of about two thousands enrolled patients (Goldstein et al., 2006). Overall, 41% of families had CKDN2A mutations, with differences in the mutation detection rates among several geographic areas. CDKN2A mutations targeting the p14 sequence only (i.e. localized mainly in exon 1β) were much less common and present in only seven families, while mutations affecting the p16 sequence were detected in 178 families and were present in both exon 1α and exon 2. Moreover, the 57 different p16 mutations included: missense mutations (65%), deletions (16%), insertions or duplications (7%), nonsense and splicing mutations (10%). Many of the most recurrent CDKN2A mutations were "founder mutations", originated from a common ancestor and dating back 100 generations (Pollock et al., 1998). Moreover, a significantly younger median age at melanoma diagnosis was observed in mutated families than in families without mutations. Furthermore, the probability to detect a CDKN2A mutation was dependent on the number of melanoma cases within each family (Kefford et al., 1999). Interestingly, the presence of pancreatic cancer was confirmed to be associated with a higher CDKN2A mutation frequency.

Finally, given a certain CDKN2A mutation, what is the risk of melanoma development in a mutation carrier? Again, a study by GenoMEL on 80 families with at least two melanoma cases in first-degree relatives, for a total of about 400 melanoma patients from Europe, Australia and United States, provided data on CDKN2A mutation penetrance (Bishop et al., 2002). Overall, CDKN2A mutation penetrance was estimated to be 30% by age 50 and 67% by age 80, without significant modifications by gender or co-presence of p14 mutations. Importantly, also in this case the penetrance was reported to be strongly influenced by geographic areas and, hence, by environmental exposure: for instance, by age 80 the penetrance was 58% in Europe, 76% in the United States and 91% in Australia, also showing that penetrance varied with melanoma incidence rates among populations.

#### 2.1.1.3 CDKN2A and melanoma/pancreatic cancer syndrome

Approximately 5-10% of pancreatic cancer (PC) cases are attributable to hereditary cancer syndromes (Habbe et al. 2006). Virtually all PCs have somatic inactivation of CDKN2A (Schutte et al., 1997), thus suggesting a critical relevance of this locus in PC pathogenesis and an association between PC and CDKN2A mutations was described. Several authors (Goldstein et al, 1995; Goldstein, 2004; Whelan et al., 1995) showed that PC was found in carriers within melanoma families harbouring CDKN2A mutations and a more recent study showed that individuals possessing the p16-Leiden mutation (a specific 19 base-pair deletion in exon 2) had an estimated cumulative risk of 17% to develop a PC with a mean age at diagnosis of 58 years (Vasen et al., 2000). In 2002, Lynch and co-workers analyzed eight families characterized by melanoma/PC association and presence of CDKN2A mutations, and they proposed the possibility of a new hereditary cancer syndrome, defined as "*F*amilial *A*typical *M*ultiple *M*ole *M*elanoma-*P*ancreatic *C*arcinoma" (FAMMM-PC) syndrome (Lynch et al., 2002).

At present, however, several questions remain, and the molecular mechanisms linking CDKN2A function and PC development need further investigations. Moreover, it is not yet clear which CDKN2A mutations are specifically associated with PC and why.

### 2.1.2 CDK4

The cyclin-dependent kinase CDK4 interacts with cyclin D and the resulting complexes catalyze the phosphorylation of target molecules that in turn promote the G1/S transition of cell cycle. As previously discussed, CDK4 activity can be regulated by p16 and mutations in CDK4 gene could perturb the cell cycle control, when they disrupt the ability of CDK4 to bind p16. CDK4 mutations are very rare compared to CDKN2A (Goldstein et al., 2006): they occur in only 2% of families analyzed to date, with a pattern of inheritance and an age of tumour onset similar to that reported for CDKN2A mutations.

The most recurrent mutations are localized in codon 24, replacing an arginine with a cysteine (Zuo et al., 1996) or a histidine (Soufir et al., 1998). These mutations, targeting the p16 binding site of CDK4, render the kinase resistant to p16 inhibition and thus convert CDK4 to a dominant oncogene, with only a single mutated allele required for tumorigenesis.

### 2.2 Moderate/low risk and modifier genes

#### 2.2.1 More on hereditary genetic risk

High-risk genes alone do not completely account for the heterogeneous genetic substrate underlying familial melanoma. Only a small fraction of melanoma-prone families, in fact, carries mutations in the highly penetrant loci described above. The remaining genetic risk could be due to high penetrance genes not yet identified or, more likely, to other less penetrant, lower risk genes. The so called "polygenic model" states that a large number of alleles, each conferring a small genotypic risk, combine additively or multiplicatively to confer a range of susceptibilities to the population (Houlston & Peto, 2004). Thus, the particular allelic pattern may influence the lifetime risk of an individual, but also expressivity and penetrance of high risk loci, acting as "modifier risk genes". Within low penetrance inheritance, the polygenic component is significantly represented by *S*ingle *N*ucleotide *P*olymorphism*s* (SNPs) that characterize each susceptibility allele. These polymorphisms could directly regulate molecular pathways involved in tumorigenesis initiation and progression (i.e., metabolism dysfunctions, cell death, inflammation, immune response and angiogenesis) or could modulate the host response to environmental factors (DNA-damage repair after sun exposure). The relevance of these numerous low penetrance genes justifies the considerable efforts that were made in their identification, mainly performed by case-control studies on candidate genes and, more recently, by GWAS. So far, several moderate/low penetrance genes were described, but for most of them the clear contribution to cancer development was not yet exhaustively elucidated. Gene functions, redundancy in the cellular pathways and protein pleiotropism represent, in fact, the main complexities in the comprehension of this field (Caporaso, 2002). For familial melanoma, different moderate/low penetrance genes were reported to influence the lifetime risk of developing the disease.

#### 2.2.2 MC1R

The *M*elano*C*ortin type-*1 R*eceptor (MC1R) is a seven-pass transmembrane G-protein-coupled receptor, specifically expressed on skin melanocytes. Functionally, MC1R is an upstream component of the intracellular pathway leading to melanin biosynthesis and skin pigmentation. The binding to its ligand α-MSH (*M*elanocyte *S*timulating *H*ormone) activates MC1R, with upregulation of intracellular cAMP levels that, in turn, modulate melanin production (Figure 3). Two melanin types are present in mammals: pheomelanin, a red-yellow pigment, typical of the so-called RHC (*R*ed *H*air *C*olour) phenotype, and eumelanin, the darker pigment that confer olive complexion and brown/black hair. MC1R engagement can shift the intracellular pheomelanin/eumelanin balance, thus increasing the production of the latter and modulating skin sensitivity to sun exposure (Sturm et al., 2001). A functional impairment in MC1R signalling alters the downstream pigmentation pathways, causing an accumulation of pheomelanin that, in turn, has reduced UV protective capacity and can produce cytotoxic and mutagenic metabolites (Sturm, 1998), accelerating melanocytic transformation. This functional impairment can result from different mechanisms: some variants fail in the stimulation of cAMP production (Beaumont et al., 2007; Garcia-Borron et al., 2005), while others show MC1R reduced affinity for its ligand α-MSH (Ringholm et al., 2004) or there are even defects in desensitization and internalization of the MC1R receptor itself (Sanchez-Laorden et al., 2007).

Given the role of MC1R on epidermal response to UV-induced damage, it is not surprising that the MC1R allelic state influences melanoma risk, by directly regulating skin pigmentation. MC1R locus is highly polymorphic in Caucasians (Savage et al., 2008) and over 100 variants have been identified so far. These include "R" alleles, found to be prevalently associated with light skin, red hair, freckles and sun sensitivity (termed RHC phenotype), all known melanoma risk factors, and "r" alleles, with a weaker or absent association with the RHC phenotype. The molecular basis discriminating between R and r alleles apparently resides in the complete (R) or partial (r) loss of the receptor signalling ability. Recently, it was demonstrated that melanocytes harbouring R alleles possessed markedly reduced surface expression and/or impaired G-protein coupling of the corresponding receptor (Newton et al., 2007).

It is important to underline that MC1R variants have also a different functional causative role on melanoma development and several studies showed that R variants were more strongly responsible for melanoma risk (Kanetsky et al., 2006). In a very recent meta-analysis, the estimated summary relative risk for R and r alleles were found to be of 2.44 and 1.29, respectively, although both estimates were associated with evidence of substantial heterogeneity across studies (Williams et al., 2010). In Italy, some R alleles, such as R151C and R160W, were reported to confer an attributable risk of 7.48 and 4.54, respectively (Raimondi et al., 2008).

By all means, correlations between MC1R allelic status, skin pigmentation features and melanoma onset are more complex. Some "R" variants could not be associated with a RHC phenotype; moreover, MC1R might influence melanoma development by acting on different molecular pathways that are pigmentation-independent such as a MC1R-induced upregulation of p38 MAPK in melanocytes, likely occurring via cAMP (Newton et al., 2007). Potential downstream outcomes of p38 activation include histone H3 phosphorylation with subsequent chromatin remodelling and altered gene regulation, relevant for non-pigmentary pathways including cell cycle regulation, differentiation, and apoptosis.

A variety of studies have reported that MC1R variants can markedly modify the penetrance of CDKN2A locus (Box et al., 2001; Fargnoli et al., 2010; Goldstein et al., 2005, 2007). To this end, a recent study performed by GenoMEL (Demenais et al., 2010) investigated the associations among host phenotype, MC1R variants and melanoma risk in CDKN2A mutation carriers. The analysis, performed on 815 mutation carriers from Europe, North America and Australia, showed interesting results: both non-RHC and RHC variants were associated with increased melanoma risk, that rose threefold in presence of at least one MC1R variant; moreover, the risk was higher in presence of RHC variants and a higher number of MC1R variants. Interestingly, the MC1R-associated risk seemed even greater when CDKN2A mutations affected p16 only, than when they involved both p16 and p14. In addition, hair colour and a high number of nevi are significantly associated with increased melanoma risk; in presence of this host phenotype, the increase in melanoma risk with anyone of the four more frequent MC1R variants (V60L, V92M, R151C and R160W) remained statistically significant. In conclusion, melanoma risk in CDKN2A mutation carriers is modified by type and number of concurrent MC1R variants, thus confirming the role of MC1R as a risk modifier gene.

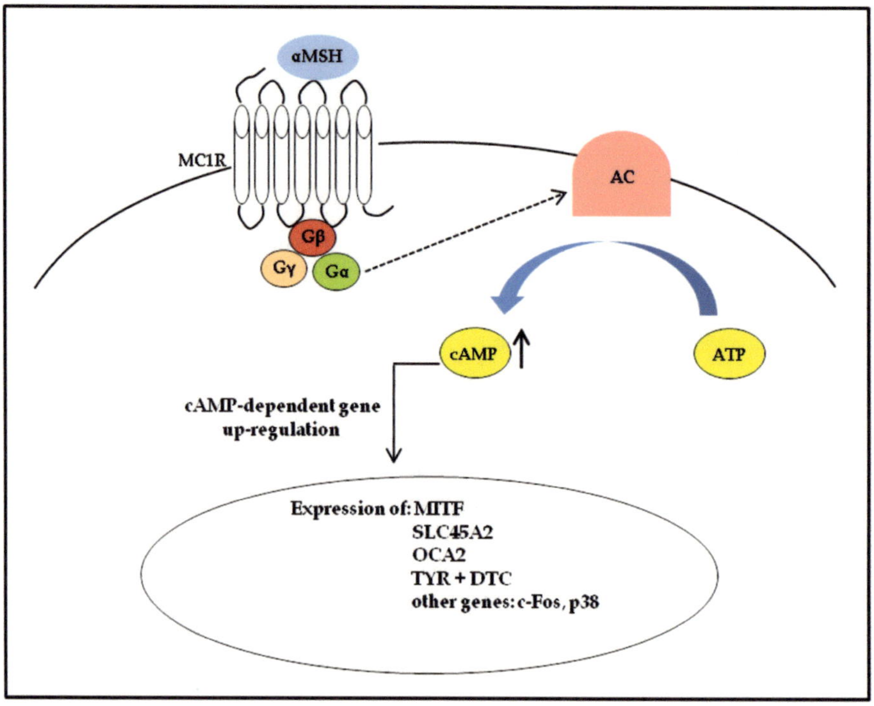


Fig. 3. MSH-MC1R signalling pathway.

The binding of the α-MSH ligand activates G-coupled MC1R, with subsequent cAMP level increase, through the catalytic activity of Adenilate Cyclase (AC). The intracellular cAMP accumulation up-regulates the expression of key genes: MITF plays a pivotal role in mediating transcriptional control of numerous other genes. Activated pigmentary genes include SLC45A2, TYR and DTC, that all modulate melanin synthesis and skin colour, and OCA2, involved in the regulation of the facultative pigmentation. Other MC1R-up-regulated non-pigmentary genes comprise c-Fos, a well-known transcription factor influencing DNA-repair, cell cycle regulation and apoptosis, and p38 MAP kinase (Newton et al., 2007).

### 2.2.3 Additional pigmentation genes

Human pigmentation is a polygenic trait influenced by a plethora of different genetic determinants. In addition to MC1R, several other pigmentation genes were described to be associated with melanoma risk. A large-scale association study investigated different loci able to influence hair, eye and skin colour (Gudbjartson et al., 2008). Variants at three of these loci showed significant association with melanoma. In particular, the strongest association was found with ASIP locus (on chromosome 20q11.22), coding for *A*gouti *SI*gnalling *P*rotein, a second ligand of MC1R and an antagonist of α-MSH. In principle, mutation in ASIP could mimic a loss-of-function of MC1R; to date, no variants have been identified in the coding regions of ASIP. The other two associated loci were TYR and TYRP1, involved in pheomelanin/eumelanin biosynthesis.

#### 2.2.4 Other genes

A GWAS carried out by the GenoMEL (Bishop et al., 2009), identified the *M*ethyl*T*hio*A*denosine *P*hosphorylase (MTAP) gene, adiacent to CDKN2A on 9p21, coding the first enzyme of the methionine salvage pathway and having a documented tumour-suppressor activity, as a melanoma-associated locus. MTAP variants were found to be strongly associated with a high melanocytic nevus number (Falchi et al., 2009), one of the strongest known melanoma risk factor.

*E*pidermal *G*rowth *F*actor (EGF) gene was also considered a reasonable risk candidate: a specific SNP, located upstream of the initiation codon of pre-pro-EGF, is more frequent in melanoma patients than in unaffected controls and it is reported to confer a 2.7 relative risk of disease development (Shahbazi et al., 2002).

*G*lutathione *S*-*T*ransferases (GSTs) are a family of isoenzymes largely involved in metabolic processes. Interestingly, GST genes are candidates for modulating CDKN2A penetrance. GST genes *M*u1 (GSTM1) and *T*heta 1 (GSTT1) are specifically expressed in the skin to detoxify products from oxidative stress reactions caused by UV irradiation. A homozygous deletion of GSTM1 (GSTM1 null) is present in about 50% of Caucasians, while about 20% of them carry a homozygous deletion of GSTT1 (GSTT1 null). In particular, combined deletions of both genes were found associated with increased UV sensitivity and UV-inducible skin cancers, and null gene variants were also proposed as melanoma risk factors (Mössner et al., 2007).

Another locus governing metabolic processes and involved in melanoma susceptibility codes for *CY*tochrome *P*450 *D*ebrisoquine Hydroxylase (CYP2D6). Different inactivating polymorphisms were found to be more recurrent in melanoma patients, who were frequently homozygous for these non-functional alleles, than in controls (Strange et al., 1999).

Additionally, it was shown that a SNP in the MDM2 gene, the SNP309 (T>G variation) was linked to the tumour onset and outcome. However, discordant results were reported on the effect of this SNP on age at diagnosis of cutaneous melanoma in Caucasian female population and no associations were found among SNP309, melanoma risk, age at diagnosis and presence of metastasis in the Italian population, although SNP309 was significantly associated with tumour Breslow thickness (Capasso et al., 2010).

It was proposed that the *V*itamin *D* *R*eceptor (VDR) gene might play a role in melanoma development as well, since its interaction with the calcitriol ligand results in antiproliferative and pro-differentiation signals on melanocytes. Rare VDR alleles were found more commonly in melanoma cases than controls, although conflicting evidence were also reported (Barroso et al., 2008; Hutchinson et al., 2000).

All these evidence stress the fact that melanoma, being a multifactorial disease, is characterized by a heterogeneous genetic background and further investigations on melanoma-predisposing genes are necessary to gain new insights into this overwhelming wealth of information and, in turn, to the comprehension of melanoma pathogenesis.

## 3. Genetic counseling and testing for familial melanoma

### 3.1 Genetic screening: how and why

In general terms, screening is a systematic attempt to identify, among apparently healthy individuals, those at higher risk for a specific disease, to finally inform them about

preventive protocols. The aim of cancer screening can be either to identify precancerous lesions, whose treatment will be truly preventive (primary prevention), or to diagnose cancer at an earlier stage and treat the tumour more efficiently (secondary prevention).
In the case of cancer syndromes, the existence of inherited alterations in tumour-predisposing genes can be detected by a genetic test, which is a DNA analysis to determine the presence of a mutation that could be responsible for the development of the disease. Thus, for hereditary cancers, genetic testing is used to predict the risk of a future health impairment (Tsao & Niendorf, 2004).
The application of each genetic test in the clinical practice should be considered in conjunction with a formal and qualified genetic counseling setting, in which an inter-disciplinary team of specialists, such as geneticists, clinicians and psychologists, provides a comprehensive consultation service, with the purpose to elicit the patient's personal and familial health history, to assess genetic risk, to discuss with patients and families about benefits, limitations, interpretations and possible implications of genetic testing and diagnosis, to assess the need of a psychological support, and to include individuals in appropriate screening programs (Niendorf & Tsao, 2006).
The methodology of genetic counseling implies, firstly, the collection of the family pedigree, which is a genealogic tree used to analyze the mendelian inheritance of a certain trait, such as the presence of a mutation in a cancer-predisposing gene. It is particularly important to include the widest amount of information about the number and type of cancer-affected patients, their age at onset, the presence of multiple cancers in the same individual and the occurrence of cancers known to be associated with the syndrome of interest (as in the association of pancreatic cancer with familial melanoma). All the collected data allow prediction of the so called "theoretical risk", given as the product between the probability to have inherited a mutation in a susceptibility gene and the mutation penetrance at a given age. In general, the presence of two or more affected first-degree relatives, an early age at onset and a personal history of multiple primary cancers are features that strongly suggest an inheritable genetic cancer predisposition. In such a case, a genetic test for the molecular characterization of a given cancer-predisposing gene can be offered to the proband, the first affected member of the family enrolled for the screening, in association with an informed consent about the predictive power and the limits of the test.

### 3.2 Genetic test for CDKN2A

The aim of genetic testing for CDKN2A is to identify which family members are mutation-carriers, in order to target these higher risk individuals to more intensive cancer prevention and surveillance.
In a recent study, the predictive value of personal and familial history of melanoma/pancreatic cancer was assessed for the identification of individuals at increased probability to harbour a CDKN2A mutation (Leachman et al., 2009). The study demonstrated that in higher melanoma incidence areas, individuals with multiple primary melanomas and/or families with at least one invasive melanoma and two or more melanoma and/or pancreatic cancer cases among first- or second-degree relatives in the same familial side represented appropriate candidates for genetic evaluation. On the other hand, in geographic areas with lower melanoma incidence rates, two melanoma and/or pancreatic cancer cases within a family could be sufficient and appropriate for a genetic investigation.

When performed, genetic testing is based on the mutational analysis of CDKN2A locus: genomic DNA, extracted from *P*eripheral *B*lood *M*ononuclear Cells (PBMCs) of the patient, is subjected to sequencing techniques to analyse the whole gene sequence, including exonic and intronic regions, splicing junctions and 3'/5'UTR. A written informed consent has to be obtained for all tested patients under local ethic committee-approved protocols.

The interpretation of the possible results of a genetic test represents one of the most delicate issues in this context (Udayakumar & Tsao, 2009) and must be done by specialists with genetics expertise. When a specific mutation is detected, the patient might develop a melanoma during life, because of his increased risk, compared to the general population, due to the occurrence of the inherited mutation. The detected mutation provides a sort of familial genetic signature and other family members could be tested for it (specific test). When the mutation occurs within the family, but it is absent in a given member (non-carrier), the result of the specific test is negative. However, even in presence of a negative specific test, an increased risk for family members still persists, due to the possible co-inheritance of other shared genetic, risk-modifier factors. On the other hand, and most often, when no mutation is detected in a melanoma-prone family, the test does not provide any new information; in this case, other types of CDKN2A mutations or other melanoma-predisposing genes could be involved in determining that specific pedigree, hampering the possibility to rule out hereditary melanoma. Of course, families comprising individuals with uninformative tests are considered at increased risk, irrespective of their DNA status. An uninformative test is also obtained when a genetic alteration with unknown functional significance (the so called "*U*nclassified *V*ariants", UVs) is identified, as later discussed in more detail.

For all these reasons, it is generally recommended that members of melanoma families should be invited to participate in screening and cancer prevention programs, regardless of their CDKN2A mutational status (Hansson, 2008; Kefford et al., 1999). Primary prevention measures mainly include education for sun protection and routine skin self-examinations, while secondary prevention is focused on monitoring pigmented skin lesions, that could be considered as melanoma precursors, since early detection and surgical excision are the only powerful means presently available to improve melanoma prognosis.

Undoubtedly, controversies on genetic tests for melanoma still exist (Kefford et al., 2002; Kefford & Mann, 2003), but the clinical utility of CDKN2A testing continues to improve and its potential benefits have been already established.

### 3.3 Clinical counseling in Italy

The variable melanoma incidence and CDKN2A mutation penetrance among countries render unfeasible the definition of international guidelines to regulate the access to genetic testing for CDKN2A, insomuch as specific selection criteria must be applied on a national scale. In Italy, one of the first countries where genetic testing for familial melanoma was offered in medical or genetics services, the Italian Society of Human Genetics (SIGU) outlined recommendations on genetic counseling and testing for familial melanoma, suggesting to offer genetic test for CDKN2A to those families with at least two first-degree affected members. A recent cooperative study, among 9 Italian centres, quantified the frequency of CDKN2A mutations in melanoma-prone families, in line with the SIGU eligibility criteria for clinical counseling, as summarized in Figure 4 (Bruno et al., 2009). This analysis, of 208 Italian families that met the SIGU criteria and underwent genetic testing, reported that 33% of the families overall carried CDKN2A mutations. More in detail, the results showed that CDKN2A mutation frequency rose with the number of affected members in the family, that the median age at diagnosis was significantly different in individuals from CDKN2A-mutated families (42 years), compared to patients from families without mutations (49 years), and that the CDKN2A mutation frequency increased with the number of patients presenting multiple primary melanomas within the family. In particular, families with two cases accounted for 71% of the entire sample and for 52% of the families harbouring CDKN2A mutations. These findings suggested that if stricter selection criteria for genetic test were applied in Italy (such as the presence of at least three affected members), a significant subset of CDKN2A mutated families would not be identified, a result that outlines how the definition of selection criteria to access to genetic testing should depend upon the particular geographic area of interest.

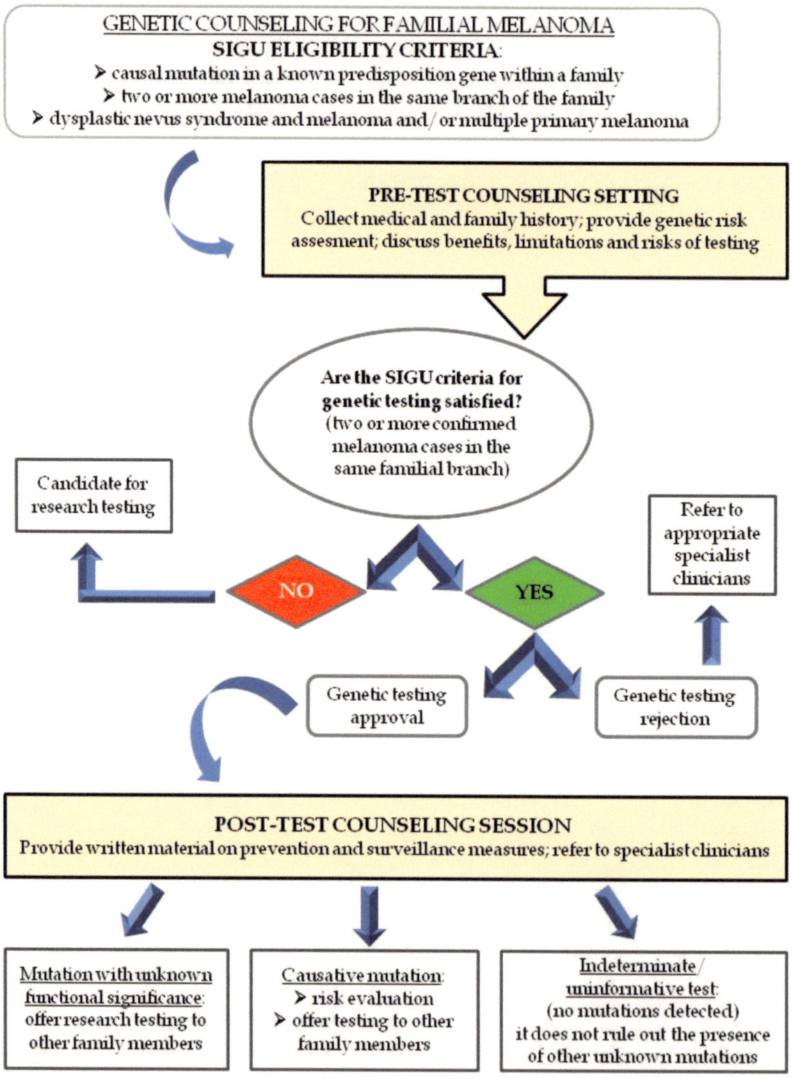


Fig. 4. Italian Society for Human Genetics (SIGU) recommendations for clinical genetic counseling and testing for familial melanoma (Bruno et al., 2009, with modifications).

## 4. The problem of CDKN2A unclassified variants

As previously anticipated, a possible outcome of genetic testing for CDKN2A can be the identification of an alteration with undetermined pathogenetic significance, that is an *U*nclassified *V*ariant (UV), a result that can complicate rather than improve cancer risk assessment. In this case, a change in the nucleotide sequence is found, but there is not enough information to decide whether it affects or not the function of the gene product and, thus, cancer predisposition. UVs are mainly represented by non-synonymous changes in a given protein position, also called "missense variants". Over 150 different UVs of CDKN2A, mostly targeting p16, were reported worldwide (Goldstein et al., 2004, 2006). The main features of these UVs were grouped together and are now also available on the *L*eiden *O*pen *V*ariation *D*atabase (LOVD; http://chromium.liacs.nl/lovd2/home.php?select_db=CDKN2A).
Obviously, an uninformative result can be a source of anxiety for individuals and their offspring because they will not be able to use this information for clinical purposes. In addition, all first-degree relatives, including non carriers, are considered at risk as long as the contribution of the variant to disease cannot be assessed, resulting in frequently unnecessary psychological stress and lifelong screening. The distinction between a true pathogenic mutation and a benign variant represents an essential prerequisite to univocally distinguish individuals at higher risk and, consequently, to enroll them in prevention protocols. In the last few years, a growing number of sequence changes of undetermined clinical significance was reported, and this issue received the attention of a large number of investigators. Recently, the *I*nternational *A*gency for *R*esearch on Cancer (IARC; the cancer research branch of the World Health Organization) convened a Working Group on UVs in high-risk cancer susceptibility genes, CDKN2A included. The Group comprised investigators of different specialties with the aim to establish a standard approach to UV evaluation. Discussions and specific recommendations of the Working Group were reported in a series of articles published in the November, 2008 special issue of *Human Mutation* (Tatvigian et al., 2008a).
Currently, there is a general agreement for UVs classification on the basis of a multicomponent model, integrating direct and indirect evidence, including genetic, bioinformatic and experimental data, thus providing the highest degree of accuracy in UVs assessment.

### 4.1 Direct evidence of pathogenicity

Various lines of evidence were proposed to address UV evaluation (Goldgar et al., 2004, 2008). Some types of evidence determine a more direct association between presence of the variant and cancer development. The most straightforward genetic evidence is the co-segregation of a given variant with the disease in pedigrees. It offers the advantage to depend only on the availability of DNA samples from several individuals belonging to families with the variant, although its power is limited by the number of informative meiosis, very low in small pedigrees, and of affected members in the family. A second direct evidence is the evaluation of the variant frequency in case-control studies, particularly suitable for common genetic variants. For most UVs, however, their rare frequency would require prohibitively wide sample sizes to demonstrate its pathogenicity. Practically, this method is mainly used to rapidly screen out potentially neutral variants.
An additional evidence relies on co-occurrence analysis: in principle, if there is a known pathogenic mutation in a melanoma family, its presence will decrease the probability that a

given variant, found in association with that mutation, could be pathogenic as well. In other terms, a probably pathogenic variant will not be found in co-occurrence with a *bona-fide* mutation.

In the case of CDKN2A, the frequency of rare variants, the low number of carriers within melanoma families and the small pedigrees make difficult the application of all the above mentioned evidences.

### 4.2 Indirect evidence of pathogenicity: *in silico* analysis

Recently, computational approaches, predicting potential effects of a missense variant on protein structure/function and activity, were developed and widely used to support the classification of UVs (Tavtigian, 2008b). Different computational tools are based on the pairwise comparison of the physico-chemical characteristics or evolutionary substitution frequencies between the wild-type and variant amino acid. The basic principle is that in almost all proteins some amino acid positions, critically relevant for protein function, are highly philogenetically conserved, and in general disease-associated variants are preferentially localized in these positions. Thus, the evolutionary conservation of the amino acidic position, at which the variant occurs, provides an indication of its putative pathogenicity. In addition to the conservation degree, the comparison of the physico-chemical characteristics between any wild-type and variant amino acid position is taken into account, in order to evaluate the biochemical severity of the substitutions. Additional tools, based on similar theoretical assumptions, operate in *P*rotein *M*ultiple *S*equence *A*lignments (PMSAs) across different species. Likewise, missense substitutions falling at gene positions that are evolutionary constrained are more likely predicted to be pathogenic.

Known examples of methods based on evolutionary fitness and/or on biochemical parameters are represented by PAM 250 and BLOSUM 62. They are amino acid substitution scoring matrices derived from the frequencies with which the 20 amino acids are observed substituting each other in PMSAs of related proteins (Henikoff & Henikoff, 1992); they assign to each variant a different score value, depending on its substitution frequency, that eventually defines the likelihood to be deleterious, rather than neutral.

Another missense substitution analysis algorithm is the Align-GVGD, based on the Grantham difference, that describes the difference in side-chain atomic composition, polarity and volume between any two amino acids (Grantham, 1974). Again, a score is attributed to the variant, according to the "conservative", "non-conservative", or "radical" substitution features.

More complex algorithms consider also protein structural properties, generally available when the three-dimensional crystal protein structure has been solved. The structural features provide information about the possible location of the variant into binding sites or enzymatic active sites, secondary structural motifs (helices, sheets, loops, etc.) or about its solvent accessibility. In these terms, an amino acid substitution that presumably perturbs or disrupts such structural conditions is predicted to be deleterious for the protein function.

Example of algorithms, based on a combination of biochemical parameters, PMSAs and structural features, include PMut (Ferrer-Costa et al., 2005), SIFT (Ng & Henikoff, 2003) and PolyPhen (Sunyaev et al., 2001).

Due to their ability to analyze the expected effects of each individual variant, they were applied to the analysis of UVs of different cancer-predisposing genes, including CDKN2A (Chan et al., 2007). A recent study on a series of CDKN2A missense variants, however, showed potential limits of these approaches: widely conflicting results, in fact, were

obtained, with several specific variants, that were paradoxically predicted to be benign or pathogenic, depending on the software used (Kannengiesser et al., 2009).
Undoubtedly, *in silico* approaches provide an excellent support for UVs classification, but their accuracy is apparently limited by the available evolutionary, mutational or structural databases and, in some cases, by intrinsic limitations of each individual method. Therefore, *in silico* analysis represents an ancillary strategy for the evaluation of UV pathogenicity, but it needs to be validated and complemented by additional, stronger evidence.

### 4.3 Indirect evidence of pathogenicity: Functional analysis

Indirect UV evaluation can be also performed by using laboratory tests that can measure the effects of a variant on the activity of the gene product (Couch et al., 2008; Olilla et al., 2008). The rationale for the use of functional assays relies on the fact that the detection of a decrease in activity of a tumour suppressor gene, due to the constitutive presence of a variant in its sequence, likely results in an increased cancer predisposition. Thus, functional assays able to quantify a reduced or altered protein function can be employed to potentially predict the outcome of the UV on protein activity and function.
A powerful assay must be designed according to the functional properties of the encoded protein and hence each single cancer-predisposing gene requires the development of a set of specific tests.
A variety of p16 missense variants were investigated by functional analysis (Kannengiesser et al., 2009; McKenzie et al., 2010; Ruas et al., 1999), since two main p16 functions can be easily measured in vitro: the CDK4/6 binding capacity and the p16 ability to arrest cell-cycle. In particular, the advantage of using cell growth inhibition assays is that they evaluate a phenotype directly involved in tumorigenesis. Other functional tests developed for p16 are discussed in the following paragraph.
Undoubtedly, several unsolved issues on the applicability of functional tests still remain. Firstly, the results obtained by various assays often disclose a relevant discordance, with the same variant showing a different behaviour, depending on the assay used. Approximately, one-half of the variants tested so far in literature possess normal CDK4/6 binding, but fail to trigger cell-cycle arrest. This indicates that a single assay is not sufficient to draw definitive conclusions, and multiple assays must be performed. To this end, a general consensus on the definition of the most suitable panel of assays to be used is still lacking. An additional complication for interpretation of test results relies on the fact that the variants show a continuum of impaired activity, ranging from UVs similar to the wild-type function to UVs with a complete loss-of-function. It is therefore necessary to establish threshold and cut-off values, for eventually distinguishing UVs with wild-type, intermediate or loss-of-function behaviours. Again, a general consensus on the degree of functional loss, which is required to classify a UV as pathogenic, is still missing. Nevertheless, there are no doubts that functional tests can provide significant information about the *in vitro* activity of an UV.

#### 4.3.1 Functional approach for a CDKN2A coding UV

Recently, an exhaustive analysis on a p16 missense variant, as an example on the use of functional methods, was performed by our group (Scaini et al., 2009). The Gly23Asp (G23D) was identified in a family with three melanoma cases, even if only one of the two tested patients was a carrier; the same variant was previously reported in a French and in another Italian melanoma family. The aa protein position 23 falls within the ankyrin consensus sequence and other variants at codon 23 were reported, with different evidence indicating some involvement in melanoma predisposition. Co-segregation of G23D with the disease was observed only in one of these three families, thus rendering this analysis to be not conclusive for the assessment of the variant pathogenicity. The presence of phenocopies, furthermore, might be likely due to the relevant role played by low penetrance genes, acting together with environmental factors within a family. Hence, the application of indirect lines of evidence, namely functional assays measuring key cellular p16 functions, was particularly useful for this variant classification. The protein ability to arrest cell cycle was evaluated by i) proliferation curves, showing the trend of cell growth in time, ii) colony efficiency assays, testing colony formation capacity when cells were seeded at low density, and iii) flow cytometric analysis, indicating a decreased percentage of G1-arrested cells, compared to p16-wild-type ones. Additionally, immunoprecipitation and mammalian two-hybrid binding assays were employed to measure p16 ability to bind CDK4, while pRb phosphorilation was analysed by Western blotting. Furthermore, we confirmed previous evidence that some p16 deleterious variants show an altered cellular localization by immunostaining followed by fluorescence microscopy, forming both cytoplasmic and nuclear aggregates, possibly due to an incorrect folding of the mutant protein during post-translational processing. The results obtained from all these functional tests, summarized in Figure 5, clearly showed an important impairment in G23D function, compared to p16 wild-type. The experimental results were also found to agree with *in silico* predictions, thus supplying sufficient evidence to classify the variant as a "loss-of-function" mutation, which most likely predisposes carriers to melanoma development.

#### 4.3.2 Beyond missense variants: CDKN2A non-coding UVs

Together with missense UVs, germline polymorphisms outside the coding regions of CDKN2A (i.e., promoter, splicing sites, 5'UTR and 3'UTR) were also detected (Hayward, 2000). The first defined pathogenic mutation was the 5'UTR -34G>T transversion, which gives rise to an alternative translation initiating codon with a decreased usage of the wild-type AUG, likely derived from a common founder in the United Kingdom (Liu et al., 1999). Two extensive studies screened more than 1kb of the p16 untranslated and promoter regions in search of mutations in English, Italian, American (Harland et al., 2000) and Australian families (Pollock et al., 2001); polymorphisms at positions -33, -191, -493, and -735, as well as three novel variants at positions -252, -347, and -981 were identified. However, these novel variants did not segregate with disease and were, thus, classified as rare polymorphisms. Rare polymorphisms or variants at the CDKN2A 5'UTR are currently defined as UVs after determining their frequency in control subjects and following co-segregation analysis, when possible. While several functional tests for determining the pathogenicity of missense germline mutations in the coding regions were developed, there are no studies addressing the possible impact of promoter/5'UTR variants on p16 transcription/translation, except for a single publication by an Italian group (Bisio et al., 2010). Reporter assays were developed to study a panel of p16 5'UTR variants, recently identified in a hospital-based series of melanoma cases selected within an ongoing case-control study from an Italian population. Polysomal profiling was also applied as a means to determine the relative impact of the 5'UTR variants on mRNA translation efficiency in heterozygous patient cells. Overall, the results provide tools to assess the functional significance of non-coding 5'UTR mutations and strongly suggest that the -21C>T non-coding variant can be of clinical significance for melanoma predisposition due to its negative impact on the post-transcriptional dynamics of p16 mRNA.

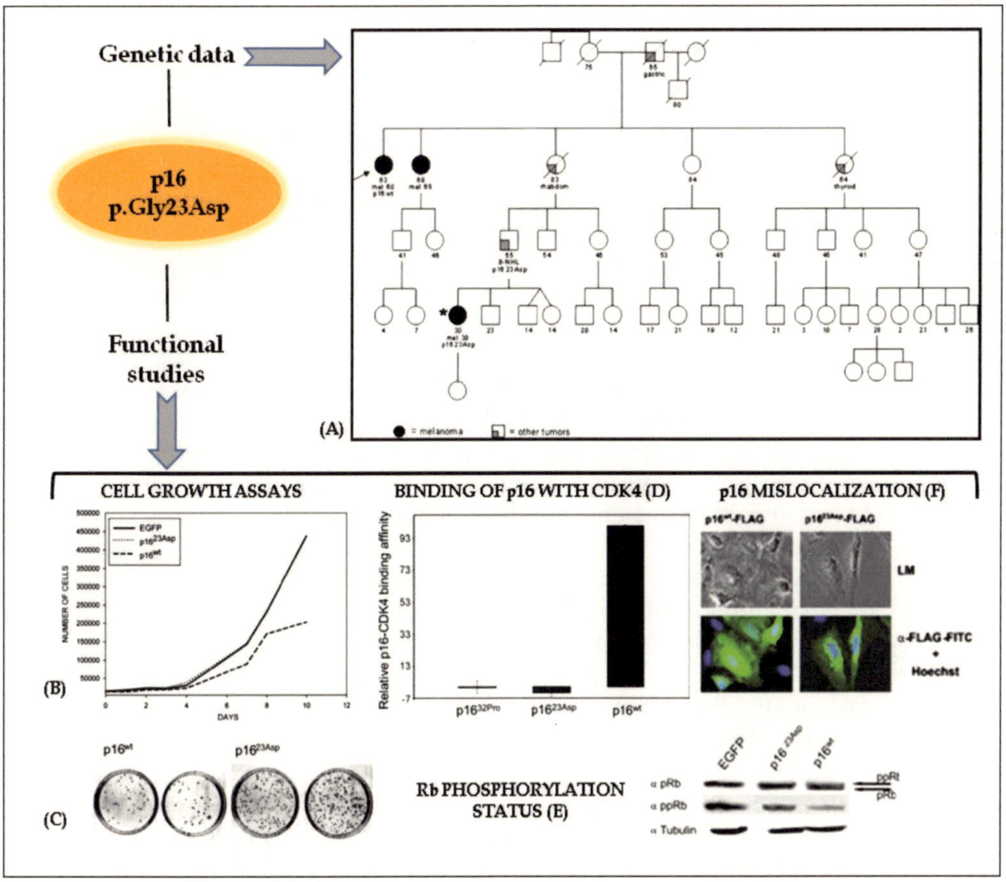


Fig. 5. Functional analysis of the G23D missense variant (Scaini et al., 2009). (A) Pedigree of the Italian family harbouring the variant. Mutational analysis of the first proband (indicated by arrow) was uninformative, while the patient marked with asterisk and her father carried the variant. (B) Proliferation curve and (C) Colony efficiency assays, showing the aberrant cell growth of p16$^{23Asp}$ transfected cells. (D) Impressive reduction in CDK4 binding of the variant, compared to wild-type p16. (E) Analysis of pRb phosphorilation status showed a variant-associated accumulation of hyper-phosphorilated pRb. (F) Mislocalization analysis revealed presence of cytoplasmic and/or nuclear p16$^{23Asp}$ aggregates. All functional tests were performed in U2-OS or NM-39 cell lines.

## 5. Mutational analysis of melanoma-predisposing genes in Italy

As previously discussed, Italy is considered a low melanoma incidence country and Italian melanoma-prone families are generally characterized by a small number of cases (mostly two affected relatives within the same family).

The estimated cumulative risk of developing melanoma over a lifetime in the Italian population is 0.5% (Balzi et al., 1997), unlike in the United States, Australia, and New Zealand, where the risks are 2.0% (Jemal et al., 2008), 3.3% (Holland et al., 1999), and 5.7% (Jones et al., 1999), respectively.

Because of this low melanoma incidence, a familial clustering in a Mediterranean country like Italy is particularly indicative of an inherited predisposition, since it seems very unlikely that such a familial aggregation could be due to chance alone. So, investigations addressing the involvement of this genetic component and the characterization of melanoma-associated gene alterations represent a relevant aspect of familial melanoma research in Italy.

Recently, a comprehensive study, reporting data on CDKN2A/CDK4 mutational analysis, was published (Bruno et al., 2009; see section 3.3). The power of this study relies on some significant characteristics: i) it merges melanoma families and patients recruited by nine different centres spread from Northern to Southern Italy, all enrolled under the same eligibility criteria; ii) it quantifies mutation frequency values on a national scale; iii) it defines how mutation frequencies relates to other familial melanoma features, including the number of affected members in the family, the age at onset, and the presence of multiple melanomas. This study estimated a CDKN2A mutation rate of 33% overall, but single studies on families from different Italian regions reported variable mutation frequencies, with high values (>35%) for Liguria (Ghiorzo et al., 1999; Mantelli et al., 2002) and low values (7.3%) for Emilia Romagna and Marche (Landi et al., 2004). Moreover, the mutation frequency in melanoma families is approximately 17-22% for Lazio and Toscana in Central Italy (Binni et al., 2010; Gensini et al., 2007). Importantly, the frequency was found to be higher in regions with founder mutations (i.e. Liguria and Toscana, as later discussed).

Further data on the genetics of familial melanoma in Italy come from a variety of different studies, heterogeneous in methodology and performed on narrow and localized regions. For this reason, each study adds relative results that need to be merged together for a better description of the mutational spectrum of familial melanoma in Italy.

### 5.1 Italian studies on high penetrance melanoma genes

Different CDKN2A germline mutations have been identified in Italy in the last two decades. As reported worldwide in other mutational studies, missense mutations are the predominant part of CDKN2A alterations and are scattered along its entire coding region. Nonsense mutations, splicing/intronic and regulatory mutations, as well as insertions/deletions, have been described with a much lower prevalence.

#### 5.1.1 Founder mutations

While some mutations were observed only once, others were repeatedly found among families. The most recurrent CDKN2A missense mutation, in Italy and worldwide, is the Gly101Trp (G101W), identified in various families from different countries and particularly prevalent in French and Italian populations. Given its high frequency, the G101W was largely investigated, and its genetic origin was assessed using several families from Italy, France and United States (Ciotti et al., 2000). The haplotype analysis, carried out by means of eight polymorphic markers spanning the CDKN2A locus, revealed no evidence for mutational heterogeneity and suggested that the genotyped families derived from a single ancestral haplotype on which the mutation firstly occurred. The authors finally stated that although it was not possible to unequivocally determine the precise geographic location where the mutation arose and how it spread around the world, it is likely that the mutation originated in South-western Europe. Subsequently, the common genetic origin of the G101W was confirmed by a French study (Auroy et al., 2001). Being a so common mutation, it gained the attention of other researchers and was also functionally characterized.

Interestingly, although the G101W showed some residual binding to CDK4/6 (McKenzie et al., 2010; Parry & Gordon, 1996), it was found to be clearly impaired in the ability to block cell cycle progression (Kannengiesser et al., 2009). These singular results obtained for the G101W emblematically represent the case of a mutation having discordant functional behaviours, on the basis of the particular assay used, as discussed before.

Another frequent founder mutation identified in Italy was the Glu27X (E27X) mutation (Ghiorzo et al., 2006). In particular the E27X, co-segregating with the disease, was found in patients living in, or originally from, a very small area on the North border of Liguria, in North-western Italy. The mutation, located in exon 1α, determines a premature termination codon with a mutant RNA transcript containing only 27 codifying codons, which results in the synthesis of a truncated protein, and possibly in p16 haploinsufficiency. Interestingly, the E27X is the first stop codon CDKN2A founder mutation detected in melanoma families presenting also PC and neuroblastoma, while PC was preferentially reported in association with exon 2 mutations, impairing both p16 and p14.

In a study addressing the frequency and spectrum of CDKN2A/CDK4 mutations in families from central Italy, a third Italian founder mutation, the Gly23Ser (G23S), was detected (Gensini et al., 2007). Again, the haplotype analysis revealed a single common origin for the G23S and several lines of evidence (co-segregation with the disease and case-control studies) suggested its pathogenicity and its involvement in melanoma predisposition.

Taken together, these data show that the major burden of CDKN2A-associated familial melanoma in Italy can be attributed to a limited number of mutations which spread nationwide through founder effects.

#### 5.1.2 Other missense mutations

More than ten years ago, when evidence for CDKN2A involvement in familial melanoma seemed still controversial, a European collaborative work headed by Fargnoli and coll (1998) was performed, to better establish the role of CDKN2A in melanoma predisposition. Four independent missense mutations in exon 1α and exon 2 were detected in four of ten tested families, while no mutations in exon 1β were found. The Gly23Asp (G23D) and the Asn71Ile (N71I) variants, showing co-segregation with the disease, were both located within consensus amino acid residues of the ankyrin repeats, crucially involved in p16 function. The Arg24Pro (R24P) and the Pro114Leu (P114L) were located in exon 1α and exon 2, respectively, and for the former a defective binding with CDK4 was previously reported (Harland et al., 1997).

Another Italian CDKN2A mutational analysis revealed a novel mutation, the Pro48Thr (P48T), showing co-segregation with the disease (Della Torre et al., 2001). The proband carrying the P48T mutation was a woman who developed 4 primary melanomas before age 56; moreover, she belonged to a large family, presenting single and multiple melanomas, oral and colon cancers, bone tumours and other additional cancer types. In the same study the P48T was functionally characterized and it was indistinguishable from wild-type p16 in its ability to interact with CDK4/6, but it had a reduced capacity to inhibit cell growth with a defect in G1/S arrest clearly detectable by flow cytometry.

Another study investigating the relations between CDKN2A mutations and single/multiple primary melanomas in North-western Italy, reported additional missense mutations detected for the first time in an Italian population and the novel Thr77Ala (T77A), never described before (Pastorino et al., 2008).

CDKN2A mutations were also analyzed in 55 families mainly from Emilia Romagna and Marche, in North-central Italy (Landi et al., 2004). A novel mutation, the Leu65Pro (L65P), was identified. Structural considerations on p16 tertiary structures suggested that the variant could disrupt secondary structures, possibly resulting in a small spatial distortion. The PolyPhen calculations failed to predict an impact of the mutation on protein function. Therefore, a yeast two hybrid system was employed and a decrease of about 50% in the binding of L65P to CDK4, compared to the wild-type p16 was observed. Being the leucine at position 65 not conserved across species and considering that molecular modelling suggested only a little effect on this amino acid substitution on protein structure, the modest reduction in CDK4 binding of L65P is very reasonable.

Obviously, not every CDKN2A missense variant necessarily predisposes to melanoma or exerts a pathogenic effect on protein function. In this regard, it was suggested that the Ala148Thr (A148T) variant, located in the fourth ankyrin repeat domain of p16, could be a low penetrance melanoma predisposing allele in a Polish population. To determine the role of the A148T on melanoma risk, this allele was genotyped in French and Italian population (Spica et al., 2006). Although discordant data were previously reported in different series of melanoma patients, the study showed no association of the A148T and melanoma risk.

Other CDKN2A missense mutations have been identified in Italy, although at low frequencies and are reported in Figure 6.

### 5.1.3 Mutations in p14

Mutations in p14 are less frequent compared to those involving p16, also in Italy. While mutations laying in exon 1β specifically target p14 only, mutations occurring in the shared exon 2 of CDKN2A can potentially affect both p16 and p14, as exemplified by the case of the Asn71Ile (N71I) missense mutation, already discussed (Fargnoli et al., 1998). The N71I is originated by the 212 A>T nucleotide substitution in exon 2, that converts an asparagine to an isoleucine, within the p16 reading frame. The A>T base change also modifies the coding region of the p14 transcript, causing the substitution of a gluthamine with a histidine.

In a case-case study matching amelanotic and pigmented melanoma, the p14 g.193+1 G>A germline mutation was detected for the first time in Italy, in a family with five melanoma cases and a neural system tumour (Ghiorzo et al., 2009). The g.193+1 G>A was previously described to occur in a mutation hotspot at the p14ARF splice site and to be associated with aberrant splicing (Harland et al., 2005). By a research group operating in Central Italy, and studying 155 either familial or sporadic multiple primary melanoma cases, p14 mutations were identified in three unrelated melanoma pedigrees, and no mutations were found in sporadic patients (Binni et al., 2010). Two of these families harboured the g.193 + 1 G>A mutation, while the third family was positive for the g.161 G>A variant, that resulted in the p.Arg54His (R54H) amino acid change. The R54H clearly showed co-segregation with the disease and was classified as deleterious by *in silico* analysis, since the substituted residue is highly conserved among species.

CDKN2A missense mutations detected in Italian melanoma-prone families are listed with their main features in Table 1.

### 5.1.4 CDKN2A rearrangements analysis

Given that point mutations have a relatively low frequency in familial melanoma, it is possible that other types of CDKN2A alterations, not detectable by routine PCR-based methods, might be involved in a fraction of melanoma cases.

To assess the role of CDKN2A large, quantitative alterations in the Italian population, 124 melanoma families without detectable CDKN2A or CDK4 point mutations were screened by *M*ultiplex *L*igation-dependent *P*robe *A*mplification (MLPA) and real-time quantitative PCR (Vignoli et al., 2008). This study, involving different Italian centres, reported that no gross rearrangements in the CDKN2A coding regions and in the p16-specific promoter were present. In five samples a 6 bp deletion was found in proximity of the promoter region of exon 1β, but further investigations likely indicated it as a low frequency polymorphism, not implicated in disease predisposition.

Similar results were obtained by Binni et al. (2010) on additional melanoma kindreds, thus confirming that CDKN2A rearrangements are an infrequent mechanism for melanoma predisposition in Italy, in agreement with data described in other European countries, reporting that only 2.1% of mutation carriers harboured large CDKN2A rearrangements (Lesueur et al., 2008).

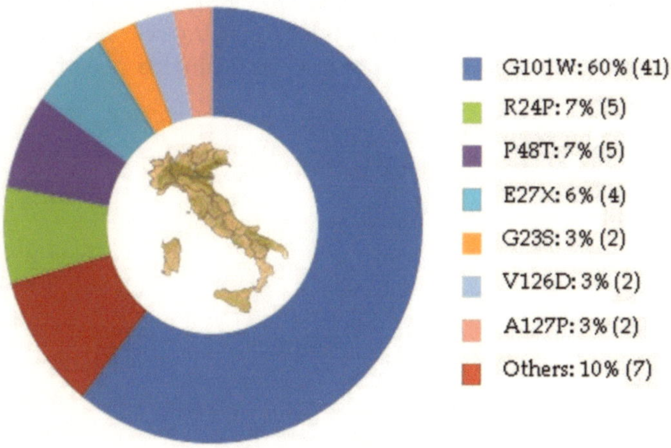


Fig. 6. CDKN2A missense mutation pattern in 208 Italian melanoma families.

An overall mutation frequency of 33% was determined. The frequency at which the single mutations occurred in positive-families is shown, with the number of carrier families in brackets (data extracted from Bruno et al., 2009).

### 5.1.5 CDK4 mutations

As mentioned before, CKD4 mutations are extremely rare: a CDK4 missense mutation in exon 7, converting the arginine 240 in glutamine (Arg240Gln), was identified (Landi et al., 2004). The mutation was found in the proband and also in two unaffected relatives. Furthermore, in a molecular analysis on subjects with familial and/or multiple primary melanoma, the Arg24His was detected in a family, presenting several melanoma cases (Majore et al., 2008).

## 5.2 Contribution of low penetrance genes and/or other risk factors to melanoma susceptibility in Italy

As already mentioned, a familial aggregation in a Mediterranean country like Italy is suggestive of an inherited predisposition (Calista et al., 2000). Moreover, melanoma in a population with a wide range of pigmentary phenotypes, small sized nevi, and intense sun exposure may reveal susceptibility pathways specific for this population. Since no evidence of linkage to other loci for melanoma susceptibility in Italian CDKN2A-negative families was reported (Kerstann et al., 2008; Landi et al., 2004), it is likely that, in some Italian regions, clustering of cutaneous malignant melanoma cases might also be the result of a combination of multiple low penetrance alleles and/or shared sun exposure habits. The MC1R gene is a major determinant of skin phototype and pigmentary characteristics, such as skin, hair and eye colour, that together with exposure to environmental ultraviolet radiation, are the main modulators of individual melanoma risk. Pigmentation and, consequently, sun sensitivity are polygenic traits and several variant alleles have been identified in different regulatory genes (Duffy et al., 2010; Fernandez et al., 2009). Up to now, a national Italian work summarizing the impact of these genes and environmental/physiological factors on melanoma risk is still lacking, while a puzzle of information coming from several Italian regions is mounting, giving only a partial description of the various contributing factors. On the other hand, despite lacking a view of the whole Italian situation, several authors suggest that this might be the right way forward for a correct estimate of low penetrance gene effects, since mutation frequency for any candidate cancer gene needs to be evaluated in each specific geographical area (Casula et al., 2007).

| Exon | DNA change | p16INK4A change | p14ARF change | References |
|---|---|---|---|---|
| 1α | c.68G>A | p.Gly23Asp | / | Fargnoli et al., 1998; Scaini et al., 2009 |
| 1α | c.67G>A | p.Gly23Ser | / | Gensini et al., 2007 |
| 1α | c.71G>C | p.Arg24Pro | / | Harland et al., 1997; Fargnoli et al., 1998 |
| 1α | c.79G>T | p.Glu27X | / | Ghiorzo et al., 2006 |
| 1α | c.142C>A | p.Pro48Thr | / | Della Torre et al., 2001 |
| 1β | g.161G>A | / | p.Arg54His | Binni et al., 2010 |
| 2 | c.172C>T | p.Arg58X | p.Pro72Leu | Bruno et al., 2009 |
| 2 | c.194T>C | p.Leu65Pro | p.= (Ala79) | Landi et al., 2004 |
| 2 | c.202_203GC>TT | p.Ala68Leu | p.Arg82Leu | Bruno et al., 2009 |
| 2 | c.212A>T | p.Asn71Ile | p.Gln85His | Fargnoli et al., 1998 |
| 2 | c.229A > G | p.Thr77Ala | p.His91Arg | Pastorino et al., 2008 |
| 2 | N.A. | p.Ala86Thr | N.A. | Bruno et al., 2009 |
| 2 | c.281T>C | p.Leu94Pro | p.= (Ala108) | Bruno et al., 2009 |
| 2 | c.301G>T | p.Gly101Trp | p.Arg115Leu | Ghiorzo et al., 1999 |
| 2 | c.341C>T | p.Pro114Leu | p.= (Ala128) | Fargnoli et al., 1998 |
| 2 | c.377T>A | p.Val126Asp | / | Bruno et al., 2009 |
| 2 | c.379G>C | p.Ala127Pro | / | Bruno et al., 2009 |

Table 1. Pathogenic CDKN2A missense mutations in Italy (N.A.: *N*ot *A*vailable in literature).

### 5.2.1 North-western Italy

The purpose of a recent study (Pastorino et al., 2008) was the analysis of the contribution of CDKN2A mutations and MC1R variants to the development of *M*ultiple *P*rimary *M*elanoma (MPM) versus *S*ingle *P*rimary *M*elanoma (SPM) in the population of two different towns of North-western Italy. As for MC1R, which is the topic of the present paragraph, thirty different non-synonymous variants were found with an overall allele frequency of 56.32% in MPM patients and 44.85% in SPM patients. In both MPM and SPM patients, V60L and R151C were the most frequently detected variants. Five novel variants (R67W, L100P, D184G, I221T and 1339 + 5 C >T) and two other novel variants (A149T and V156A) were detected in the MPM and in the SPM cases, respectively. No association was observed between the presence of MC1R variants and age at diagnosis. Compared to the SPM patients, MPM cases had a 2-fold increased likelihood of being MC1R variant carriers and a higher probability of carrying two or more variants, as reported by Kanetsky et al. (2006) in their large multicenter population-based study.

Finally, the analysis showed no specific association between the variant type and the number of CMs (one, two or more). This finding suggested that the presence of at least one MC1R variant, regardless of whether it is a R or a r variant, may influence the probability of developing two or more CMs, independently of the CDKN2A mutation status. This consideration was supported also by the results on the association between phenotypic characteristics and prevalence and type of MC1R variants: unexpectedly, the r rather than the R variants were associated with light eyes and hair. Fair skin was significantly associated with both r and R variants. At the very end, the results on MC1R variants in SPM/MPM patients suggest that, in this population, the number rather than the type of MC1R variants increases the risk of developing MPM.

### 5.2.2 North-eastern Italy

A case-control study including 183 incident cases of any stage and 179 controls was conducted in North-eastern Italy to identify important risk factors and determine how their combinations affected risk in a Mediterranean population (Landi et al., 2001). Presence of dysplastic nevi, low propensity to tan, light eye, and light skin colour were significantly associated with melanoma risk after adjustment for age, gender and pigmentation characteristics, showing the need of preventive advice against melanoma in these populations. According to the combination of these factors, a relative risk range from 1 to 98.5 was found. Moreover, light skin colour, high number of sunburns with blistering, and low propensity to tan were significantly associated with melanoma thickness, possibly indicating that individuals with these characteristics underestimate their risk and seek attention when their lesion is already advanced.

### 5.2.3 Central Italy

A work by Fargnoli and coll. (2006) investigated the contribution of the MC1R genotype to the risk of sporadic cutaneous melanoma in a population of Central Italy composed by 100 patients with sporadic cutaneous melanoma of any stage and 100 unrelated controls. All high-penetrance R variants of MC1R combined conferred a 2.5-fold increased risk of melanoma, and a significant increase in melanoma risk associated with high-penetrance R variants was observed mainly in the presence of clinically atypical nevi, more than 50 melanocytic nevi and prolonged UV exposure habits. Consistent with other studies, the R151C allele was significantly associated with melanoma risk, conferring a 2.9-fold higher risk. Interestingly, D294H was detected only in melanoma patients, and not in controls, although a larger sample size would be required to achieve statistical significance. Finally, the data confirmed the role of high penetrance R variants in the genetic predisposition to sporadic melanoma in an Italian population.

### 5.2.4 Southern Italy

Oncogenic BRAF signalling was demonstrated to interfere with the CDKN2A activity. A sustained expression of the mutated BRAF protein induces p16 expression and cell cycle arrest, indicating that both BRAF and CDKN2A pathways are functionally associated (Michaloglou et al., 2005). Finally, inherited mutations of the BRCA2 gene give rise to a multi-site cancer phenotype which includes ocular and cutaneous melanomas in addition to the main predisposition to breast (in females and males) and ovarian cancers. The work of Casula and coll. (2007) tried to assess the likelihood of identifying CDKN2A mutations in patients, belonging to Southern Italy or Sardinia, with histologically-proven diagnosis of melanoma, included regardless of age at diagnosis, family history status, and disease features.

The authors made also a final comparison between prevalence of CDKN2A germline mutations within different Italian regions, pooling together data coming from different publications: in contrast to a higher frequency of CDKN2A germline mutations observed in non-familial cases from Northern Italy, their findings among the same type of patients from Southern Italy strongly suggest that the discrepancy in CDKN2A mutation frequency may be due to patient origin and/or to the different 'genetic background' of the population.

Molecular analysis was also performed in order to identify any correlation between genetic alterations and phenotypic parameters: CDKN2A mutations were more frequent in patients with familial history of melanoma compared to patients without. Moreover, age at diagnosis was significantly correlated with the presence of a CDKN2A mutation: the mean age of onset was significantly lower in carriers of mutations compared to non-carriers.

To evaluate whether additional candidate genes might be involved in melanoma susceptibility, prevalence of germline mutations in BRAF and BRCA2 genes (the other two major genes related to melanoma pathogenesis) was assessed in subsets of patients originating from different geographical areas within Southern Italy.

Germline mutations in BRAF and BRCA2 genes were found in Sardinian patients only (altogether, 3/116; 2.6%), with no additional alterations in the remaining cases from Southern Italy. These findings strongly confirmed that mutation frequency for any candidate cancer gene needs to be evaluated in each geographical area.

## 6. Conclusions

Familial melanoma has proven to be a disease with a heterogeneous etiology, associated with mutations in susceptibility genes. Several high and moderate/low risk genes have now been identified. CDKN2A remains the most important high risk gene in melanoma development; other predisposition genes comprise CDK4, MC1R, and a variety of risk modifier genes including MTAP, EGF, GST, MDM2 and many others. There is a great interest in the identification of high risk individuals harbouring melanoma-associated gene mutations to offer clinical screening and follow up, since early detection and diagnosis are the most significant tools in improving melanoma prognosis and outcome. Undoubtedly, the identification of new predisposition loci, together with further investigations on gene-gene and gene-environment interactions will shed light on molecular mechanisms involved in melanocyte transformation. Of course, the real challenge of melanoma research relies in converting the growing body of information on the disease into effective strategies to implement melanoma prevention and treatment in the near future.

## 7. Acknowledgements

Research work from our laboratory was supported by Ministero della Salute: Programma Integrato Oncologia N.5, Alleanza contro il Cancro (N.ACC2/R6.9), Lega Italiana per la Lotta contro i Tumori (LILT), Associazione Italiana per la Ricerca sul Cancro (AIRC), Fondazione Cassa di Risparmio di Padova e Rovigo and "Piccoli Punti" Charity. LE and MCS are fellows from FSE (*E*uropean *S*ocial *F*und) and University of Padua, respectively.

## 8. References

Armstrong, BK. & Kricker, A. (1994). Cutaneous melanoma. *Cancer Surveys: Trends Cancer Incidence,* 19, 219-239

Auroy, S.; Avril, MF.; Chompret, A.; Pham, D.; Goldstein, AM.; Bianchi Scarrà, G.; Frebourg, T.; Joly, P.; Spatz, A.; Rubino, C.; Demenais, F. & Bressac-de-Paillerets, B. (2001). Sporadic multiple primary melanoma cases: *CDKN2A* germline mutations with a founder effect. *Genes, Chromosome & Cancer,* 32, 195-202

Autier, P.; Dore, JF.; Gefeller, O.; Cesarini, JP.; Lejeune, F.; Koelmel, KF.; Lienard, D. & Kleeberg, UR. (1997). Melanoma risk and residence in sunny areas. EORTC Melanoma Co-operative Group. European Organization for Research and Treatment of Cancer. *British Journal of Cancer,* 76, 1521-1524

Balzi, D.; Bidoli, E.; Franceschini, S.; Pisani, P. & Geddes, M. (1997). Estimates of cancer incidence and mortality in Italian regions. Aviano, Italia: Centro di Riferimento Oncologico di Aviano, 48-49

Barroso, E.; Fernandez, LP.; Milne, RL.; Pita, G.; Sendagorta, E.; Floristan, U.; Feito, M.; Aviles, JA.; Martin-Gonzalez, M.; Arias, JI.; Zamora, P.; Blanco, M.; Lazaro, P.; Benitez, J.; & Ribas, G. (2008). Genetic analysis of the vitamin D receptor gene in two epithelial cancers: melanoma and breast cancer case-control studies. *BioMed Central Cancer,* 8, 385-392

Bataille, V.; Grulich, A.; Sasieni, P.; Swerdlow, A.; Newton-Bishop, J.; McCarthy, W.; Hersey, P. & Cuzick, J. (1998). The association between naevi and melanoma in populations with different levels of sun exposure: a joint case-control study of melanoma in the UK and Australia. *British Journal of Cancer,* 77, 505-510

Bates, S.; Phillips, AC.; Clarke, PA.; Stott, F.; Peters, G.; Ludwig, RL. & Vousden, KH. (1998). p14ARF links the tumour suppressors RB and p53. *Nature,* 395, 124–125

Beaumont, KA.; Shekar, SN.; Newton, RA.; James, MR.; Stow, JL.; Duffy, DL. & Sturm, RA. (2007). Receptor function, dominant negative activity and phenotype correlations for MC1R variant alleles. *Human Molecular Genetics,* 16, 2249-2260

Bennett, DC. (1993). Genetics, development and malignancy of melanocytes. *International Review of Cytology*, 146, 191-260

Berwick, M.; Orlow, I.; Hummer, AJ.; Armstrong, BK.; Kricker, A.; Marrett, LD.; Millikan, RC.; Gruber, SB.; Anton-Culver, H.; Zanetti, R.; Gallagher, RP.; Dwyer, T.; Rebbeck, TR.; Kanetsky, PA.; Busam, K.; From, L.; Mujumdar, U.; Wilcox, H. & Begg, CB. (2006). The Prevalence of CDKN2A Germ-Line Mutations and Relative Risk for Cutaneous Malignant Melanoma: An International Population-Based Study. *Cancer Epidemiology, Biomarkers & Prevention*, 15, 1519-1525

Bishop, DT.; Demenais, F.; Goldstein, AM.; Bergman, W.; Newton Bishop, J.; Bressac-de-Paillerets, B.; Chompret, A.; Ghiorzo, P.; Gruis, N.; Hansson, J.; Harland, M.; Hayward, N.; Holland, EA.; Mann, GJ.; Mantelli, M.; Nancarrow, D.; Platz, A. & Tucker, MA. (2002). Geographical Variation in the Penetrance of CDKN2A Mutations for Melanoma. *Journal of the National Cancer Institute*, 94, 894-903

Bishop, DT.; Demenais, F.; Iles, MM.; Harland, M.; Taylor, JC.; Corda, E.; Randerson-Moor, J.; Aitken, JF.; Avril, MF.; Azizi, E.; Bakker, E.; Bianchi-Scarrà, G.; Bressac-de-Paillerets, B.; Calista, D.; Cannon-Albright, LA.; Chin-A-Woeng, T.; Dębniak, T.; Galore-Haskel, G.; Ghiorzo, P.; Gut, I.; Hansson, J.; Hočevar, M.; Höiom, V.; Hopper, JL.; Ingvar, C.; Kanetsky, PA.; Kefford, RF.; Landi, MT.; Lang, J.; Lubiński, J.; Mackie, R.; Malvehy, J.; Mann, GJ.; Martin, NG.; Montgomery, NG.; Van Nieuwpoort, FA.; Novakovic, S.; Olsson, H.; Puig S.; Weiss, M.; Van Workum, W.; Zelenika, D.; Brown, KM.; Goldstein, AM.; Gillanders, EM.; Boland, A.; Galan, P.; Elder, DE.; Gruis, NA.; Hayward, NK.; Lathrop, GM.; Barrett, JH. & Newton Bishop, JA. (2009). Genome-wide association study identifies three loci associated with melanoma risk. *Nature Genetics*, 41, 920-925

Binni, F.; Antigoni, I.; De Simone, P.; Majore, S.; Silipo, V.; Crisi, A.; Amantea, A.; Pacchiarini, D.; Castori, M.; De Bernardo, C.; Catricalà, C. & Grammatico, P. (2010). Novel and recurrent $p14^{ARF}$ mutations in Italian familial melanoma. *Clinical Genetics*, 77, 581-586

Bisio, A.; Nasti, S.; Jordan, JJ.; Gargiulo, S.; Pastorino, L.; Provenzani, A.; Quattrone, A.; Queirolo, P.; Bianchi-Scarrà, G.; Ghiorzo, P. & Inga, A. (2010). Functional analysis of CDKN2A/p16INK4a 5′-UTR variants predisposing to melanoma. *Human Molecular Genetics*, 19, 1479-1491

Boi, S.; Cristofolini, M.; Micciolo, R.; Polla, E. & Dalla Palma, P. (2003). Epidemiology of skin tumors: data from the cutaneous cancer registry in Trentino, Italy. *Journal of Cutaneous Medicine and Surgery*, 7, 300-305

Box, NF.; Duffy, DL.; Chen, W.; Stark, M.; Martin, NG.; Sturm, RA.; & Hayward, NK. (2001). MC1R genotype modifies risk of melanoma in families segregating CDKN2A mutations. *American Journal of Human Genetics*, 69, 765-773

Bruno, W.; Ghiorzo, P.; Battistuzzi, L.; Ascierto, PA.; Barile, M.; Gargiulo, S.; Gensini, F.; Gliori, S.; Guida, M.; Lombardo, M.; Manoukian, S.; Menin, C.; Nasti, S.; Origone, P.; Pasini, B.; Pastorino, L.; Peissel, B.; Pizzichetta MA.; Queirolo, P.; Rodolfo, M.; Romanini, A.; Scaini, MC.; Testori, A.; Tibiletti, MG.; Turchetti, D.; Leachman, SA. & Bianchi-Scarrà, G. (2009). Clinical genetic testing for familial melanoma in Italy: A cooperative study. *Journal of the American Academy of Dermatology*, 61, 775-782

Calista, D.; Goldstein, AM. & Landi, MT. (2000). Familial melanoma aggregation in north-eastern Italy. *Journal of Investigative Dermatology,* 115, 764-765

Campisi, J. (1997). The biology of replicative senescence. *European Journal of Cancer,* 33, 703-709

Capasso, M.; Ayala, F.; Avvisati, RA.; Russo, R.; Gambale, A.; Mozzillo, N.; Ascierto, PA. & Iolascon, A. (2010). MDM2 SNP309 and p53 Arg72Pro in cutaneous melanoma: association between SNP309 GG genotype and tumor Breslow thickness. *Journal of Human Genetics,* 55, 518-524

Caporaso, NE. (2002). Why have we failed to find the low penetrance genetic constituents of common cancers? *Cancer Epidemiology, Biomarkers & Prevention,* 11, 1544-1549

Casula, M.; Colombino, M.; Satta, MP.; Cossu, A.; Lissia. A.; Budroni, M.; Simeone, E.; Calemma, R.; Loddo, C.; Caracò, C.; Mozzillo. N.; Daponte, A.; Comella, G.; Canzanella, S.; Guida, M.; Castello, G.; Ascierto, PA. & Palmieri, G. (2007). Factors predicting the occurrence of germline mutations in candidate genes among patients with cutaneous malignant melanoma from South Italy. *European Journal of Cancer,* 43, 137-143

Chan, PA.; Duraisamy, S.; Miller, PJ.; Newell, JA.; McBride, C.; Bond,JP.; Raevaara, T.; Ollila, S.; Nyström, M.; Grimm, AJ.; Christodoulou, J.; Oetting, WS. & Greenblatt, MS. (2007). Interpreting Missense Variants: Comparing Computational Methods in Human Disease Genes CDKN2A, MLH1, MSH2, MECP2, and Tyrosinase (TYR). *Human Mutation,* 28, 683-693

Chin, L. (2003). The genetics of malignant melanoma: lessons from mouse and man. *Nature Reviews,* 3, 559-570

Ciotti, P.; Struewing, JP.; Mantelli, M:, Chompret, A.; Avril, MF.; Santi, PL.; Tucker, MA.; Bianchi-Scarrà, G.; Bressac-de-Paillerets, B. & Goldstein, AM. (2000). A single genetic origin for the G101W mutation in 20 melanoma-prone families. *American Journal of Human Genetics,* 67, 311-319

Couch, FJ.; Rasmussen, LJ.; Hofstra, R.; Monteiro, ANA.; Greenblatt, MS. & de Wind, N. (2008). Assessment of Functional Effects of Unclassified Genetic Variants. *Human Mutation,* 29, 1314–1326

Della Torre, G.; Pasini, B.; Frigerio, S.; Donghi, R.; Rovini, D.; Delia, D.; Peters, G.; Huot, TJG.; Bianchi Scarrà, G.; Lantieri, F.; Rodolfo, M.; Parmiani, G. & Pierotti, MA. (2001). *CDKN2A* and *CDK4* mutation analysis in Italian melanoma-prone families: functional characterization of a novel *CDKN2A* germ line mutation. *British Journal of Cancer,* 85, 836-844

Demenais, F.; Mohamdi, H.; Chaudru, V.; Goldstein, AM.; Newton Bishop, JA.; Bishop, DT.; Kanetsky, PA.; Hayward, NK.; Gillanders, E.; Elder, DE.; Avril, MF.; Azizi, E.; van Belle, P.; Bergman, W.; Bianchi-Scarrà, G.; Bressac-de-Paillerets, B.; Calista, D.; Carrera, C.; Hansson, J.; Harland, M.; Hogg, D.; Höiom, V.; Holland, EA.; Ingvar, C.; Landi, MT.; Lang, JM.; Mackie, RM.; Mann, GJ.; Ming, ME.; Njauw, CJ.; Olsson, H.; Palmer, J.; Pastorino, L.; Puig, S.; Randerson-Moor, J.; Stark, M.; Tsao, H.; Tucker, MA.; van der Velden, P.; Yang, XR. & Gruis, N. (2010). Association of MC1R Variants and Host Phenotypes With Melanoma Risk in CDKN2A Mutation Carriers: a GenoMEL Study. *Journal of the National Cancer Institute,* 102, 1568-1583

Dennis, LK. (1999). Analysis of the melanoma epidemic, both apparent and real: data from 1973 through 1994 surveillance, epidemiology and end results program registry. *Archives of Dermatology*, 135, 275-280

Duffy, DL.; Zhao, ZZ.; Sturm, RA.; Hayward, NK.; Martin, NG. & Montgomery, GW. (2010). Multiple pigmentation gene polymorphisms account for a substantial proportion of risk of cutaneous malignant melanoma. *Journal of Investigative Dermatology*, 130, 520-528

Eymin, B.; Leduc, C.; Coll, JL.; Brambilla, E. & Gazzeri, S. (2003). p14ARF induces G2 arrest and apoptosis independently of p53 leading to regression of tumours established in nude mice. *Oncogene*, 22, 1822–1835

Falchi, M.; Bataille, V.; Hayward, NK.; Duffy, DL.; Newton Bishop, JA.; Pastinen, T.; Cervino, A.; Zhao, ZZ.; Deloukas, P.; Soranzo, N.; Elder, DE.; Barrett, JH.; Martin, NG.; Bishop, DT.; Montgomery, GW. & Spector, TD. (2009). Genome-wide association study identifies variants at 9p21 and 22q13 associated with development of cutaneous nevi. *Nature Genetics*, 41, 915-921

Fargnoli, MC.; Chimenti, S.; Keller, G.; Soyer, HP.; Dal Pozzo, V.; Höfler, H. & Peris, K. (1998). CDKN2a/p16INK4a mutations and lack of p19$^{ARF}$ involvment in familial melanoma kindreds. *Journal of Investigative Dermatology*, 111, 1202-1206

Fargnoli, MC.; Altobelli, E.; Keller, G.; Chimenti, S.; Hofler, H. & Peris, K. (2006). Contribution of melanocortin-1 receptor gene variants to sporadic cutaneous melanoma risk in a population in central Italy: a case-control study. *Melanoma Research*, 16, 175-182

Fargnoli, MC.; Gandini, S.; Peris, K.; Maisonneuve, P. & Raimondi, S. (2010). MC1R variants increase melanoma risk in families with CDKN2A mutations: a meta-analysis. *European Journal of Cancer*, 46, 1413-1420

Fernandez, LP.; Milne, RL.; Pita, G.; Floristan, U.; Sendagorta, E.; Feito, M.; Aviles, JA.; Martin-Gonzalez, M.; Lazaro, P.; Benitez, J. & Ribas, G. (2009). Pigmentation-related genes and their implication in malignant melanoma susceptibility. *Experimental Dermatology*, 18, 634-642

Ferrer-Costa, C.; Gelpi, JL.; Zamakola, L.; Parraga, I.; de la Cruz, X. & Orozco, M. (2005). PMUT: a web-based tool for the annotation of pathological mutations on proteins. *Bioinformatics*, 21, 3176-3178

Fortes, C.; Mastroeni, S.; Melchi, F.; Pilla, MA.; Antonelli, G.; Camaioni, D.; Alotto, M. & Pasquini, P. (2008). A protective effect of the Mediterranean diet for cutaneous melanoma. *International Journal of Epidemiology*, 37, 1018-1029

Gandini, S.; Sera, F.; Cattaruzza, MS.; Pasquini, P.; Picconi, O.; Boyle, P. & Melchi, CF. (2005a). Meta-analysis of risk factors for cutaneous melanoma: II. Sun exposure. *European Journal of Cancer*, 41, 45-60

Gandini, S.; Sera, F.; Cattaruzza, MS.; Pasquini, P.; Zanetti, R.; Masini, C.; Boyle, P. & Melchi, CF. (2005b). Meta-analysis of risk factors for cutaneous melanoma: III. Family history, actinic damage and phenotypic factors. *European Journal of Cancer*, 41, 2040-2059

Garcia-Borron, JC.; Sanchez-Laorden, BL. & Jimenez-Cervantes, C. (2005). Melanocortin-1 receptor structure and functional regulation. *Pigment Cell & Melanoma Research*, 18, 393–410

Gensini, F.; Sestini, R.; Piazzini, M.; Vignoli, M.; Chiarugi, A.; Brandani, P.; Ghiorzo, P.; Salvini, C.; Borgognoni, L.; Palli, D.; Bianchi Scarrà, G.; Carli, P. & Genuardi, M. (2007). The p.G23S CDKN2A founder mutation in high-risk melanoma families from Central Italy. *Melanoma Research*, 17, 387-392

Ghiorzo, P.; Ciotti, P.; Mantelli, M.; Heouaine, A.; Queirolo, P.; Rainero, ML.; Ferrari, C.; Santi, PL.; De Marchi, R.; Farris, A.; Ajmar, F.; Bruzzi, P. & Bianchi Scarrà, G. (1999). Characterization of ligurian melanoma families and risk of occurrence of other neoplasia. *International Journal of Cancer*, 83, 441-448

Ghiorzo, P.; Gargiulo, S.; Pastorino, L.; Nasti, S.; Cusano, R.; Bruno, W.; Gliori, S.; Sertoli, MR.; Burroni, A.; Savarino, V.; Gensini, F.; Sestini, R.; Queirolo, P.; Goldstein, AM. & Bianchi Scarrà, G. (2006). Impact of E27X, a novel CDKN2A germline mutation, on p16 and p14ARF expression in Italian melanoma families displaying pancreatic cancer and neuroblastoma. *Human Molecular Genetics*, 15, 2682-2689

Ghiorzo, P.; Pastorino, L.; Pizzichetta, MA.; Bono, R.; Queirolo, P.; Talamini, R.; Annessi, G.; Bruno, W.; Nasti, S.; Gargiulo, S.; Battistuzzi, L.; Sini, MC.; Palmieri, G. & Bianchi Scarrà, G. (2009). CDKN2A and MC1R analysis in amelanotic and pigmented melanoma. *Melanoma Research*, 19, 142-145

Gil, J. & Peters, G. (2006). Regulation of the *INK4b-ARF-INK4a* tumour suppressor locus: all for one or one for all. *Molecular and Cellular Biology*, 7, 667-677

Goldgar, DE.; Easton, DF.; Deffenbaugh, AM.; Monteiro, AN.; Tavtigian, SV. & Couch, FJ. (2004). Integrated Evaluation of DNA Sequence Variants of Unknown Clinical Significance: Application to *BRCA1* and *BRCA2*. *American Journal of Human Genetics*, 75, 535–544

Goldgar, DE.; Easton, DF.; Byrnes, GB.; Spurdle, AB.; Iversen, ES. & Greenblatt, MS. (2008). Genetic Evidence and Integration of Various Data Sources for Classifying Uncertain Variants Into a Single Model. *Human Mutation*, 29, 1265-1272

Goldstein, AM.; Fraser, MC.; Struewing, JP.; Hussussian, CJ.; Ranade, K.; Zametkin, DP.; Fontaine, LS.; Organic, SM.; Dracopoli, NC.; Clark, WH. Jr. & Tucker, MA. (1995). Increased risk of pancreatic cancer in melanoma-prone kindreds with p16INK4 mutations. *New England Journal of Medicine*, 333, 970–974

Goldstein, AM. (2004). Familial Melanoma, Pancreatic Cancer and Germline CDKN2A Mutations. *Human Mutation* 23, 630-641

Goldstein, AM.; Struewing, JP.; Fraser, MC.; Smith, MW. & Tucker, MA. (2004). Prospective Risk of Cancer in CDKN2A Germline Mutation Carriers. *Journal of Medical Genetics*, 41, 421-424

Goldstein, AM.; Landi, MT.; Tsang, S.; Fraser, MC.; Munroe, DJ. & Tucker, MA. (2005). Association of MC1R variants and risk of melanoma in melanoma-prone families with CDKN2A mutations. *Cancer Epidemiology, Biomarkers & Prevention*, 14, 2208-2212

Goldstein, AM.; Chan, M.; Harland, M.; Gillanders, EM.; Hayward, NK.; Avril, MF.; Azizi, E.; Bianchi-Scarrà, G.; Bishop, DT.; Bressac-de-Paillerets, B.; Bruno, W.; Calista, D.; Cannon Albright, LA.; Demenais, F.; Elder, DE.; Ghiorzo, P.; Gruis, NA.; Hansson, J.; Hogg, D.; Holland, EA.; Kanetsky, PA.; Kefford, RF.; Landi, MT.; Lang, J.; Leachman, SA.; Mackie, RM.; Magnusson, V.; Mann, GJ.; Niendorf, K.; Newton Bishop, JA.; Palmer, JM.; Puig, S.; Puig-Butille, JA.; de Snoo, FA.; Stark,

M.; Tsao, H.; Tucker, MA.; Whitaker, L. & Yakobson, E. (2006). High-Risk Melanoma Susceptibility Genes and Pancreatic Cancer, Neural System Tumors, and Uveal Melanoma Across GenoMEL. *Cancer Research*, 66, 9818-9828

Goldstein, AM.; Chaudru, V.; Ghiorzo, P.; Badenas, C.; Malvehy, J.; Pastorino, L.; Laud, K.; Hulley, B.: Avril, MF. Puig-Butille, JA.; Miniere, A.; Marti, R,; Chompret, A.; Cuellar, F.; Kolm, I.; Mila, M.; Tucker, MA.; Demenais, F.; Bianchi-Scarrà, G.; Puig, S. & Bressac-de-Paillerets, B. (2007). Cutaneous phenotype and MC1R variants as modifying factors for the development of melanoma in CDKN2A G101W mutation carriers from 4 countries. *International Journal of Cancer*, 121, 825-831

Grantham, R. (1974). Amino acid difference formula to help explain protein evolution. *Science*, 185, 862-864

Gudbjartsson, DF.; Sulem, P.; Stacey, SN.; Goldstein, AM.; Rafnar, T.; Sigurgeirsson, B.; Benediktsdottir, KR.; Thorisdottir, K.; Ragnarsson, R.; Sveinsdottir, SG.; Magnusson, V.; Lindblom, A.; Kostulas, K; Botella-Estrada, R.; Soriano, V.; Juberias, P.; Grasa, M.; Saez, B.; Andres, R.; Scherer, D.; Rudnai, P.; Gurzau, E.; Koppova, K.; Kiemeney, LA.; Jakobsdottir, M.; Steinberg, S.; Helgason, A.; Gretarsdottir, S.; Tucker, MA.; Mayordomo, JI.; Nagore, E.; Kumar, R.; Hansson, J.; Olafsson, JH; Gulcher, J.; Kong, A.; Thorsteinsdottir, U. & Stefansson, K. (2008). ASIP and TYR pigmentation variants associate with cutaneous melanoma and basal cell carcinoma. *Nature Genetics*, 40, 886–891

Habbe, N.; Langer, P.; Sina-Frey, M. & Bartsch, DF. (2006). Familial Pancreatic Cancer Syndromes. *Endocrinology Metabolism Clinics of North America*, 35 417–430

Hansson, J. (2008). Familial Melanoma. *Surgical Clinics of North America*, 88, 897-916

Harland, M.; Meloni, R.; Gruis, N.; Pinney, E.; Brookes, S.; Spurr, NK.; Frischauf, AM.; Bataille, V.; Peters, G.; Cuzick, J.; Selby, P.; Bishop, DT. & Newton Bishop, J. (1997). Germline mutations of the CDKN2 gene in UK melanoma families. *Human Molecular Genetics*, 6, 2061–2067

Harland, M.; Holland, EA.; Ghiorzo, P.; Mantelli, M.; Bianchi-Scarrà, G.; Goldstein, AM.; Tucker, MA.; Ponder, BAJ.; Mann, GJ.; Bishop, DT. & Bishop, JN. (2000). Mutation Screening of the *CDKN2A* Promoter in Melanoma Families. *Genes, Chromosomes & Cancer*, 28, 45–57

Harland, M.; Taylor, CF.; Chambers, PA.; Kukalizch, K.; Randerson-Moor, JA.; Gruis, NA.; de Snoo, FA.; ter Huurne, JA.; Goldstein, AM.; Tucker, MA.; Bishop, DT. & Newton Bishop, JA. (2005). A mutation hotspot at the p14ARF splice site. *Oncogene*, 24, 4604–4608

Hayward, N. (2000). New developments in melanoma genetics. *Current Oncology Reports*, 2, 300-306

Holland, EA.; Schmid, H.; Kefford, RF. & Mann, GJ. (1999). CDKN2A (p16) and CDK4 mutation analysis in 131 Australian melanoma probands: effect of family history and multiple primary melanomas. *Genes, Chromosomes & Cancer*, 25, 339-348

Houlston, RS. & Peto, J. (2004). The search for low penetrance cancer susceptibility alleles. *Oncogene*, 23, 6471-6476

Henikoff, S. & Henikoff, J. (1992). Amino acid substitutions matrices from protein blocks. *Proceedings of the National Academy of Science USA*, 89, 10915-10919

Hutchinson, PE.; Osborne, JE.; Lear, JT.; Smith, AG.; Bowers, PW.; Morris, PN.; Jones, PW.; York, C.; Strange, RC. & Fryer, AA. (2000). Vitamin D Receptor Polymorphisms Are Associated with Altered Prognosis in Patients with Malignant Melanoma. *Clinical Cancer Research,* 6, 498-504

Jemal, A.; Devesa, SS.; Hartge P. & Tucker, MA. (2001). Recent trends in cutaneous melanoma incidence among whites in the United States. *Journal of the National Cancer Institute,* 3, 678-683

Jemal, A.; Siegel, R.; Ward, E.; Hao, Y.; Xu, J.; Muttay, T. & Thun, MJ. (2008). Cancer statistics, 2008. *California Cancer Journal of Clinics,* 58, 71–96

Jones, WO.; Harman, CR.; Ng, AK. & Shaw JH. (1999). Incidence of malignant melanoma in Auckland, New Zealand: highest rates in the world. *World Journal of Surgery,* 23, 732-735

Kanetsky, PA.; Rebbeck, TR.; Hummer, AJ.; Panossian, S.; Armstrong, BK.; Kricker, A.; Marrett, LD.; Millikan, RC.; Gruber, SB.; Culver, HA.; Zanetti, R.; Gallagher, RP.; Dwyer, T.; Busam, K.; From, L.; Mujumdar, U.; Wilcox, H.; Begg, CB. & Berwick, M. (2006). Population-based study of natural variation in the melanocortin-1 receptor gene and melanoma. *Cancer Research,* 66, 9330-9337

Kannengiesser, C.; Brookes, S.; Gutierrez del Arroyo, A.; Pham, D.; Bombled, J.; Barrois, M.; Mauffret, O.; Avril, MF.; Chompret, A.; Lenoir, GM.; Sarasin, A.; Peters, G. & Bressac-de-Paillerets, B. (2009). Functional, Structural, and Genetic Evaluation of 20 CDKN2A Germ Line Mutations Identified in Melanoma-Prone Families or Patients. *Human Mutation,* 30, 564–574

Kaskel, P.; Sander, S.; Kron, M. Kind, P.; Peter, RU. & Krähn, G. (2001). Outdoor activities in childhood: a protective factor for cutaneous melanoma? Results of a case-control study in 271 matched pairs. *British Journal of Dermatology,* 145, 602-609

Kefford, RF.; Newton Bishop, JA.; Bergman, W. & Tucker, MA. (1999). Counseling and DNA testing for individuals perceived to be genetically predisposed to melanoma: a consensus statement of the Melanoma Genetics Consortium. *Journal of Clinical Oncology,* 17, 3245-3251

Kefford, RF.; Newton Bishop, J.; Tucker, M.; Bressac-de Paillerets, B.; Bianchi-Scarrà, G.; Bergman, W.; Goldstein, A.; Puig, S.; Mackie, R.; Elder, D.; Hansson, J.; Hayward, N.; Hogg, D. & Olsson, H. (2002). Genetic testing for melanoma. *Lancet Oncology,* 3, 653-654

Kefford, RF. & Mann, GJ. (2003). Is there a role for genetic testing in patients with melanoma? *Current Opinion in Oncology,* 15, 157-161

Kerstann, KF.; Bradford, PT.; Steighner, R.; Calista, D.; Fargnoli, MC.; Peris. K.; Scaini, MC.; Menin, C.; Ghiorzo, P.; Bianchi-Scarrà, G.; Goldstein, AM. & Landi, MT. (2008). No evidence for linkage with melanoma in Italian melanoma-prone families. *Cancer Epidemiology, Biomarkers & Prevention,* 17, 1838-1840

Kopf, AW.; Hellman, LJ.; Rogers, GS.; Gross, DF.; Rigel, DS.; Friedman, RJ.; Levenstein, M.; Brown, J.; Golomb, FM.; Roses, DF.; Gumport, SL. & Mintzis, MM. (1986). Familial malignant melanoma. *Jama,* 256, 1915-1919

Landi, MT.; Baccarelli, A.; Calista, D.; Pesatori, A.; Fears, T.; Tucker, MA. & Landi, G. (2001). Combined Risk Factors for Melanoma in a Mediterranean Population. *British Journal of Cancer,* 85, 1304-1310

Landi, MT.; Goldstein, AM.; Tsang, S.; Munroe, D.; Modi, W.; Ter-Minassian, M.; Steighner, R.; Dean, M.; Metheny, N.; Staats, B.; Agatep, R.; Hogg, D. & Calista, D. (2004). Genetic susceptibility in familial melanoma from northeastern Italy. *Journal of Medical Genetics,* 41, 557-566

Leachman, SA.; Carucci, J.; Kohlmann, W.; Banks, KC.; Asgari, MM.; Bergman, W.; Bianchi-Scarrà, G.; Brentnall, T.; Bressac-de Paillerets, B.; Bruno, W.; Curiel-Lewandrowski, C.; de Snoo, FA.; Debniak, T.; Demierre, MF.; Elder, D.; Goldstein, AM.; Grant-Kels, J.; Halpern, AC.; Ingvar, C.; Kefford, RF.; Lang, J.; MacKie, RM.; Mann, GJ.; Mueller, K.; Newton-Bishop, J.; Olsson, H.; Petersen, GM.; Puig, S.; Rigel, D.; Swetter, SM.; Tucker, MA.; Yakobson, E.; Zitelli, JA. & Tsao, H. (2009) Selection criteria for genetic assessment of patients with familial melanoma. *Journal of American Academy of Dermatology,* 61, 677e.1-14

Liu, L.; Dilworth, D.; Gao, L.; Monzon, J.; Summers, A.; Lassam, N. & Hogg, D. (1999). Mutation of the CDKN2A 5′ UTR creates an aberrant initiation codon and predisposes to melanoma. *Nature Genetics,* 21, 128–132

Lukas, J.; Parry, D.; Aagaard, L.; Mann, DJ.; Bartkova, J.; Strauss, M.; Peters, G. & Bartek J. (1995) Retinoblastoma-protein-dependent cell-cycle inhibition by the tumour suppressor p16. *Nature,* 375, 503 - 506

Lesueur, F.; de Lynch, M.; Barrois, M.; Durand, G.; Bombled, J.; Avril, MF.; Chompret, A.; Boitier, F.; Lenoir, GM. & Bressac-de Paillerets, B. (2008). The contribution of large genomic deletions at the *CDKN2A* locus to the burden of familial melanoma. *British Journal of Cancer,* 99, 364-370

Lynch, HT.; Brand, RE.; Hogg, D.; Deters, CA.; Fusaro, RM.; Lynch, JF.; Liu, L.; Knezetic, J.; Lassam, NJ.; Goggins, M. & Kern, S. (2002). Phenotypic Variation in Eight Extended *CDKN2A* Germline Mutation Familial Atypical Multiple Mole Melanoma–Pancreatic Carcinoma–Prone Families: the familial atypical mole melanoma-pancreatic carcinoma syndrome. *American Cancer Society,* 94, 84-96

MacKie, RM.; McHenry, P. & Hole, D. (1993). Accelerated detection with prospective surveillance for cutaneous malignant melanoma in high-risk groups. *Lancet,* 341, 1618-1620

Majore, S.; De Simone, P.; Crisi, A.; Eibenschutz, L.; Binni, F, Antigoni, I.; De Bernardo, C.; Catricalà, C. & Grammatico, P. (2008). CDKN2A/CDK4 molecular study on 155 Italian subjects with familial and/or primary multiple melanoma. *Pigment Cell & Melanoma Research,* 21, 209-211

Mantelli, M., Barile, M., Ciotti, P., Ghiorzo, P., Lantieri, F., Pastorino, L., Catricala, C., Torre, G. D., Folco, U., Grammatico, P., et al. (2002). High prevalence of the G101W germline mutation in the CDKN2A (P16(ink4a)) gene in 62 Italian malignant melanoma families. *American Journal of Medical Genetics,* 107, 214-21

McKenzie, HA.; Fung, C.; Becker, TM.; Irvine, M.; Mann, JG.; Kefford, RF. & Rizos, H. (2010). Predicting functional significance of cancer-associated $p16^{INK4A}$ in *CDKN2A*. *Human Mutation,* 31, 1-10

Michaloglou, C.; Vredeveld, LC.; Soengas, MS.; Denoyelle, C.; Kuilman, T.; Van der Horst, CM.; Majoor, DM.; Shay, JW.; Mooi, WJ. & Peeper, DS. (2005). BRAFE600-associated senescence-like cell cycle arrest of human naevi. *Nature,* 436, 720-724

Mössner, R.; Anders, N.; König, IR.; Krüger, U.; Schmidt, D.; Berking, C.; Ziegler, A.; Brockmöller. J.; Kaiser, R.; Volkenandt, M.; Westphal, GA. & Reich, K. (2007). Variation of the melanocortin-1 receptor and the glutathione-S transferase T1 and M1 genes in cutaneous malignant melanoma. *Archives of Dermatological Research*, 298, 371-379

Naldi, L.; Imberti, GL.; Parazzini, F.; Gallus, S. & La Vecchia, C. (2000). Pigmentary traits, modalities of sun reaction, history of sunburns, and melanocytic nevi as risk factors for cutaneous malignant melanoma in the Italian population. *Cancer*, 88, 2703-2710

Newton, RA.; Roberts, DW.; Leonard, JH. & Sturm, RA. (2007). Human melanocytes expressing MC1R variant alleles show impaired activation of multiple signalling pathways. *Peptides*, 28, 2387-2396

Ng, PC. & Henikoff, S. (2003). SIFT: predicting amino acid changes that affect protein function. *Nucleic Acids Research*, 31, 3812-3814

Niendorf, KB. & Tsao, H. (2006). Cutaneous melanoma: family screening and genetic testing. *Dermatologic Therapy*, 19, 1–8

Ollila, S.; Dermadi Bebek, D.; Jiricny, J. & Nystrom, M. (2008). Mechanisms of pathogenicity in human MSH2 missense mutants. *Human Mutation*, 29, 1355–1363

Oliveria, SA.; Saraiya, M.; Geller, AC.; Heneghan, MK. & Jorgensen, C. (2006). Sun exposure and risk of melanoma. *Archives of Disease in Childhood*, 91, 131-138

Parry, D. & Gordon, P. (1996). Temperature sensitive mutants of p16CDKN2 associated with familial melanoma. *Molecular and Cellular Biology*, 16, 3844-3852

Pastorino, L.; Bonelli, L.; Ghiorzo, P.; Queirolo, P.; Battistuzzi, L.; Balleari, E.; Nasti, S.; Gargiulo, S.; Gliori, S.; Savoia, P.; Abate Osella, S.; Bernengo, MG. & Bianchi Scarrà G. (2008). CDKN2A mutations and MC1R variants in Italian patients with single or multiple primary melanoma. *Pigment Cell & Melanoma Research*, 21, 700-709

Pfahlberg, A.; Kolmel, KF. & Gefeller, O. (2001). Timing of excessive ultraviolet radiation and melanoma: epidemiology does not support the existence of a critical period of high susceptibility to solar ultraviolet radiation-induced melanoma. *British Journal of Dermatology*, 144, 471-475

Pollock, PM.; Spurr, N.; Bishop, T.; Gruis, N.; van der Velden, PA.; Golstein, AM.; Tucker, MA.; Foulkes, WD.; Barnhill, R.; Haber, D.; Fountain, J. & Hayward, NK. (1998). Haplotype analysis of two recurrent CDKN2A mutations in 10 melanoma families: evidence for common founders and independent mutations. *Human Mutation*, 11, 424-431

Pollock, PM.; Stark, MS.; Palmer, JM.; Walters, MK.; Aitken, JF.; Martin, NG. & Hayward, NK. (2001). Mutation analysis of the CDKN2A promoter in Australian melanoma families. *Genes, Chromosomes & Cancer*, 32, 89-94

Raimondi, S.; Sera, F.; Gandini, S.; Iodice, S.; Caini, S.; Maissonneuve, P. & Fargnoli, MC. (2008). MC1R variants, melanoma and red hair color phototype: a meta-analysis. *International Journal of Cancer*, 122, 2753-2760

Ringholm, A.; Klovins, J.; Rudzish, R.; Phillips, S.; Rees, JL.; & Schiöth, HB. (2004). Pharmacological characterization of loss of function mutations of the human melanocortin 1 receptor that are associated with red hair. *Journal of Investigative Dermatology*, 123, 917–923

Robsahm, TE. & Tretli, S. (2001). Cutaneous malignant melanoma in Norway: variation by region of residence before and after the age of 17. *Cancer Causes & Control,* 12, 569-576

Ruas, M.; Brookes, S.; McDonald, N.Q. & Peters, G. (1999). Functional evaluation of tumour-specific variants of p16$^{INK4A}$/CDKN2A: correlation with protein structure information. *Oncogene,* 18, 5423-5434

Sanchez-Laorden, BL.; Jimenez-Cervantes, C.; & Garcia-Borron, JC. (2007). Regulation of human melanocortin 1 receptor signaling and trafficking by Thr-308 and Ser-316 and its alteration in variant alleles associated with red hair and skin cancer. *Journal of Biological Chemistry,* 282, 3241–3251

Savage, SA.; Gerstenblith, MR.; Goldstein, AM.; Mirabello, L.; Fargnoli, MC.; Peris, K. & Landi, MT. (2008). Nucleotide diversity and population differentiation of the melanocortin 1 receptor gene, MC1R. *BioMed Central Genetics,* 9, 31-38

Scaini, MC.; Rossi, E.; Lobao Antunes de Siqueira Torres, P.; Zullato, D.; Callegaro, M.; Casella, C.; Quaggio, M.; Agata, S.; Malacrida, S.; Chiarion-Sileni, V.; Vecchiato, A.; Alaibac, M.; Montagna, M.; Mann, GJ.; Menin, C. & D'Andrea, E. (2009). Functional impairment of p16INK4A due to CDKN2A p.Gly23Asp missense mutation. *Mutation Research,* 671, 26–32

Schutte, M.; Hruban, RH.; Geradts, J.; Maynard, R.; Hilgers, W.; Rabindran, SK.; Moskaluk, CA.; Hahn, SA.; Schwarte-Waldhoff, I.; Schmiegel, W.; Baylin, SB.; Kern, SE. & Herman, JG. (1997) Abrogation of the Rb/p16 tumor-suppressive pathway in virtually all pancreatic carcinomas. *Cancer Research,* 57, 3126–3130

Shahbazi, M.; Pravica, V.; Nasreen, N.; Fakhoury, H.; Fryer, AA.; Strange, RC.; Hutchinson, PE.; Osborne, JE.; Lear, JT.; Smith, AG. & Hutchinson, IV. (2002). Association between functional polymorphism in EGF gene and malignant melanoma. *Lancet,* 359, 397-401

Sherr, CJ. (2001). The INK4a/ARF network in tumour suppression. *Nature Reviews Molecular Cell Biology,* 2, 731-737

Sherr, CJ. & McCormick, F. (2002) The RB and p53 pathways in cancer. *Cancer Cell,* 2, 102-112

Soufir N.; Avril MF.; Chompret A.; Demenais, F.; Bombled, J.; Spatz, A.; Stoppa-Lyonnet, D.; Bénard, J. & Bressac-de-Paillerets, B. (1998). Prevalence of p16 and CDK4 germline mutations in 48 melanoma-prone families in France. *Human Molecular Genetics,* 7, 209–216

Spica, T.; Portela, M.; Gérard, B.; Formicone, F.; Descamps, V.; Crickx, B.; Ollivaud, L.; Archimbaud, A.; Dupin, N.; Wolkenstein, P.; Vitoux, D.; Lebbe, C.; Saiag, P.; Basset-Segui, N.; Fargnoli, MC.; Grandchamp, B.; Peris, K. & Soufir, N. (2006). The A148T variant of the *CDKN2A* gene is not associated with melanoma risk in the French and Italian populations. *Journal of Investigative Dermatology,* 126, 1658-1660

Stott, FJ.; Bates, S.; James, MC.; McConnell, BB.; Starborg, M.; Brookes, S.; Palmero, I.; Ryan, K.; Hara, E.; Vousden, KH.; & Peters, G. (1998). The alternative product from the human CDKN2A locus, p14(ARF), participates in a regulatory feedback loop with p53 and MDM2. *Embo Journal,* 17, 5001–5014

Strange, RC. & Ellison, T.; Ichii-Jones, F.; Bath, J.; Hoban, P.; Lear, JT.; Smith AG.; Hutchinson, PE.; Osborne, J.; Bowers, B.; Jones, PW. & Fryer, AA. (1999).

Cytochrome P450 CYP2D6 genotypes: association with hair colour, Breslow thickness and melanocyte stimulating hormone receptor alleles in patients with malignant melanoma. *Pharmacogenetics*, 9, 269-276

Sturm, RA. (1998). Human pigmentation genes and their response to solar UV radiation. *Mutation Research*, 422, 68-76

Sturm, RA.; Teasdale, RD. & Box, NF. (2001). Human pigmentation genes: identification, structure and consequences of polymorphic variation. *Gene*, 277, 49-62

Sunyaev, S.; Ramensky, V.; Koch, I.; Lathe, W. 3rd.; Kondrashov, AS. & Bork, P. (2001) Prediction of deleterious human alleles. *Human Molecular Genetics*, 10, 591-587

Sviderskaya, EV.; Hill, SP.; Evans-Whipp, TJ.; Chin, L.; Orlow, SJ.; Easty, DJ.; Cheong, SC.; Beach, D.; DePinho, RA. & Benett, DC. (2002). p16(Ink4a) in melanocyte senescence and differentiation. *Journal of the National Cancer Institute*, 94, 446-454

Swerlick, RA. & Chen, S. (1997). The melanoma epidemic: more apparent than real? *Mayo Clinic Proceedings*, 72, 559-564

Tavtigian, SV.; Greenblatt, MS.; Goldgar, DE. & Boffetta, P. (2008a). Assessing Pathogenicity: Overview of Results from the IARC Unclassified Genetic Variants Working Group. *Human Mutation*, 29, 1261-1264

Tavtigian, SV.; Greenblatt, MS.; Lesueur, F. & Byrnes, GB. (2008b). In silico analysis of missense substitutions using sequence-alignment based methods. *Human Mutation*, 29, 1327-1336

Tsao, H. & Niendorf, K. (2004). Genetic testing in hereditary melanoma. *Journal of the American Academy of Dermatology*, 51, 803-808

Tucker, MA.; Halpern, A.; Holly, EA; Hartge, P.; Elder, DE.; Sagebiel, RW.; Guerry, D. 4th. & Clark, WH. Jr. (1997). Clinically recognized dysplastic nevi. A central risk factor for cutaneous melanoma. *Jama*, 277, 1439-1444

Udayakumar, D. & Tsao, H. (2009). Melanoma Genetics: An Update on Risk-Associated Genes. *Hematology/Oncology Clinics of North America*, 23, 415-429

Vasen, HFA.; Gruis, NA.; Frants, RR.; van der Velden, PA.; Hille, ETM. & Bergman, W. (2000). Risk of developing pancreatic cancer in families with familial atypical multiple mole melanoma associated with a specific 19 deletion of p16 (p16-Leiden). *International Journal of Cancer*, 87, 809–811

Vignoli, M.; Scaini, MC.; Ghiorzo, P.; Sestini, R., Bruno, W.; Menin, C.; Gensini, F.; Piazzini, M.; Testori, A.; Manoukian, S.; Orlando, C.; D'Andrea, E.; Bianchi Scarrà, G. & Genuardi, M. (2008). Genomic rearrangements of the *CDKN2A* locus are infrequent in Italian malignant melanoma families without evidence of *CDKN2A/CDK4* point mutations. *Melanoma Research*, 18, 431-437

Whelan, AJ.; Bartsch, D. & Goodfellow, PJ. (1995). Brief report: a familial syndrome of pancreatic cancer and melanoma with a mutation in the *CDKN2* tumor-suppressor gene. *New England Journal of Medicine*, 333, 975–977

Williams, PF.; Olsen, CM.; Hayward, NK. & Whitemen, DC. (2010). Melanocortin-1-receptor and risk of cutaneous melanoma: a meta-analysis and estimates of population burden. *International Journal of Cancer*, in press

Zhang, B. & Peng, Z. (2000). A Minimum Folding Unit in the Ankyrin Repeat Protein p16INK4. *Journal of Molecular Biology*, 299, 1121-1132

Zuo, L.; Weger, J.; Yang, Q.; Goldstein, AM.; Tucker, MA.; Walker, GJ.; Hayward, N. & Dracopoli, NC. (1996). Germline mutations in the p16INK4a binding domain of CDK4 in familial melanoma. *Nature Genetics*, 12, 97-99

http://chromium.liacs.nl/lovd2/home.php?select_db=CDKN2A (Leiden Open Variation Database)

# 7

# Genetics of Uveal Melanoma

Thomas van den Bosch, Jackelien van Beek, Emine Kiliç,
Nicole Naus, Dion Paridaens and Annelies de Klein
*Rotterdam Ocular Melanoma Studygroup (ROMS)*
*Erasmus University Medical Center & Rotterdam Eye Hospital*
*The Netherlands*

## 1. Introduction

Uveal melanoma is the most common type of primary eye cancer in adults, affecting 0.7/100,000 of the Western population yearly (Egan et al., 1988). The melanoma originates from neural crest derived melanocytes of the uvea (choroid, ciliary body and iris) and despite enucleation or conservative treatment half of patients die of, most often late appearing, metastatic disease (15-year survival: 53%) (Diener-West et al., 1992; Gamel et al., 1993; Kujala et al., 2003). To detect these (micro) metastasising cells in an early phase is one of the main challenges in the (uveal melanoma) oncology field and a prerequisite for proper patient selection in future therapeutic interventions. Several clinical, histological and genetic markers have been identified to predict poor prognosis in uveal melanoma patients. Genetic markers as chromosome 3 loss or the expression of a specific set of genes have proven to be far out the most significant prognostic markers. This will not only facilitate diagnosis and prediction of prognosis but will also assist in selecting patients for adjuvant therapy and the monitoring of circulating tumour cells. Alternatively, some of the tumour markers as *GNAQ/GNA*11, or *BAP*1 may serve as targets for new types of intervention tackling that specific pathway.
In this chapter, the most recent cytogenetic and molecular genetic approaches will be discussed along with the most important findings and their value for current and future management of patients with uveal melanoma.

## 2. Clinical aspects of uveal melanoma

### 2.1 Diagnosis

The diagnosis of uveal melanoma is based on ophthalmic examination using ancillary tests (ultrasonography, transillumination, optical coherence tomography) and occasionally fluorescein angiography, computed tomography and magnetic resonance imaging) and photography for follow-up. (Figure 1). Approximately 30% of patients have no symptoms at time of diagnosis (Damato 2010). Upon diagnosis of the primary tumour, patients are screened for metastases by liver enzyme tests and liver ultrasound and at that moment, less than 2% patients have detectable metastases (Shields, J. A. et al., 1991).
The primary uveal melanoma is located either in the choroid (72%), in the ciliary body (23%) or in the iris (5%). Choroidal melanomas usually present as a discoid, dome-shaped or mushroom-shaped subretinal mass, whereas ciliary-body melanomas regularly present as sessile or dome-shaped lesions. Iris melanomas may also present as dome-shaped

lesions or diffuse lesions and are the least common type of uveal melanoma. Iris melanomas tend to present at a smaller size, probably because pigmented lesions of the iris are usually visible to the patient at an early stage, which adds to a favourable prognosis. Iris melanomas may cause blockage of the drainage angle and lead to secondary elevation of intraocular pressure (Shields, C. L. et al., 2001). In contrast to iris melanomas, melanomas located in the ciliary body are associated with a high metastatic potential (Schmittel et al., 2004).

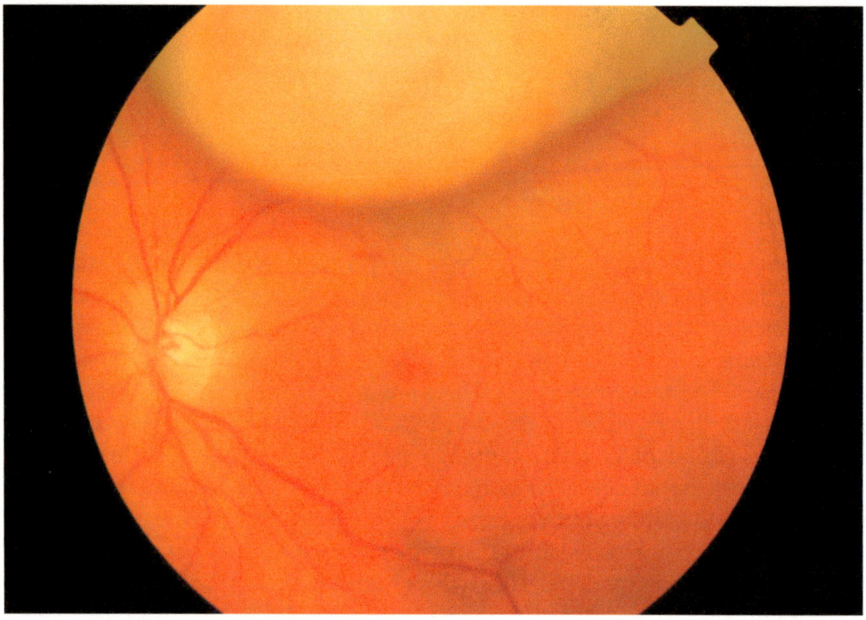

Fig. 1. Fundus photography showing a superiorly located uveal melanoma in the left eye.

If enucleation or biopsy is performed, the diagnosis is confirmed by histopathological examination (Figure 2). Melanomas consist of spindle, epitheloid cells or a mix of both cell types, and haematoxylin and eosin (H&E) staining is used to differentiate between these cell types. Periodic-acid Schiff (PAS) staining helps to identify microvascular patterns (three closed loops located back to back). Additional melanocytic markers that can be used in immunohistochemistry are S-100 or HMB-45.

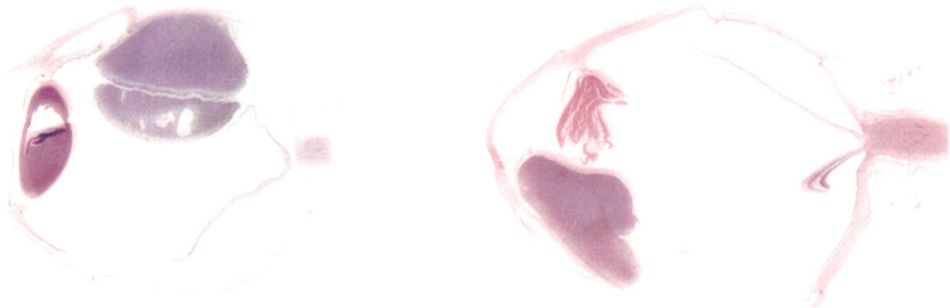

Fig. 2. Haematoxylin and eosin (H&E) staining of 2 tumour sections showing choroidal melanoma (left) and ciliary body melanoma (right).

### 2.2 Predisposing factors

Men and women are equally affected by uveal melanoma and most patients are 60 years of age and older. Certain phenotypes have been described, predisposing to uveal melanoma. Caucasian race for instance, is the most important known to date: uveal melanoma is approximately 150 times more common in Caucasians than in Africans (Margo et al., 1998; Singh et al., 2005). Furthermore, blue or gray eyes as well as fair skin type and inability to tan have been suggested to predispose to uveal melanoma (Gallagher et al., 1985; Schmidt-Pokrzywniak et al., 2009; Tucker et al., 1985). Although these facts may point towards a possible role of UV-radiation in the development of uveal melanoma, current evidence regarding UV-radiation is still inconclusive (Li et al., 2000; Manning et al., 2004; Marshall et al., 2006; Singh et al., 2004; Vajdic et al., 2002). There is however a tendency for iris melanomas to occur in the lower half of the iris, which has been explained by the increased sunlight exposure of this area (Shields, J.A. & Shields 2007).

Specific conditions as ocular and oculodermal melanocytosis (Nevus of Ota) (Gonder et al., 1982; Singh et al., 1998), neurofibromatosis type I (Wiznia et al., 1978), dysplastic nevus syndrome (Albert et al., 1985) are all associated with an increased incidence of uveal melanoma. Although uveal melanoma is rarely hereditary, several familial cancer syndromes have been reported: xeroderma pigmentosa, Li-Fraumeni syndrome and familial breast and ovarian cancer (Travis et al., 1996; Wooster et al., 1994). The low incidence of familial uveal melanoma cases limits approaches such as linkage analysis for the identification of susceptibility genes (Singh et al., 1996; Triozzi et al., 2008).

### 2.3 Clinical prognostic factors

The predictive value of classic prognostic parameters such as age, tumour size, tumour location, histological cell type and presence of vascular loops has been analysed in several retrospective studies (Coleman et al., 1993; Mooy & De Jong 1996). These parameters were complemented by the more recent identification of other histological (tumour-infiltrating lymphocytes, protein biomarkers) and genetic parameters (chromosomal aberrations, expression profiling) (Kujala et al., 2003; Naus et al., 2002; Patel, B. C. et al., 1998; Petrausch et al., 2008; Sisley et al., 2006; Tschentscher et al., 2003; van den Bosch et al., 2010; van Gils et al., 2008b). Tumour size (largest tumour diameter) is the most important clinical prognostic parameter and because of its ease of determination with ultrasonography, most often used for therapy planning. The 5-year mortality rate in patients with tumours below 10 mm in diameter is approximately 15% and increases to 53% for tumours larger than 15 mm in diameter (Gamel et al., 1993). Tumours located in the ciliary body correlate with progressive disease (Schmittel et al., 2004). The same holds true for tumours that show scleral invasion, optic nerve invasion, or extraocular extension (Damato 2010; McLean et al., 2004).

Histological presence of epitheloid cells and closed vascular patterns are also strongly associated with early death from uveal melanoma (Folberg et al., 1993; Maniotis et al., 1999; Seddon et al., 1983). These histological prognostic factors as well as genetic factors are less frequently used for primary therapy planning as tumour tissue is required for the pathological and genetic assessment of risk factors. In most cases, enucleation enables research on tumour tissue from relatively large-sized tumours. More frequent use of in-vivo biopsy prior to therapy may help assessing genetic risk factors, also in smaller tumours that may be treated conservatively. Several groups have already proven fine-needle biopsy to be a reliable technique yielding sufficient tumour tissue for cytogenetic analysis (Midena et al., 2006; Naus et al., 2002; Shields, C. L. et al., 2011).

Clinical, histological, and cytogenetic factors can be used to identify patients with high risk of metastases from uveal melanoma (Eskelin et al., 2000). As micrometastases are thought to arise early in the disease and precede clinically detectable macro metastases, present prognostic factors may thus be used to identify patients with micrometastatic disease.

### 2.4 Metastasis

Uveal melanomas metastasise almost exclusively by haematogenous route, and about 90% of patients with metastatic disease have hepatic metastases (Bedikian et al., 1995; Gragoudas et al., 1991). Other, less frequent sites for metastases include lung, skin, bone and brain (Collaborative Ocular Melanoma Study 2001; Diener-West et al., 2004; Gragoudas 2006; Landreville et al., 2008). Involvement of regional lymph nodes is rare and is attributed to the absence of draining lymphatics of the eye. Extraocular extension of tumour tissue though, may result in occasional metastatic involvement of lymph nodes.

The 15-year disease specific survival rates for patients with uveal melanoma is: 53% (Gamel et al., 1993). Shields et al (Shields, C. L. et al., 2011) recently reported a 3-year peak mortality of 24%. This could indicate a possible state of tumour dormancy or latency where circulating tumour cells remain silent and undetectable for the first 2 years after diagnosis (Klein 2011). Metastatic disease only rarely responds to treatment, and is usually fatal within 2-9 months after onset of symptoms (Diener-West et al., 2005; Eskelin et al., 2003). If the liver is involved, survival is most of the time shorter than 3 months. Treatment by systemic or intra-hepatic chemotherapy or partial hepatectomy rarely prolongs life (Augsburger et al., 2009). This highlights the urgent need for new and more effective therapies.

### 2.5 Fine needle biopsies and tumour heterogeneity

In previous research we have substantiated that specific regions on chromosome 1 and 3 are important in the aetiology of uveal melanoma (Kilic et al., 2005). Both our genetic and expression profiling studies point towards certain areas of the genome, that are important in tumour development and progression (van Gils et al., 2008a; van Gils et al., 2008b). As most cytogenetic and molecular genetic studies up till now involve patient samples from large tumours treated by enucleation, no specific knowledge is currently available for patients who receive conservative treatment such as stereotactic radiation therapy. Even though the melanomas treated by stereotactic radiotherapy are smaller than those treated by enucleation, still 25% of these tumours metastasise (van den Bosch T, manuscript in preparation). This implies that also smaller-sized tumours have the typical chromosomal aberrations required for dissemination of the disease. Cytogenetic and molecular genetic analyses of smaller tumours will most likely give more insight into tumour evolution and may enable identification of less complex chromosomal aberrations in uveal melanoma. In-vivo biopsy will be crucial for gaining tissue of small-sized tumours.

Previous results, with Fluorescent in situ hybridisation (McGill et al., ) (FISH) on Fine-needle aspiration biopsies (FNAB) acquired tumour tissue, showed that adequate FNAB material can be collected in a reliable and safe way for FISH analysis (Naus et al., 2002). The risk of local metastasis due to biopsy taking was found not to be increased with the FNAB technique (Char et al., 1996), and even a lower risk is reported if a transvitreal route is chosen for FNAB (Glasgow et al., 1988; Karcioglu et al., 1985). Tissue structure is also recognisable next to the single cells that have been aspirated with FNAB. Bechrakis et al. combined a vitrectomy with a biopsy and showed that in 97% of the biopsies histological diagnosis was possible (Bechrakis et al., 2002). So there is a growing preference using this technique, especially since it is a more controllable approach and yields more material, on which in addition to cytogenetic and molecular genetic techniques histological examination will be possible.

Heterogeneity of monosomy 3 (complete loss of chromosome 3) in uveal melanoma has been studied by FISH analysis on paraffin embedded tumour material, and on single-cell suspensions of fresh tumor tissue and showed that a difference in percentage of monosomy 3 may be present in some cases. However, our earlier results, where FISH on FNAB and tumour samples were compared, showed this to lead to misclassification in less than 1% (Naus et al., 2002). Tumour heterogeneity was further investigated and it was concluded that analysis of tumour biopsies in uveal melanoma gives an accurate prediction of the high-risk characteristics (Mensink et al., 2009b). In a more thorough study, we showed that hyperdiploidy (60-70 chromosomes) often resulted in copy number loss of chromosome 3, with loss of heterozygosity of one allele (Mensink manuscript submitted).

### 2.6 Therapy

Until the late eighties, the only treatment available was enucleation of the affected eye. Nowadays, conservative treatment protocols such as brachytherapy, thermotherapy, or radiation therapy may be used to treat small and medium-sized tumours with conservation of the eye additionally. Large-sized melanomas however are preferably still treated by enucleation (Shields, J. A. et al., 1996). The survival rate of patients with metastatic disease remains extremely poor as none of the current therapies proves to be effective. Several different cytotoxic agents such as dacarbazine have been administered alone, or in combination with other chemotherapeutic drugs or interferon-alfa-2b to high-risk patients after primary therapy. These regimens however, have not led to improved outcomes for these patients yet (Triozzi et al., 2008).

Despite improvements in treatment protocols for primary tumour and metastatic disease, and despite the fact that hardly any of the patients have clinical detectable metastasis at presentation, still half of all patients die of metastatic disease (Kujala et al., 2003).

Unfortunately no effective therapy exists for the treatment of metastatic disease at this moment, but new protocols involving combinations of chemotherapy and immunotherapy have been initiated recently. Systemic therapy may be more effective if administered early after diagnosis treating micrometastatic rather than macrometastatic disease. In the latter case, multiple mechanisms of resistance against systemic interventions may be present (Triozzi et al., 2008). With this in mind a new adjuvant immunotherapy protocol has been developed, where clinical, histological, and cytogenetic factors are used to identify high-risk uveal melanoma patients and treat these by immunization with their own trained dendritic cells to prevent future metastatic disease. This multicenter trial is performed by the ROMS in collaboration with Radboud University Nijmegen.

## 3. Molecular aspects of uveal melanoma

Cancer development is often associated with genomic instability and acquisition of genomic heterogeneity (Bayani et al., 2007), generating both clonal and non-clonal tumour cell populations ( Katona et al., 2007; Ye et al., 2007). Several mutations in the cell cycle can lead to aneuploidy: during mitosis, spindle checkpoint processes such as chromosome attachment to the spindle and chromosome segregation are vulnerable to changes leading to single point mutations or even gross chromosomal rearrangements (Kops et al., 2005; Olaharski et al., 2006). There is delicate balance between a possible benefit from the accumulation of genetic and epigenetic alterations and a lethal genetically unstable state of the cells (Nguyen & Ravid 2006). Polyploidy is also well known in cancer and it tends to occur in tumours with a more aggressive phenotype (Castedo et al., 2006; Kaneko & Knudson 2000).

Research is focusing on finding pathways involved in carcinogenesis, thereby trying to understand tumour onset and early development and transition to metastatic disease. Highly invasive tumours are compared with poorly invasive ones, primary tumours with its metastases, and therapy-resistant tumours with responsive ones in order to search for differentially expressed genes and specific chromosomal regions or genes involved in these processes.

### 3.1 Cytogenetic and molecular genetic techniques

A wide variety of cytogenetic and molecular genetic techniques are available and others still in development. Short term cultured uveal melanoma specimens are very suitable for classic cytogenetic analysis and spectral karyotyping (SKY), and these generally display display a relatively simple karyotype with recurrent chromosomal anomalies. (Figure 3)

Fluorescent in situ hybridisation, comparative genomic hybridisation (CGH) and quantitative PCR techniques can be applied to fresh or frozen tissues, cell lines, and archival formalin-fixed paraffin-embedded samples.

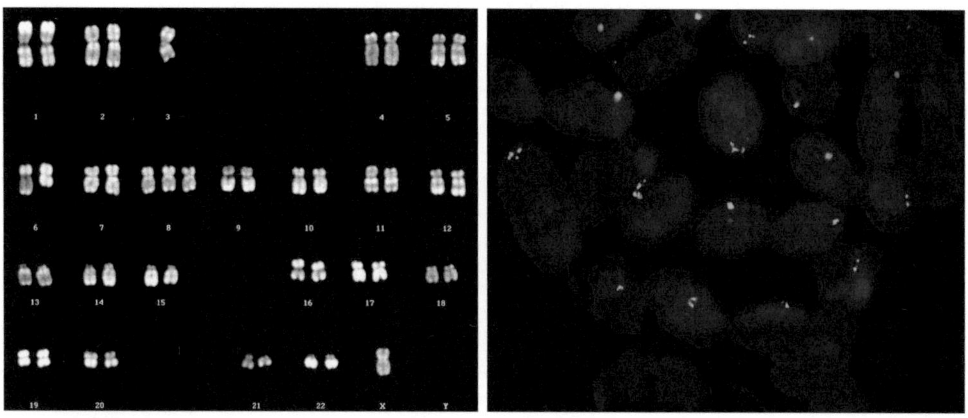

Fig. 3. Karyogram showing loss of chromosome 3, isodisomy of 6p, and gain of chromosome 8 (left). FISH: nuclei showing one signal for chromosome 3p (red) and centromere 3 (green) (right).

Currently microarray based CGH, SNP analysis and gene expression analysis are the most frequently applied techniques. A drawback of array-based approaches is that the analysed signal represents the average value of all cells in the tumour sample, requiring a high signal-to-noise ratio to quantitatively and reliably detect low-level DNA copy number changes on individual array elements (Albertson et al., 2003). The great advantage is that expression and copy number information on thousands of gene and chromosome locations can be obtained from a single mRNA or DNA sample in just one experiment.

Recently Next Generation Sequencing (NGS) has been applied on primary uveal melanoma samples resulting in the detection of mutations, showing single or multiple base pair changes.

A brief summary of the current findings is outlined below (The technical aspects of these techniques have been reviewed by us (Mensink et al., 2009a) and others (Harbour 2009) recently.

### 3.2 Chromosomal anomalies as prognostic markers

Specific chromosomal anomalies, as deletion of chromosome 1p, monosomy of chromosome 3 or gain of chromosome 8q, strongly correlate with decreased survival in uveal melanoma.
Monosomy of chromosome 3 is the most frequently found non-random chromosomal aberration in uveal melanoma and is predominantly found in metastasising tumours (Prescher et al., 1996). In univariate analysis, monosomy 3 was the most significant predictor ($p < 0.0001$) of poor prognosis in uveal melanoma, followed by tumour location and diameter (Prescher et al., 1996). It is considered to be a primary event, because it is seen in combination with all other chromosomal aberrations in uveal melanoma such as loss of chromosome 1p, gain of 6p and gain of 8q (Prescher et al., 1995). In the majority of tumours with chromosome 3 losses there is complete monosomy, although occasionally isodisomy is acquired (Aalto et al., 2001; Scholes et al., 2001; White, V. A. et al., 1998). Rarely, melanomas with partial aberrations on chromosome 3 or translocations have been described, making it difficult to map putative tumour suppressor genes. Loss of heterozygosity studies demonstrate common regions of allelic loss located on 3p25 and on the long arm spanning from 3q24 to 3q26 (Onken et al., 2007; Parrella et al., 2003).
Concomitant loss of chromosomes 1p and 3 has a stronger correlation with metastasising disease than either one of them separately (Figure 4) (Kilic et al., 2005). The common deleted region on chromosome 1 ranges from 1p34.3 to 1p36.2 (Aalto et al., 2001; Hausler et al., 2005; Hughes et al., 2005).

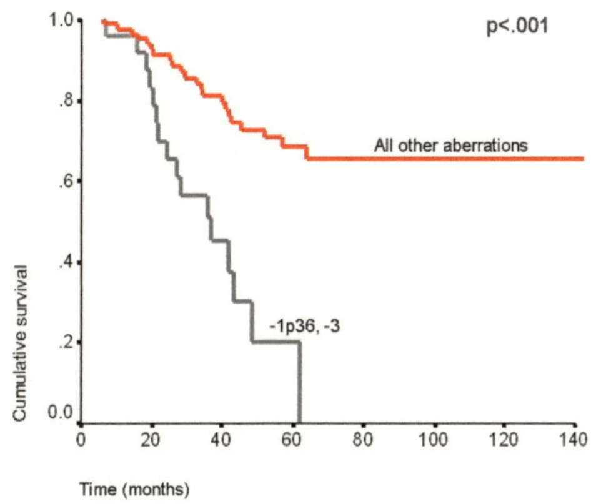


Fig. 4. Kaplan-Meier survival curve of UM patients with tumours showing loss of chromosome 1p36 and chromosome 3. Figure adapted from (Kilic et al., 2005).

The association with chromosome 8q gain was slightly less significant than for monosomy 3, but a strong inverse correlation ($p < 0.0001$) of dosage effect of additional copies of 8q on survival was observed (Sisley et al., 1997). Gain of chromosome 8, or acquisition of an isochromosome 8q, is suggested to be a secondary event in uveal melanoma, because variable copy numbers of 8q can be present in one tumour (Horsman & White 1993; Prescher et al., 1994). It occurs frequently in tumours that have lost one copy of chromosome

3 and it is an independent prognostic factor of progressive disease (Patel, K. A. et al., 2001; Sisley et al., 1997; White, V. A. et al., 1998). The shortest region of overlapping gain spans from 8q24.1 to 8qter (Hughes et al., 2005; Sisley et al., 2006).

In a series of large posterior uveal melanomas, presence of a chromosome 6p abnormality was predictive of good outcome (White, V. A. et al., 1998). These tumours with gain of chromosome 6p have been proposed to represent a separate group of uveal melanoma with an alternative genetic pathway in carcinogenesis, because gain of 6p is frequently found in tumours with disomy 3 (Ehlers et al., 2008; Hoglund et al., 2004; Landreville et al., 2008; Sisley et al., 1997).

Abnormalities of other chromosomes have also been detected in uveal melanoma. However, they often lead to contradictory results regarding the prognostic impact. Chromosome 18q22 has been suggested to play a prognostic role(White, J. S. et al., 2006), but this could not be confirmed by other groups (Mensink et al., 2008). Chromosome 9p21( Scholes et al., 2001) and chromosome 16q (Vajdic et al., 2003) have been described to be important in uveal melanoma as well.

SNP arrays can simultaneously be used to define copy number changes in tumours from signal intensities reflecting the amount of hybridised DNA (Bignell et al., 2004), and for determining and mapping of chromosomal regions with loss of heterozygosity. The great advantage is that information on thousands of locations or genes can be obtained in a single experiment with a high resolution. With SNP-array we and others were able to confirm the frequently found alterations by FISH on chromosomes 1p, 3, 6p, 6q, 8p and 8q (Figure 5). Other chromosomal alterations were found by FISH: +7, -9p, -10 or +10, -11q23-q25 (van den Bosch et al., 2010).

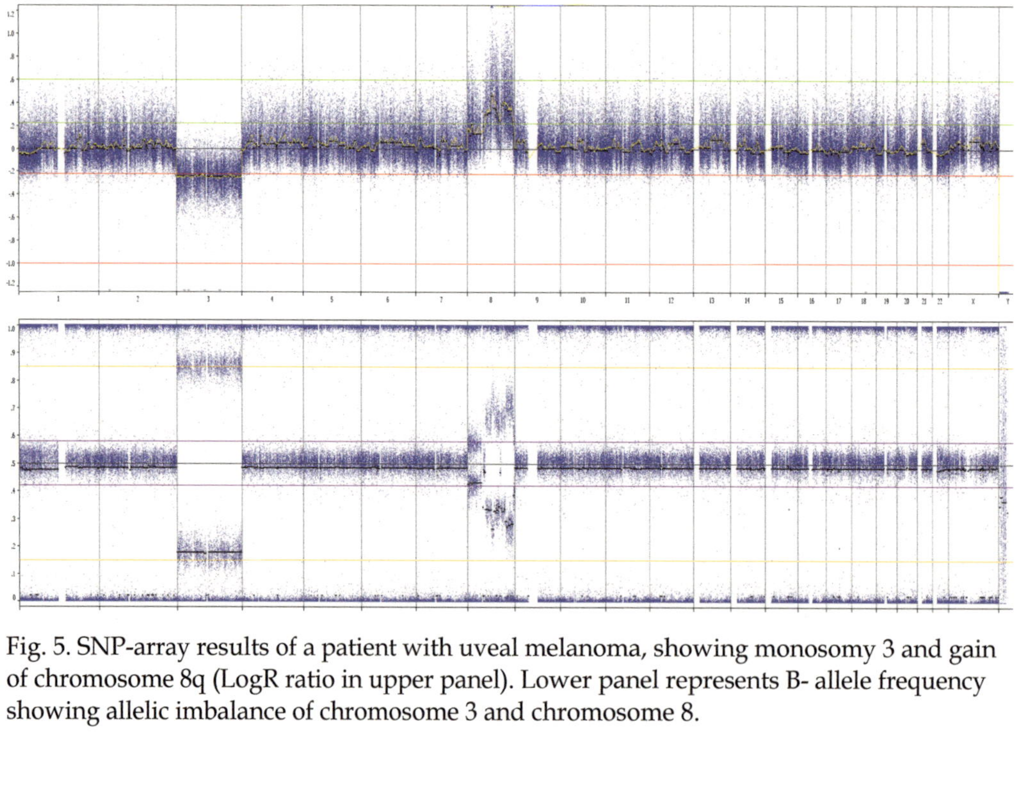

Fig. 5. SNP-array results of a patient with uveal melanoma, showing monosomy 3 and gain of chromosome 8q (LogR ratio in upper panel). Lower panel represents B- allele frequency showing allelic imbalance of chromosome 3 and chromosome 8.

Partial losses of chromosome 3 are very rare and therefore also rarely reported in the available literature (Parrella et al., 2003; Trolet et al., 2009; Tschentscher et al., 2001). In nearly all cases, complete loss of one copy of chromosome 3 is found, even in the smaller-sized melanomas that had been enucleated. With the recent high-resolution SNP-array's, no specific small regions of loss on chromosome 3 have been found.

For the fact that most uveal melanomas have complete loss of chromosome 3, either FISH, q-PCR or SNP-array may be used for analysing chromosome status in patients with uveal melanoma. There is thus no advantage of either SNP-array or FISH for only detecting chromosome 3 alterations in uveal melanoma. SNP-array though, allows for testing of multiple loci on different chromosomes compared to just one or two loci per chromosome with FISH or q-PCR. SNP-array is a fast measure for genome-wide assessment of chromosomal aberrations whereas FISH takes more time as multiple experiments would be necessary to assess multiple chromosomes or loci. There is one major difference between SNP-array and FISH, being that SNP-array enables assessment of heterozygosity, potentially revealing regions with loss of heterozygosity or allelic imbalances. This feature may provide us with information especially in disomic chromosome 3 cases where one allele is lost and the remaining one is copied by mistake (isodisomy) or uniparental disomic states. These processes may lead to loss of heterozygosity and analysis of these cases may help find an answer for patients with disomy 3 who still developed metastasis.

### 3.3 Gene-expression profiling

Based on expression data uveal melanomas can be divided in two classes. We and others showed these two classes to correspond remarkably well with the ability of the tumour to metastasize. When compared to clinico-pathologic or genetic prognostic markers, this classification on basis of a set of classifier genes is far-out superior (Petrausch et al., 2008; Tschentscher et al., 2003; Worley et al., 2007). In general the top classifier list revealed a global down-regulation of neural crest and melanocyte-specific genes and an up-regulation of epithelial genes in "metastatic" class II. These tumours exhibit epithelial features, such as cell morphology, and up-regulation of the E-cadherin pathway (Worley et al., 2007). RNA extraction from enucleated tumour or a fine needle biopsy is feasible and can be used for transcriptomic analysis on uveal melanoma samples, this service is in fact currently commercially available (Onken et al., 2010). Mentioned expression studies yielded similar sets of classifier genes however these classifier genes are merely markers of the underlying cause whereas genes involved in tumour progression and metastatic potential still have to be discovered. (van Gils et al., 2008b), If these are genes encoding cell surface markers, they could be a target for cell therapy aimed at an immunological response to eliminate tumour cells.

### 3.4 Next Generation Sequencing

The introduction of Next Generation Sequencing provides chromosomal mutational analysis up to the base-pair level. This sequencing technique therefore has the highest resolution possible and with the possibility for fast genome-wide testing in multiple tumour samples at once, is a very precise and reliable technique for mutational analysis. A limitation is the fact that preceding PCR amplification is required most of the time, which may introduce mutations due to the error rate of polymerase enzyme. The most recent genes involved in uveal melanoma however were found by sequence analysis, such as *BAP*1 and *GNAQ*. These genes are discussed in more detail further on.

### 3.5 Epigenetic regulation

Epigenetic mechanisms are known to alter genomes by other ways than direct changes in DNA sequence. For example, genes and promoters may have their functions silenced by methylation processes. In uveal melanoma, methylation of *CDKN2A* is present in 4 to 32% (Merbs & Sidransky 1999), *RASSF1* in 13 to 70% (Maat et al., 2007), *RARB* up to 7% and *TIMP3* in 9% (van der Velden et al., 2003; van Gils et al., 2008b). *RASEF* is targeted by loss of heterozygosity in combination with methylation in primary uveal melanoma; there is only low percentage methylation (Maat et al., 2008). *hTERT*, an important gene in carcinogenesis, is methylated in up to 52% of uveal melanoma, whereas *FHIT* and *APC* are never hypermethylated (Merhavi et al., 2007; Moulin et al., 2008; Zeschnigk et al., 2003). In none of these studies hypermethylation of a gene correlated with metastatic disease. When we looked for regions containing blocks of up or downregulated genes using LAP analysis specific regions with significantly low or high expression on the genome were apparent (van Gils et al., 2008b). These local over or underexpression could be the result of small deletions or amplifications. Alternatively epigenetic mechanisms as hyper or hypomethylation could be an explanation.

### 3.6 Genes involved in uveal melanoma

Deregulation of the RAS-RAF-MEK-ERK or mitogen-activated protein kinase (MAPK) pathway is common in many human malignancies (Inamdar et al., 2010). Mutations of specific members of these key molecular signaling pathways have been implicated in tumourigenesis of cutaneous melanoma. Many of these often well known oncogenes (e.g. *NRAS*, *BRAF*) or tumour suppressor genes (*PTEN*, *CDKN2A*) have also been analysed in uveal melanoma and occasionally mutations in these genes were found. Although no relation with development of metastatic disease was found, the presence of somatic mutations in these genes can provide a starting point for early detection of metastatic cells in blood or therapeutic intervention.

More promising are the recent findings of two frequently mutated members of the MAP-kinase pathway, *GNAQ* and *GNA11*, and the *BAP1* gene.

#### 3.6.1 The MAP-kinase pathway: GNAQ and GNA11

Recently Van Raamsdonk and coworkers demonstrated that approximately 80% of uveal melanomas carried activating mutations in either *GNAQ* or *GNA11*, turning these into oncogenes (Herlyn & Nathanson 2010; Van Raamsdonk et al., 2009; Van Raamsdonk et al., 2010). These genes belong to a subfamily of genes encoding for the G-protein α subunit involved in MAPK cell signaling. Mutations in the G-protein α stimulatory subunit of *GNAQ* were found in 46% of uveal melanoma cases, wheras mutations of *GNA11* were found in 35% of uveal melanoma cases. Both of these genes showed to be mutually exclusive and were by their oncogenic conversion suggested to be the cause of constitutive MAP-kinase pathway activation. This in turn leads to cell proliferation even in the absence of extracellular stimuli.

Activating somatic mutations of *GNAQ* at codon 209 were found by Onken et al, in 31 of 58 (54%) posterior uveal melanomas, and in two of nine (22%) iris melanomas(Onken et al., 2008; Romano et al., 2011). Iris melanomas thus less often show *GNAQ* mutations, but can occasionally have mutant *BRAF* (Henriquez et al., 2007; Onken et al., 2008; Sisley et al., 2011; Van Raamsdonk et al., 2009). Conjunctival melanomas on the other hand often have *BRAF* involvement but do not frequently have *GNAQ* mutations(Dratviman-Storobinsky et al., 2010).

These specific *GNAQ*/*GNA*11 mutations are also found in 83% of blue naevi of the skin (Van Raamsdonk et al., 2009) and are present in all stages of progression (Sisley et al., 2011). These mutations therefore are thought to occur early in tumourigenesis, which is underlined by the fact they are not correlated with either molecular class or metastasis in general (Bauer et al., 2009; Onken et al., 2008).

### 3.6.2 The RAS-RAF-MEK-ERK pathway

Mutations in the RAS-RAF-MEK-ERK (MAPK) pathway are thought to be early or initiating events in tumorigenesis (Onken et al., 2008). In general, this pathway is activated by autocrine growth factor stimulation or by mutation of *BRAF* or *RAS* genes (Dhomen & Marais 2009; Fensterle 2006; Mercer & Pritchard 2003; Zuidervaart et al., 2005) resulting in excessive cell proliferation. A single substitution (p.V600E) appears to account for more than 90% of all *BRAF* mutations in cutaneous melanoma and this mutation is also frequently found in benign and premalignant nevi thereby suggesting these to be early events in tumourigenesis (Davies et al., 2002; Pollock et al., 2003). *BRAF* and *NRAS* are both activators of the MAPK pathway though mutations of these genes are very rare in uveal melanoma (Cohen et al., 2003; Kilic et al., 2004; Mooy et al., 1991; Saldanha et al., 2004).

Activation of the MAPK pathway appears to be a common event through *GNAQ*/ *GNA*11-mutation induced G-protein signaling and possibly also by activation of ERK, a downstream kinase of this pathway (Calipel et al., 2006; Weber et al., 2003).

It has been suggested that MAPK activation in uveal melanoma may also arise via crosstalk with the PI3K-PTEN-AKT pathway (Zuidervaart et al., 2005).

### 3.6.3 The PI3K-PTEN-AKT pathway

The tumour suppressor gene phosphatase and tensin homolog (*PTEN*), is involved in the PI3K pathway as negative regulator of AKT. Loss of function of *PTEN* by deletion or mutation, leads to activation of AKT and overexpression of the PI3K-PTEN-AKT pathway preventing apoptosis (Ehlers et al., 2008; Ibrahim & Haluska 2009). Inactivation of *PTEN* is reported in 15% of uveal melanoma cases and has been linked to an increase in aneuploidy but also poor clinical outcome (Abdel-Rahman et al., 2006; Ehlers et al., 2008). This may suggest a role in later stages of tumour growth and development. Activating mutations of *AKT3* may also lead to activation of this pathway, though mutations of *AKT3* have not been reported in uveal melanoma up till now.

### 3.6.4 The metastasis-associated gene BAP1

Somatic mutations in the ubiquitin carboxyl-terminal hydrolase of BRCA1-associated protein 1 (BAP1) were found in 84% of gene-expression class II uveal melanomas (Harbour et al., 2010). The *BAP*1-gene is located on chromosome 3p21.1 and the encoded protein is part of the ubiquitin proteasome system that has been implicated in other cancer types as well, such as lung, breast and renal cell carcinoma (Harbour et al., 2010; Jensen et al., 1998; Patel, M. et al., 2011; Wood et al., 2007). *BAP*1 is reported to participate in multiprotein complexes involved in regulation of expression of several other genes that regulate cellular processes (Patel, M. et al., 2011). Somatic *BAP*1 mutation was only found in 1 out of 26 investigated class I tumours against 26 out of 31 class II tumours. These mutations are thus suggested to occur later in uveal melanoma progression than for instance *GNAQ* mutations (Harbour et al., 2010).

### 3.6.5 Other investigated genes

Several candidate genes were proposed in uveal melanoma recently, such as *DDEF*1, *NBS*1, *HDM*2, *LZST*-1, *APITD*1, *CCND*1 and *BCL*-2 (van den Bosch et al., 2010). For most of these genes, a definite role in tumourigenesis or progression towards metastasis has to be validated.

In 65% of uveal melanoma cases, *CCND*1 is reported to be overexpressed resulting in activation of cyclin dependent kinases (Coupland et al., 1998; Coupland et al., 2000; Ehlers & Harbour 2006). The *CCND*1 overexpression is associated with large tumour size, epitheloid cytology, and poor prognosis (Coupland et al., 2000).

Elevated expression of *BCL*-2 is observed in uveal melanomas but also in normal melanocytes. This overexpression is reported to block apoptosis (Brantley & Harbour 2000; Chana et al., 1999; Coupland et al., 2000; Jay et al., 1996) and suggested to be responsible for the resistance to chemotherapy or irradiation therapy (Ehlers & Harbour 2006; McGill et al., 2002).

### 3.7 Gene targeted therapy

The survival rates for patients with metastasised uveal melanoma, treated by chemotherapeutic drugs or combination chemotherapy regimens remain disappointingly low and toxicity may be significant (Sullivan & Atkins 2010). Conventional cytotoxic chemotherapeutics are toxic to all cells including normal cells, and therefore targeted therapy may be more valuable in the treatment of these patients. As the molecular basis for tumour development and progression is emerging, therapy aimed at interfering with specific molecular pathways may be important (Triozzi et al., 2008).

MAPK pathway activation appears to be important in uveal melanoma, therefore inhibition of this pathway or intermediates of this pathway represent a promising target (Sisley et al., 2011). *GNAQ*$^{Q209}$ mutations are exclusive to melanocytic tumour cells thereby enabling therapy specifically targeted at mutant cells only. *GNAQ* mutant cell lines appeared highly sensitive to inhibitors of MEK (Van Raamsdonk et al., 2009) and phase II clinical trials testing this hypothesis are currently underway (Sullivan & Atkins 2010).

Inhibitors of members of the RAS-RAF-MEK-ERK pathway such as the small-molecule inhibitor PLX4032, showed promising results in patients with cutaneous melanoma containing *BRAF* mutations. Tumour shrinkage was found in 80% of patients who received PLX4032 and progression-free survival was found to increase by an average of 7 months (Bollag et al., 2010; Flaherty et al., 2010; Herlyn & Nathanson 2010). These mutations are however rarely encountered in uveal melanoma patients. Downstream effectors of GNAQ and GNA11 remain to be elucidated and are highly potential targets for therapy. Care needs to be taken as interference with the normal function of these proteins, could be harmful. GNAQ protein activity for instance, appeared to be crucial for cardiomyocyte survival in animal models (Sisley et al., 2011). This problem may however be solved if inhibitors could be designed that specifically interfere with mutant *GNAQ* only. As MEK inhibitors proved to be of value for uveal melanoma, other ways to circumvent the *GNAQ*-protein blocking problem may lie in designing inhibitors of intermediates of the MAPK pathway such as BRAF, RAS, MEK and ERK.

IGF-1R and the downstream molecule mTOR, may also be involved in the PI3K-PTEN-AKT pathway and RAS-RAF-MEK-ERK pathway, and also serve as potential targets for inhibitor-therapy, which is currently being tested (Patel, M. et al., 2011).

New immunotherapeutic approaches are also currently tested, such as those administering patients immunomodulatory monoclonal antibodies (e.g. CTLA4 antibodies) or vaccinating patients with their own dendritic cells trained to identify (circulating) tumour cells and initiate tumour cell desctruction by presenting tumour particles to cytotoxic T cells. We use this Dendritic Cell Therapy to treat high-risk patients after they have received local therapy, such as enucleation or irradiation, in order to eliminate circulating tumour cells and micrometastatic lesions. Results have to be awaited from this phase I study that already showed promising results in cutaneous melanoma patients (De Vries et al, 2005). Combination strategies such as immmunotherapy gene therapy may be more effective than single therapy regimes but these combinations have to be researched in the future.

## 4. Conclusion

Uveal melanoma is a rare but aggressive intraocular malignancy leading to metastatic spread in approximately 50% of patients. Current therapies have up till now unfortunately not resulted in improved survival. Patients with metastases from uveal melanoma still have a poor prognosis, with no effective adjuvant therapy available yet. Even chemotherapeutic agents administered alone or in combination, have not resulted in a change in survival rates for these patients. Recent cytogenetic and molecular genetic research identified several genetic prognostic factors, capable of making reliable predictions of prognosis in patients with uveal melanoma. These genetic factors prove to be even more important predictors than clinical and pathological factors and have already been implemented in the current ocular oncology clinical practice.

Next generation genetic techniques such as SNP-array, Next Generation Sequencing and gene-expression profiling shed light on chromosomal regions, genes, gene-expression, and molecular pathways involved in uveal melanoma tumour progression and development. More knowledge has been gained by these recent techniques combined with fine-needle aspiration biopsy tumour sampling, identifying the molecular genetic make-up of small and medium-sized melanomas as well as large melanomas. Uveal melanoma has hereby been identified as a heterogeneous type of malignancy showing variations in chromosome 3 alterations within tumours and variation in genes altered in different patients. With the molecular background of large and smaller-sized uveal melanoma emerging, patients may be selected on this molecular basis for future therapy.

Gene-targeted therapy is recently been tested in the clinical setting, facilitating interference with specific molecular pathways or signaling molecules, either as single agent or in combination with immunotherapy or chemotherapy. These developments may serve as first steps towards more specific and patient-tailored therapy not limited to treatment of patients with metastatic disease alone. These therapies may also be valuable for patients with recent diagnosis of uveal melanoma, attacking micrometastatic disease as early as possible.

There is great optimism that more specific and thus more effective therapies in the next several years will lead to advanced patient management, and thereby improved survival rates for patients with this deadly disease.

## 5. References

Aalto, Y., Eriksson, L., Seregard, S., et al. (2001). Concomitant loss of chromosome 3 and whole arm losses and gains of chromosome 1, 6, or 8 in metastasizing primary uveal melanoma. *Invest Ophthalmol Vis Sci*, Vol. 42, No. 2, pp. 313-317.

Abdel-Rahman, M.H., Yang, Y., Zhou, X.P., et al. (2006). High frequency of submicroscopic hemizygous deletion is a major mechanism of loss of expression of PTEN in uveal melanoma. *J Clin Oncol,* Vol. 24, No. 2, pp. 288-295.

Albert, D.M., Chang, M.A., Lamping, K., et al. (1985). The dysplastic nevus syndrome. A pedigree with primary malignant melanomas of the choroid and skin. *Ophthalmology,* Vol. 92, No. 12, pp. 1728-1734.

Albertson, D.G., Collins, C., McCormick, F., et al. (2003). Chromosome aberrations in solid tumors. *Nat Genet,* Vol. 34, No. 4, pp. 369-376.

Augsburger, J.J., Correa, Z.M. & Shaikh, A.H. (2009). Effectiveness of treatments for metastatic uveal melanoma. *Am J Ophthalmol,* Vol. 148, No. 1, pp. 119-127.

Bauer, J., Kilic, E., Vaarwater, J., et al. (2009). Oncogenic GNAQ mutations are not correlated with disease-free survival in uveal melanoma. *Br J Cancer,* Vol. 101, No. 5, pp. 813-815.

Bayani, J., Selvarajah, S., Maire, G., et al. (2007). Genomic mechanisms and measurement of structural and numerical instability in cancer cells. *Semin Cancer Biol,* Vol. 17, No. 1, pp. 5-18.

Bechrakis, N.E., Foerster, M.H. & Bornfeld, N. (2002). Biopsy in indeterminate intraocular tumors. *Ophthalmology,* Vol. 109, No. 2, pp. 235-242.

Bedikian, A.Y., Legha, S.S., Mavligit, G., et al. (1995). Treatment of uveal melanoma metastatic to the liver: a review of the M. D. Anderson Cancer Center experience and prognostic factors. *Cancer,* Vol. 76, No. 9, pp. 1665-1670.

Bignell, G.R., Huang, J., Greshock, J., et al. (2004). High-resolution analysis of DNA copy number using oligonucleotide microarrays. *Genome Res,* Vol. 14, No. 2, pp. 287-295.

Bollag, G., Hirth, P., Tsai, J., et al. (2010). Clinical efficacy of a RAF inhibitor needs broad target blockade in BRAF-mutant melanoma. *Nature,* Vol. 467, No. 7315, pp. 596-599.

Brantley, M.A., Jr. & Harbour, J.W. (2000). Deregulation of the Rb and p53 pathways in uveal melanoma. *Am J Pathol,* Vol. 157, No. 6, pp. 1795-1801.

Calipel, A., Mouriaux, F., Glotin, A.L., et al. (2006). Extracellular signal-regulated kinase-dependent proliferation is mediated through the protein kinase A/B-Raf pathway in human uveal melanoma cells. *J Biol Chem,* Vol. 281, No. 14, pp. 9238-9250.

Castedo, M., Coquelle, A., Vitale, I., et al. (2006). Selective resistance of tetraploid cancer cells against DNA damage-induced apoptosis. *Ann N Y Acad Sci,* Vol. 1090, No. pp. 35-49.

Chana, J.S., Wilson, G.D., Cree, I.A., et al. (1999). c-myc, p53, and Bcl-2 expression and clinical outcome in uveal melanoma. *Br J Ophthalmol,* Vol. 83, No. 1, pp. 110-114.

Char, D.H., Kroll, S.M., Miller, T., et al. (1996). Irradiated uveal melanomas: cytopathologic correlation with prognosis. *Am J Ophthalmol,* Vol. 122, No. 4, pp. 509-513.

Cohen, Y., Goldenberg-Cohen, N., Parrella, P., et al. (2003). Lack of BRAF mutation in primary uveal melanoma. *Invest Ophthalmol Vis Sci,* Vol. 44, No. 7, pp. 2876-2878.

Coleman, K., Baak, J.P., Van Diest, P., et al. (1993). Prognostic factors following enucleation of 111 uveal melanomas. *Br J Ophthalmol,* Vol. 77, No. 11, pp. 688-692.

Collaborative Ocular Melanoma Study, G. (2001). Assessment of metastatic disease status at death in 435 patients with large choroidal melanoma in the Collaborative Ocular

Melanoma Study (COMS): COMS report no. 15. *Arch Ophthalmol,* Vol. 119, No. 5, pp. 670-676.

Coupland, S.E., Anastassiou, G., Stang, A., et al. (2000). The prognostic value of cyclin D1, p53, and MDM2 protein expression in uveal melanoma. *J Pathol,* Vol. 191, No. 2, pp. 120-126.

Coupland, S.E., Bechrakis, N., Schuler, A., et al. (1998). Expression patterns of cyclin D1 and related proteins regulating G1-S phase transition in uveal melanoma and retinoblastoma. *Br J Ophthalmol,* Vol. 82, No. 8, pp. 961-970.

Damato, B. (2010). Does ocular treatment of uveal melanoma influence survival? *Br J Cancer,* Vol. 103, No. 3, pp. 285-290.

Davies, H., Bignell, G.R., Cox, C., et al. (2002). Mutations of the BRAF gene in human cancer. *Nature,* Vol. 417, No. 6892, pp. 949-954.

de Vries IJ, Bernsen MR, Lesterhuis WJ, Scharenborg NM, Strijk SP, Gerritsen MJ, Ruiter DJ, Figdor CG, Punt CJ, Adema GJ. Immunomonitoring tumor-specific T cells in delayed-type hypersensitivity skin biopsies after dendritic cell vaccination correlates with clinical outcome. *J Clin Oncol.* 2005 Aug 20;23(24):5779-87.

Dhomen, N. & Marais, R. (2009). BRAF signaling and targeted therapies in melanoma. *Hematol Oncol Clin North Am,* Vol. 23, No. 3, pp. 529-545, ix.

Diener-West, M., Hawkins, B.S., Markowitz, J.A., et al. (1992). A review of mortality from choroidal melanoma. II. A meta-analysis of 5-year mortality rates following enucleation, 1966 through 1988. *Arch Ophthalmol,* Vol. 110, No. 2, pp. 245-250.

Diener-West, M., Reynolds, S.M., Agugliaro, D.J., et al. (2004). Screening for metastasis from choroidal melanoma: the Collaborative Ocular Melanoma Study Group Report 23. *J Clin Oncol,* Vol. 22, No. 12, pp. 2438-2444.

Diener-West, M., Reynolds, S.M., Agugliaro, D.J., et al. (2005). Development of metastatic disease after enrollment in the COMS trials for treatment of choroidal melanoma: Collaborative Ocular Melanoma Study Group Report No. 26. *Arch Ophthalmol,* Vol. 123, No. 12, pp. 1639-1643.

Dratviman-Storobinsky, O., Cohen, Y., Frenkel, S., et al. (2010). Lack of oncogenic GNAQ mutations in melanocytic lesions of the conjunctiva as compared to uveal melanoma. *Invest Ophthalmol Vis Sci,* Vol. 51, No. 12, pp. 6180-6182.

Egan, K.M., Seddon, J.M., Glynn, R.J., et al. (1988). Epidemiologic aspects of uveal melanoma. *Surv Ophthalmol,* Vol. 32, No. 4, pp. 239-251.

Ehlers, J.P. & Harbour, J.W. (2006). Molecular pathobiology of uveal melanoma. *Int Ophthalmol Clin,* Vol. 46, No. 1, pp. 167-180.

Ehlers, J.P., Worley, L., Onken, M.D., et al. (2008). Integrative genomic analysis of aneuploidy in uveal melanoma. *Clin Cancer Res,* Vol. 14, No. 1, pp. 115-122.

Eskelin, S., Pyrhonen, S., Hahka-Kemppinen, M., et al. (2003). A prognostic model and staging for metastatic uveal melanoma. *Cancer,* Vol. 97, No. 2, pp. 465-475.

Eskelin, S., Pyrhonen, S., Summanen, P., et al. (2000). Tumor doubling times in metastatic malignant melanoma of the uvea: tumor progression before and after treatment. *Ophthalmology,* Vol. 107, No. 8, pp. 1443-1449.

Fensterle, J. (2006). [A trip through the signaling pathways of melanoma]

Ein Streifzug durch die (Signal-)Wege des malignen Melanoms. *J Dtsch Dermatol Ges,* Vol. 4, No. 3, pp. 205-217.

Flaherty, K.T., Puzanov, I., Kim, K.B., et al. (2010). Inhibition of mutated, activated BRAF in metastatic melanoma. *N Engl J Med,* Vol. 363, No. 9, pp. 809-819.

Folberg, R., Rummelt, V., Parys-Van Ginderdeuren, R., et al. (1993). The prognostic value of tumor blood vessel morphology in primary uveal melanoma. *Ophthalmology,* Vol. 100, No. 9, pp. 1389-1398.

Gallagher, R.P., Elwood, J.M., Rootman, J., et al. (1985). Risk factors for ocular melanoma: Western Canada Melanoma Study. *J Natl Cancer Inst,* Vol. 74, No. 4, pp. 775-778.

Gamel, J.W., McLean, I.W. & McCurdy, J.B. (1993). Biologic distinctions between cure and time to death in 2892 patients with intraocular melanoma. *Cancer,* Vol. 71, No. 7, pp. 2299-2305.

Glasgow, B.J., Brown, H.H., Zargoza, A.M., et al. (1988). Quantitation of tumor seeding from fine needle aspiration of ocular melanomas. *Am J Ophthalmol,* Vol. 105, No. 5, pp. 538-546.

Gonder, J.R., Shields, J.A., Albert, D.M., et al. (1982). Uveal malignant melanoma associated with ocular and oculodermal melanocytosis. *Ophthalmology,* Vol. 89, No. 8, pp. 953-960.

Gragoudas, E.S. (2006). Proton beam irradiation of uveal melanomas: the first 30 years. The Weisenfeld Lecture. *Invest Ophthalmol Vis Sci,* Vol. 47, No. 11, pp. 4666-4673.

Gragoudas, E.S., Egan, K.M., Seddon, J.M., et al. (1991). Survival of patients with metastases from uveal melanoma. *Ophthalmology,* Vol. 98, No. 3, pp. 383-389; discussion 390.

Harbour, J.W. (2009). Molecular prognostic testing and individualized patient care in uveal melanoma. *Am J Ophthalmol,* Vol. 148, No. 6, pp. 823-829 e821.

Harbour, J.W., Onken, M.D., Roberson, E.D., et al. (2010). Frequent mutation of BAP1 in metastasizing uveal melanomas. *Science,* Vol. 330, No. 6009, pp. 1410-1413.

Hausler, T., Stang, A., Anastassiou, G., et al. (2005). Loss of heterozygosity of 1p in uveal melanomas with monosomy 3. *Int J Cancer,* Vol. 116, No. 6, pp. 909-913.

Henriquez, F., Janssen, C., Kemp, E.G., et al. (2007). The T1799A BRAF mutation is present in iris melanoma. *Invest Ophthalmol Vis Sci,* Vol. 48, No. 11, pp. 4897-4900.

Herlyn, M. & Nathanson, K.L. (2010). Taking the guesswork out of uveal melanoma. *N Engl J Med,* Vol. 363, No. 23, pp. 2256-2257.

Hoglund, M., Gisselsson, D., Hansen, G.B., et al. (2004). Dissecting karyotypic patterns in malignant melanomas: temporal clustering of losses and gains in melanoma karyotypic evolution. *Int J Cancer,* Vol. 108, No. 1, pp. 57-65.

Horsman, D.E. & White, V.A. (1993). Cytogenetic analysis of uveal melanoma. Consistent occurrence of monosomy 3 and trisomy 8q. *Cancer,* Vol. 71, No. 3, pp. 811-819.

Hughes, S., Damato, B.E., Giddings, I., et al. (2005). Microarray comparative genomic hybridisation analysis of intraocular uveal melanomas identifies distinctive imbalances associated with loss of chromosome 3. *Br J Cancer,* Vol. 93, No. 10, pp. 1191-1196.

Ibrahim, N. & Haluska, F.G. (2009). Molecular pathogenesis of cutaneous melanocytic neoplasms. *Annu Rev Pathol,* Vol. 4, No. pp. 551-579.

Inamdar, G.S., Madhunapantula, S.V. & Robertson, G.P. (2010). Targeting the MAPK pathway in melanoma: why some approaches succeed and other fail. *Biochem Pharmacol,* Vol. 80, No. 5, pp. 624-637.

Jay, V., Yi, Q., Hunter, W.S., et al. (1996). Expression of bcl-2 in uveal malignant melanoma. *Arch Pathol Lab Med,* Vol. 120, No. 5, pp. 497-498.

Jensen, D.E., Proctor, M., Marquis, S.T., et al. (1998). BAP1: a novel ubiquitin hydrolase which binds to the BRCA1 RING finger and enhances BRCA1-mediated cell growth suppression. *Oncogene,* Vol. 16, No. 9, pp. 1097-1112.

Kaneko, Y. & Knudson, A.G. (2000). Mechanism and relevance of ploidy in neuroblastoma. *Genes Chromosomes Cancer,* Vol. 29, No. 2, pp. 89-95.

Karcioglu, Z.A., Gordon, R.A. & Karcioglu, G.L. (1985). Tumor seeding in ocular fine needle aspiration biopsy. *Ophthalmology,* Vol. 92, No. 12, pp. 1763-1767.

Katona, T.M., Jones, T.D., Wang, M., et al. (2007). Genetically heterogeneous and clonally unrelated metastases may arise in patients with cutaneous melanoma. *Am J Surg Pathol,* Vol. 31, No. 7, pp. 1029-1037.

Kilic, E., Bruggenwirth, H.T., Verbiest, M.M., et al. (2004). The RAS-BRAF kinase pathway is not involved in uveal melanoma. *Melanoma Res,* Vol. 14, No. 3, pp. 203-205.

Kilic, E., Naus, N.C., van Gils, W., et al. (2005). Concurrent loss of chromosome arm 1p and chromosome 3 predicts a decreased disease-free survival in uveal melanoma patients. *Invest Ophthalmol Vis Sci,* Vol. 46, No. 7, pp. 2253-2257.

Klein, C.A. (2011). Framework models of tumor dormancy from patient-derived observations. *Curr Opin Genet Dev,* Vol. 21, No. 1, pp. 42-49.

Kops, G.J., Weaver, B.A. & Cleveland, D.W. (2005). On the road to cancer: aneuploidy and the mitotic checkpoint. *Nat Rev Cancer,* Vol. 5, No. 10, pp. 773-785.

Kujala, E., Makitie, T. & Kivela, T. (2003). Very long-term prognosis of patients with malignant uveal melanoma. *Invest Ophthalmol Vis Sci,* Vol. 44, No. 11, pp. 4651-4659.

Li, W., Judge, H., Gragoudas, E.S., et al. (2000). Patterns of tumor initiation in choroidal melanoma. *Cancer Res,* Vol. 60, No. 14, pp. 3757-3760.

Maat, W., Beiboer, S.H., Jager, M.J., et al. (2008). Epigenetic regulation identifies RASEF as a tumor-suppressor gene in uveal melanoma. *Invest Ophthalmol Vis Sci,* Vol. 49, No. 4, pp. 1291-1298.

Maat, W., van der Velden, P.A., Out-Luiting, C., et al. (2007). Epigenetic inactivation of RASSF1a in uveal melanoma. *Invest Ophthalmol Vis Sci,* Vol. 48, No. 2, pp. 486-490.

Maniotis, A.J., Folberg, R., Hess, A., et al. (1999). Vascular channel formation by human melanoma cells in vivo and in vitro: vasculogenic mimicry. *Am J Pathol,* Vol. 155, No. 3, pp. 739-752.

Manning, W.S., Jr., Greenlee, P.G. & Norton, J.N. (2004). Ocular melanoma in a Long Evans rat. *Contemp Top Lab Anim Sci,* Vol. 43, No. 1, pp. 44-46.

Margo, C.E., Mulla, Z. & Billiris, K. (1998). Incidence of surgically treated uveal melanoma by race and ethnicity. *Ophthalmology,* Vol. 105, No. 6, pp. 1087-1090.

Marshall, J.C., Gordon, K.D., McCauley, C.S., et al. (2006). The effect of blue light exposure and use of intraocular lenses on human uveal melanoma cell lines. *Melanoma Res,* Vol. 16, No. 6, pp. 537-541.

McGill, G.G., Horstmann, M., Widlund, H.R., et al. (2002). Bcl2 regulation by the melanocyte master regulator Mitf modulates lineage survival and melanoma cell viability. *Cell,* Vol. 109, No. 6, pp. 707-718.

McLean, I.W., Saraiva, V.S. & Burnier, M.N., Jr. (2004). Pathological and prognostic features of uveal melanomas. *Can J Ophthalmol,* Vol. 39, No. 4, pp. 343-350.

Mensink, H.W., Kilic, E., Vaarwater, J., et al. (2008). Molecular cytogenetic analysis of archival uveal melanoma with known clinical outcome. *Cancer Genet Cytogenet,* Vol. 181, No. 2, pp. 108-111.

Mensink, H.W., Paridaens, D. & De Klein, A. (2009a). Genetics of uveal melanoma. *Expert Review of Ophthalmology,* Vol. 4, No. 6, pp. 607-616.

Mensink, H.W., Vaarwater, J., Kilic, E., et al. (2009b). Chromosome 3 intratumor heterogeneity in uveal melanoma. *Invest Ophthalmol Vis Sci,* Vol. 50, No. 2, pp. 500-504.

Merbs, S.L. & Sidransky, D. (1999). Analysis of p16 (CDKN2/MTS-1/INK4A) alterations in primary sporadic uveal melanoma. *Invest Ophthalmol Vis Sci,* Vol. 40, No. 3, pp. 779-783.

Mercer, K.E. & Pritchard, C.A. (2003). Raf proteins and cancer: B-Raf is identified as a mutational target. *Biochim Biophys Acta,* Vol. 1653, No. 1, pp. 25-40.

Merhavi, E., Cohen, Y., Avraham, B.C., et al. (2007). Promoter methylation status of multiple genes in uveal melanoma. *Invest Ophthalmol Vis Sci,* Vol. 48, No. 10, pp. 4403-4406.

Midena, E., Bonaldi, L., Parrozzani, R., et al. (2006). In vivo detection of monosomy 3 in eyes with medium-sized uveal melanoma using transscleral fine needle aspiration biopsy. *Eur J Ophthalmol,* Vol. 16, No. 3, pp. 422-425.

Mooy, C.M. & De Jong, P.T. (1996). Prognostic parameters in uveal melanoma: a review. *Surv Ophthalmol,* Vol. 41, No. 3, pp. 215-228.

Mooy, C.M., Van der Helm, M.J., Van der Kwast, T.H., et al. (1991). No N-ras mutations in human uveal melanoma: the role of ultraviolet light revisited. *Br J Cancer,* Vol. 64, No. 2, pp. 411-413.

Moulin, A.P., Clement, G., Bosman, F.T., et al. (2008). Methylation of CpG island promoters in uveal melanoma. *Br J Ophthalmol,* Vol. 92, No. 2, pp. 281-285.

Naus, N.C., Verhoeven, A.C., van Drunen, E., et al. (2002). Detection of genetic prognostic markers in uveal melanoma biopsies using fluorescence in situ hybridization. *Clin Cancer Res,* Vol. 8, No. 2, pp. 534-539.

Nguyen, H.G. & Ravid, K. (2006). Tetraploidy/aneuploidy and stem cells in cancer promotion: The role of chromosome passenger proteins. *J Cell Physiol,* Vol. 208, No. 1, pp. 12-22.

Olaharski, A.J., Sotelo, R., Solorza-Luna, G., et al. (2006). Tetraploidy and chromosomal instability are early events during cervical carcinogenesis. *Carcinogenesis,* Vol. 27, No. 2, pp. 337-343.

Onken, M.D., Worley, L.A., Long, M.D., et al. (2008). Oncogenic mutations in GNAQ occur early in uveal melanoma. *Invest Ophthalmol Vis Sci,* Vol. 49, No. 12, pp. 5230-5234.

Onken, M.D., Worley, L.A., Person, E., et al. (2007). Loss of heterozygosity of chromosome 3 detected with single nucleotide polymorphisms is superior to monosomy 3 for predicting metastasis in uveal melanoma. *Clin Cancer Res,* Vol. 13, No. 10, pp. 2923-2927.

Onken, M.D., Worley, L.A., Tuscan, M.D., et al. (2010). An accurate, clinically feasible multi-gene expression assay for predicting metastasis in uveal melanoma. *J Mol Diagn,* Vol. 12, No. 4, pp. 461-468.

Parrella, P., Fazio, V.M., Gallo, A.P., et al. (2003). Fine mapping of chromosome 3 in uveal melanoma: identification of a minimal region of deletion on chromosomal arm 3p25.1-p25.2. *Cancer Res,* Vol. 63, No. 23, pp. 8507-8510.

Patel, B.C., Egan, C.A., Lucius, R.W., et al. (1998). Cutaneous malignant melanoma and oculodermal melanocytosis (nevus of Ota): report of a case and review of the literature. *J Am Acad Dermatol,* Vol. 38, No. 5 Pt 2, pp. 862-865.

Patel, K.A., Edmondson, N.D., Talbot, F., et al. (2001). Prediction of prognosis in patients with uveal melanoma using fluorescence in situ hybridisation. *Br J Ophthalmol,* Vol. 85, No. 12, pp. 1440-1444.

Patel, M., Smyth, E.C., Chapman, P.B., et al. (2011). Therapeutic Implications of the Emerging Molecular Biology of Uveal Melanoma. *Clin Cancer Res,* Vol. No. pp.

Petrausch, U., Martus, P., Tonnies, H., et al. (2008). Significance of gene expression analysis in uveal melanoma in comparison to standard risk factors for risk assessment of subsequent metastases. *Eye (Lond),* Vol. 22, No. 8, pp. 997-1007.

Pollock, P.M., Harper, U.L., Hansen, K.S., et al. (2003). High frequency of BRAF mutations in nevi. *Nat Genet,* Vol. 33, No. 1, pp. 19-20.

Prescher, G., Bornfeld, N. & Becher, R. (1994). Two subclones in a case of uveal melanoma. Relevance of monosomy 3 and multiplication of chromosome 8q. *Cancer Genet Cytogenet,* Vol. 77, No. 2, pp. 144-146.

Prescher, G., Bornfeld, N., Friedrichs, W., et al. (1995). Cytogenetics of twelve cases of uveal melanoma and patterns of nonrandom anomalies and isochromosome formation. *Cancer Genet Cytogenet,* Vol. 80, No. 1, pp. 40-46.

Prescher, G., Bornfeld, N., Hirche, H., et al. (1996). Prognostic implications of monosomy 3 in uveal melanoma. *Lancet,* Vol. 347, No. 9010, pp. 1222-1225.

Romano, E., Schwartz, G.K., Chapman, P.B., et al. (2011). Treatment implications of the emerging molecular classification system for melanoma. *Lancet Oncol,* Vol. No. pp.

Saldanha, G., Purnell, D., Fletcher, A., et al. (2004). High BRAF mutation frequency does not characterize all melanocytic tumor types. *Int J Cancer,* Vol. 111, No. 5, pp. 705-710.

Schmidt-Pokrzywniak, A., Jockel, K.H., Bornfeld, N., et al. (2009). Positive interaction between light iris color and ultraviolet radiation in relation to the risk of uveal melanoma: a case-control study. *Ophthalmology,* Vol. 116, No. 2, pp. 340-348.

Schmittel, A., Bechrakis, N.E., Martus, P., et al. (2004). Independent prognostic factors for distant metastases and survival in patients with primary uveal melanoma. *Eur J Cancer,* Vol. 40, No. 16, pp. 2389-2395.

Scholes, A.G., Liloglou, T., Maloney, P., et al. (2001). Loss of heterozygosity on chromosomes 3, 9, 13, and 17, including the retinoblastoma locus, in uveal melanoma. *Invest Ophthalmol Vis Sci,* Vol. 42, No. 11, pp. 2472-2477.

Seddon, J.M., Albert, D.M., Lavin, P.T., et al. (1983). A prognostic factor study of disease-free interval and survival following enucleation for uveal melanoma. *Arch Ophthalmol,* Vol. 101, No. 12, pp. 1894-1899.

Shields, C.L., Ganguly, A., Bianciotto, C.G., et al. (2011). Prognosis of uveal melanoma in 500 cases using genetic testing of fine-needle aspiration biopsy specimens. *Ophthalmology,* Vol. 118, No. 2, pp. 396-401.

Shields, C.L., Shields, J.A., Materin, M., et al. (2001). Iris melanoma: risk factors for metastasis in 169 consecutive patients. *Ophthalmology,* Vol. 108, No. 1, pp. 172-178.

Shields, J.A., Shields, C.L., De Potter, P., et al. (1996). Diagnosis and treatment of uveal melanoma. *Semin Oncol,* Vol. 23, No. 6, pp. 763-767.

Shields, J.A., Shields, C.L. & Donoso, L.A. (1991). Management of posterior uveal melanoma. *Surv Ophthalmol,* Vol. 36, No. 3, pp. 161-195.

Shields, J.A. & Shields, S.C. (2007). *Intraocular Tumors: An Atlas and Textbook,* (second edition), Lippincott Williams & Wilkins, ISBN 978-0-7817-7580-9, Philadelphia, PA.

Singh, A.D., Bergman, L. & Seregard, S. (2005). Uveal melanoma: epidemiologic aspects. *Ophthalmol Clin North Am,* Vol. 18, No. 1, pp. 75-84, viii.

Singh, A.D., De Potter, P., Fijal, B.A., et al. (1998). Lifetime prevalence of uveal melanoma in white patients with oculo(dermal) melanocytosis. *Ophthalmology,* Vol. 105, No. 1, pp. 195-198.

Singh, A.D., Rennie, I.G., Seregard, S., et al. (2004). Sunlight exposure and pathogenesis of uveal melanoma. *Surv Ophthalmol,* Vol. 49, No. 4, pp. 419-428.

Singh, A.D., Wang, M.X., Donoso, L.A., et al. (1996). Familial uveal melanoma, III. Is the occurrence of familial uveal melanoma coincidental? *Arch Ophthalmol,* Vol. 114, No. 9, pp. 1101-1104.

Sisley, K., Doherty, R. & Cross, N.A. (2011). What hope for the future? GNAQ and uveal melanoma. *Br J Ophthalmol,* Vol. 95 No. 5 pp. 620-623.

Sisley, K., Rennie, I.G., Parsons, M.A., et al. (1997). Abnormalities of chromosomes 3 and 8 in posterior uveal melanoma correlate with prognosis. *Genes Chromosomes Cancer,* Vol. 19, No. 1, pp. 22-28.

Sisley, K., Tattersall, N., Dyson, M., et al. (2006). Multiplex fluorescence in situ hybridization identifies novel rearrangements of chromosomes 6, 15, and 18 in primary uveal melanoma. *Exp Eye Res,* Vol. 83, No. 3, pp. 554-559.

Sullivan, R.J. & Atkins, M.B. (2010). Molecular targeted therapy for patients with melanoma: the promise of MAPK pathway inhibition and beyond. *Expert Opin Investig Drugs,* Vol. 19, No. 10, pp. 1205-1216.

Travis, L.B., Curtis, R.E., Boice, J.D., Jr., et al. (1996). Second malignant neoplasms among long-term survivors of ovarian cancer. *Cancer Res,* Vol. 56, No. 7, pp. 1564-1570.

Triozzi, P.L., Eng, C. & Singh, A.D. (2008). Targeted therapy for uveal melanoma. *Cancer Treat Rev,* Vol. 34, No. 3, pp. 247-258.

Trolet, J., Hupe, P., Huon, I., et al. (2009). Genomic profiling and identification of high-risk uveal melanoma by array CGH analysis of primary tumors and liver metastases. *Invest Ophthalmol Vis Sci,* Vol. 50, No. 6, pp. 2572-2580.

Tschentscher, F., Husing, J., Holter, T., et al. (2003). Tumor classification based on gene expression profiling shows that uveal melanomas with and without monosomy 3 represent two distinct entities. *Cancer Res,* Vol. 63, No. 10, pp. 2578-2584.

Tschentscher, F., Prescher, G., Horsman, D.E., et al. (2001). Partial deletions of the long and short arm of chromosome 3 point to two tumor suppressor genes in uveal melanoma. *Cancer Res,* Vol. 61, No. 8, pp. 3439-3442.

Tucker, M.A., Shields, J.A., Hartge, P., et al. (1985). Sunlight exposure as risk factor for intraocular malignant melanoma. *N Engl J Med,* Vol. 313, No. 13, pp. 789-792.

Vajdic, C.M., Hutchins, A.M., Kricker, A., et al. (2003). Chromosomal gains and losses in ocular melanoma detected by comparative genomic hybridization in an Australian population-based study. *Cancer Genet Cytogenet,* Vol. 144, No. 1, pp. 12-17.

Vajdic, C.M., Kricker, A., Giblin, M., et al. (2002). Sun exposure predicts risk of ocular melanoma in Australia. *Int J Cancer,* Vol. 101, No. 2, pp. 175-182.

van den Bosch, T., Kilic, E., Paridaens, D., et al. (2010). Genetics of uveal melanoma and cutaneous melanoma: two of a kind? *Dermatol Res Pract,* Vol. 2010, No. pp. 360136.

van der Velden, P.A., Zuidervaart, W., Hurks, M.H., et al. (2003). Expression profiling reveals that methylation of TIMP3 is involved in uveal melanoma development. *Int J Cancer,* Vol. 106, No. 4, pp. 472-479.

van Gils, W., Kilic, E., Bruggenwirth, H.T., et al. (2008a). Regional deletion and amplification on chromosome 6 in a uveal melanoma case without abnormalities on chromosomes 1p, 3 and 8. *Melanoma Res,* Vol. 18, No. 1, pp. 10-15.

van Gils, W., Lodder, E.M., Mensink, H.W., et al. (2008b). Gene expression profiling in uveal melanoma: two regions on 3p related to prognosis. *Invest Ophthalmol Vis Sci,* Vol. 49, No. 10, pp. 4254-4262.

Van Raamsdonk, C.D., Bezrookove, V., Green, G., et al. (2009). Frequent somatic mutations of GNAQ in uveal melanoma and blue naevi. *Nature,* Vol. 457, No. 7229, pp. 599-602.

Van Raamsdonk, C.D., Griewank, K.G., Crosby, M.B., et al. (2010). Mutations in GNA11 in uveal melanoma. *N Engl J Med,* Vol. 363, No. 23, pp. 2191-2199.

Weber, A., Hengge, U.R., Urbanik, D., et al. (2003). Absence of mutations of the BRAF gene and constitutive activation of extracellular-regulated kinase in malignant melanomas of the uvea. *Lab Invest,* Vol. 83, No. 12, pp. 1771-1776.

White, J.S., McLean, I.W., Becker, R.L., et al. (2006). Correlation of comparative genomic hybridization results of 100 archival uveal melanomas with patient survival. *Cancer Genet Cytogenet,* Vol. 170, No. 1, pp. 29-39.

White, V.A., Chambers, J.D., Courtright, P.D., et al. (1998). Correlation of cytogenetic abnormalities with the outcome of patients with uveal melanoma. *Cancer,* Vol. 83, No. 2, pp. 354-359.

Wiznia, R.A., Freedman, J.K., Mancini, A.D., et al. (1978). Malignant melanoma of the choroid in neurofibromatosis. *Am J Ophthalmol,* Vol. 86, No. 5, pp. 684-687.

Wood, L.D., Parsons, D.W., Jones, S., et al. (2007). The genomic landscapes of human breast and colorectal cancers. *Science,* Vol. 318, No. 5853, pp. 1108-1113.

Wooster, R., Neuhausen, S.L., Mangion, J., et al. (1994). Localization of a breast cancer susceptibility gene, BRCA2, to chromosome 13q12-13. *Science,* Vol. 265, No. 5181, pp. 2088-2090.

Worley, L.A., Onken, M.D., Person, E., et al. (2007). Transcriptomic versus chromosomal prognostic markers and clinical outcome in uveal melanoma. *Clin Cancer Res,* Vol. 13, No. 5, pp. 1466-1471.

Ye, C.J., Liu, G., Bremer, S.W., et al. (2007). The dynamics of cancer chromosomes and genomes. *Cytogenet Genome Res,* Vol. 118, No. 2-4, pp. 237-246.

Zeschnigk, M., Tschentscher, F., Lich, C., et al. (2003). Methylation analysis of several tumour suppressor genes shows a low frequency of methylation of CDKN2A and RARB in uveal melanomas. *Comp Funct Genomics,* Vol. 4, No. 3, pp. 329-336.

Zuidervaart, W., van Nieuwpoort, F., Stark, M., et al. (2005). Activation of the MAPK pathway is a common event in uveal melanomas although it rarely occurs through mutation of BRAF or RAS. *Br J Cancer,* Vol. 92, No. 11, pp. 2032-2038.

# Part 3

# Investigational Treatments for Melanoma and Pigmentary Disorders

8

# Melanoma Immunotherapy

HT Duc
*Université Paris XI, Regulation de la Survie Cellulaire et des Allogreffes, Groupe Hospitalier Paul-Brousse, Villejuif, France*

## 1. Introduction

Although the mortality due to melanoma or malignant mutated pigment cell cancer has begun to stabilize in developed country (1, 2), the disease shows, however a substantial increased incidence which, in term of public health, represents a high burden (3-5). As well known, among the risk factors leading to melanoma there is exposition to solar ultraviolet radiation associated to sensitive genetic background (6-9). Numerous reports have shown that important key genes such as MC1R or melanocortin-1 receptor, BRAF, NRAS as well as IDH1 were mutated in melanoma (10-16). Once metastases occur, the rate of patients'5 year survival is low (17), at this stage, it was shown that melanoma develops a resistance to current chemotherapy associated to high level of apoptosis inhibition (18, 19). Treatment is becoming difficult, useless and even futile. Although new generation of drugs is in development aiming to target mutated gene expression product sustaining tumor cell proliferation, i.e., BRAF (20) there is an urgent need for novel therapeutic approaches such as cancer immunotherapy involving immune effectors specifically activated for killing tumor cells.

## 2. Stimulating antimelanoma immune effectors

Efforts toward development of cancer immunotherapy have mainly focused on the possibility to vaccinate patients for obtaining specific immune response against their own cancer. The characterization of numerous tumor associated antigens or TAAs, especially in the context of melanoma with melanoma associated antigens (MAAs) such as gp100, MAGE-1, MAGE-3, MART-1 as well as tyrosinase has allowed to derive epitopes used for inducing CTLs (cytotoxic T lymphocytes) (21-28). In most of the case, the tumor associated antigens which belong to the group of differentiation antigens shared with normal tissue, are less immunogenic than those derived from pathogen (virus, bacteria). Thus several procedures were used in order to increase the MAA's immunogenicity such as amino-acid sequence alteration, cytokine boosting. As well known, the immunogenic peptide, in general, harboring anchor residues that bind to the MHC (major histocompatibility complex) antigen presenting molecule forming a stable complex that is essential for immune cognate recognition (29). As an example, the human MHC class I, HLA-A2 bind with high affinity peptides with either leucine/methionine at position 2 or valine at position 9 in the 9-10 amino-acid sequence. Thus a substitution of anchor residues at the indicated position (2 and/or 9) by high affinity binding ones will render the modified peptide, i.e., gp100 209-217 2M (IMDQVFSV) more immunogenic than the native sequence, i.e., gp100 209-217 (ITDQVFSV) (30). In clinical trials, vaccination of patients with the modified peptide, gp100 209-217 2M has been shown to increase the number of CTL precursors recognizing not only the modified peptide, but also the native one (31). It is worth to note that, although alteration in amino-acid sequence has led to increasing the immunogenicity of the tumor associated antigenic peptide, other factors were necessary to achieve objective clinical response, i.e., the use of adjuvant and cytokine. Thus, the oil-based montanide ISA 51 or IFA (incomplete Freund's adjuvant) (32,33) being shown to stimulate immune response was frequently used (34,35) contributing to the overall T cell immune stimulation. However, as reported by Rosenberg and colleagues, the immune response leading to objective clinical response was observed only when patients received also IL-2 along with the vaccine (31). Likewise, Weber and colleagues (36), Lee and colleagues (37), have shown the implication of GMCSF (granulocyte-macrophage-colony stimulating factor) and IL-12, respectively as boosting factors that stimulated CTL response to melanoma peptides gp100, tyrosinase and MART-1.

## 3. Immune and clinical response to melanoma vaccination

Results from numerous vaccine trials using melanoma peptides in patients with either primary or metastatic resected tumors showed the presence of CTLs as measured by the release of IFN-gamma (ELISA, Elispot tests), Cr 51 cytotoxicity assay, TCR specificity assay with tetramer analysis, skin test, among other assays. However, as far as could be observed, the generated CTLs from immunization approaches were variable in their antimelanoma potency which could be ranged, in the case of gp100 vaccine, from cytotoxic only to modified peptide pulsed target, to cytotoxic to both native and modified peptide sensitized target but not melanoma, or recognizing HLA matched melanoma peptide pulsed target and finally recognizing melanomas HLA-A2+ gp100+ (38). Furthermore, the immune response did not always correlate with tumor regression, although there were indications that positive immune response obtained in ELISA and Elispot assays correlated better with prolonged relapse-free survival (35). Overall, the lack of correlation between the high proportion of positive immune response among immunized melanoma patients and objective clinical effects could be explained by the difficulty in obtaining CD8+CTLs with specific high avidities. Another possibility is that tumor cells might express low number of specific epitopes on their cell surface, or simply down regulated the MHC I presenting antigenic peptide. Another approach developed by the group led by Rosenberg consisting to isolate reactive immune effectors infiltrating the tumor (TILs or tumor infiltrating lymphocytes) which have shown to produce objective cancer regression in treated patients (39-42). The prior lymphodepletion by treatment with cyclophosphamide and fludarabine has probably enabled the persistence and the function of adoptive transferred cells. The onset of autoimmune melanocyte destruction that accompanied cancer regression is considered as the hallmark of efficient reactive effector cells that have targeted also normal tissue expressing melanocyte differentiation antigen. The efficacy of T cell transfer as reported by the Rosenberg's group in comparison with the active immunization of patients with melanoma could be explained by the fact that reactive T cells were already selected in the work of the former and the lymphodepletion has, in addition, contributed to disrupt and overcome some tolerogenic and normal homeostatic regulation.

## 4. Targeting IGF-1 based melanoma immunotherapy

### 4.1 IGF-1 as target in melanoma immunotherapy

Beside the above strategies that are essentially based on activation of immune effectors through antigenic differentiation peptides, other strategy has been explored by means of gene transfection aiming to increase tumor immunogenicity in disrupting its immune tolerance/suppression. There were for example experimental models in which gene coding for either immunogenic foreign protein such as OVA (egg albumin) or MHC-I were introduced into tumor cells making them sensitive to immune effectors (CTLs)(43-48). In the following chapter we reported results concerning the strategy that consisted to inhibit melanoma autocrine growth factor IGF-1 expression and its consequences upon the recruitment of antimelanoma immune effectors. The strategy is thus based on the use of antisense episomal vector as well as specific antibody targeting melanoma IGF-1 expression. Concerning the experimental model, the B16 melanoma cell line originated from the mouse strain C57Bl/6 (H-2b) was used (49). There are several variants derived from the B16 cell line. The most studied melanoma variants are the highly metastatic B16-F10, BL6 and the subline B78H1 (50-52). The latter one is mainly devoid of TAP2 gene as well as MHC-I K b and D b which are weakly expressed in the formers and whose expression is inducible by IFN-γ (interferon gamma).

Although widely used the B16 melanoma was subject to critics according to which it was not a good experimental model due to differences with the human counterparts, particularly the lack of some key mutations such as those found in *PTEN* and *BRAF* (53,54). In general, cancer cells are heterogeneous with constant developmental evolution and adaptation, leading to regular acquisition of several new emerging mutant phenotypes (55,56), it is therefore difficult to find out a best defined one model for studying all complex aspects relevant to the cancer biology. Nevertheless, approaches through a well known model would allow to analyze and dissect the mechanisms underlying the deregulated growth of the relevant malignant cancer type. In the present work we focused on IGF-1 expressed in melanoma which is known as the most prominent growth factor produced by the majority of cancer types. Thus, as a pleotrophic growth factor, IGF-1 plays an essential role in cellular proliferation and apoptosis inhibition (57,58). Therefore, targeting IGF-1 appeared as an effective strategy for the control of tumor development and tumor invasiveness. This strategy had been already applied to experimental models of glioma and hepatocarcinoma, leading to prevent the tumorigenicity of the former and rendering the latter less tumorigenic (59,60). In these reported studies the control exerted on tumor development as well as on tumor rejection was undoubtedly due to the action of immune effectors, since it was reported the presence of CD8+ T cells at the site of tumor rejection.

### 4.2 In vitro analyses of inhibited IGF-1 melanoma cells

As stated above, the two procedures used for inhibiting IGF-1 expression in B16 melanoma cells were transfection of tumor cells with antisense episomal vector as well as treatment with specific antibodies. The IGF-1 episomal vector harboring IGF-1 antisense cDNA was constructed as depicted in the work reported by the group led by J.Ilan from Case Western Reserve University, Cleveland, Ohio (USA) (61). Briefly, the expression vector construct, a gift from Dr Ilan, incorporated EBV (Epstein-Bar virus) replicative signals, an IGF-1 cDNA transcriptional cassette, a gene encoding nuclear antigen 1 and a metallothionein-I promoter. This construct is episomal and drive extrachrosomal replication. The vector was transfected to B16 melanoma cells by electroporation giving rise to subclones selected according to their resistance to the selective pressure of hygromycin B. It was shown that activation of the transgene leading to extinguish IGF-1 expression did not affect the viability of transfected melanoma cells (62). Concerning the treatment using specific antibodies, the B16 melanoma cells were submitted to anti-IGF-1 antibodies that were made, in the present work, from goat and available commercially (Abcys, France). Two treatment cycles in the presence of heterologous complement (rabbit) were performed and the cells that have survived were subcloned. The two IGF-1 inhibitory procedures have led to obtention of subclones showing abrogated IGF-1 expression as ascertained by immunocytochemical assays (62). Thereafter, the inhibited IGF- 1 melanoma cells were submitted to analyses concerning mainly their morphology as well as the expression of their cell surface molecules in comparison to parental cells. It was shown that the inhibited IGF-1 B16 did not reveal noticeable difference with parental cells relevant to their morphology, their in vitro growth in culture as well as their adherence properties. It is worth to note that results reported from studies of C6 glioma have indicated a slight difference in the morphology between wild-type and transfected cells, at least in the early period of cell culture (61). Concerning the expression of cell surface molecules, studies were focused on those involved in immune activation, mainly the MHC-I and B7.1, as well as in cellular interactions such as the family members of integrin and tetraspanin molecules. From the results obtained, it was shown that the expression of molecules known for their implication in the immune activation processes remained unmodified (62). The results obtained were thus different from previously observed when glioblastoma C6 and hepatoma LF were transfected with antisense IGF-1 vector. Indeed, in these studies, the IGF-1 modified cells exhibited either an upregulation of MHC-I and B7.1 expression (glioma C6 cells) (63) or a strong increase of MHC-I expression (hepatoma LF cells) (62).

Among the group of molecules involved in cellular interaction, an alteration in the expression of the tetraspanin CD9 but not CD81 was essentially observed. The expression of the integrin α4/CD49d remained unchanged. The fact that only one member of the tetraspanin family molecules was affected is of interest and suggested that the tetraspanin CD9 and CD81 followed different pathways in their expression. It is worth to note the implication of CD9 but not CD81 in the cancer process as reported elsewhere (64).

### 4.3 In vivo tumor development of inhibited IGF-1 melanoma cells

The potential of inhibited IGF-1 B16 modified melanoma cells to develop into solid tumors in vivo were assessed (62). 25X1000 cells from either inhibited IGF-1 or parental cells were thus subscutaneously injected to C57BL/6 mice, their syngeneic host. The development of injected cell suspensions into solid tumors was followed up by regular examination and measures using a caliper. It was shown that solid tumors were developed in syngeneic hosts with a delay when modified B16 cells inhibited in their IGF-1 expression were injected as compared to the parental counterparts. The difference was significant and resulted in tumors with a mean size smaller than that of parental cells in the interval of time starting from the cell injection to the first apparition of lethal tumors which were observed in all recipients of injected parental cells. On the other hand, a proportion of 40-50% of recipients injected with modified B16 cells (IGF-1 inhibited) survived free of tumor for more than three months while no survival was observed among the recipients of parental cells.

### 4.4 Characterization of immune effectors stimulated by modified melanoma cells exhibiting inhibited IGF-1 expression

The fact that modified (IGF-1 inhibited) B16 cells developed solid tumors in syngeneic hosts with an aggressiveness lesser than parental cells suggested the presence of effector elements in host organisms controlling the outgrowth of modified cells (62). Since there was no difference between parental and inhibited IGF-1 B16 modified cells related to their in vitro cell culture expansion and their in vivo growth in immunocompromised recipients (NOD-SCID mice) (Nguyen et.al., unpublished results), it was assumed that tumor development from modified B16 cells in syngeneic host was regulated by adaptive immune effectors. In order to characterize the immune effectors controlling in vivo tumor development, experiments were performed using melanoma cells, either from inhibited IGF-1 or parental type, for vaccinating syngeneic immunocompetent hosts (65). The two types of melanoma cells were first blocked by mytomycin C treatment or by several frozen and thawed cycles. The blocked cells were subsequently injected to C57Bl/6 mice in vaccination purpose. The spleen cells and the sera from vaccinated animals harvested 10-15 days after were assessed for their effects upon B16 tumor cells in comparison to that of control untreated animals . The results obtained with the serum collected from mice vaccinated with parental cells showed no difference with the control serum from untreated animals. On the contrary, the serum collected from mice vaccinated with modified (IGF-1 inhibited) cells revealed the presence of antibodies that recognized not only modified, IGF-1 inhibited B16 cells but also their parental counterparts. This aspect was essentially observed in cytometry (FACS) analyses as well as in cytotoxic assays. Thus, in cytometry analyses the mean fluorescence obtained with serum from mice vaccinated with modified cells was 7-9 fold higher as compared to that obtained with serum from mice injected with parental B16 cells which was not different to the results from normal serum. Moreover, only serum collected from mice vaccinated with modified B16 cells exhibited cytotoxic activities against melanoma cells in the presence of heterologous (rabbit) complement, while practically no cytotoxic effects were observed with serum from mice injected with parental cells. Concerning the cellular effectors, in vitro cytotoxic assays showed that spleen cells harvested from mice injected with modified, IGF-1 inhibited B16 cells were able to kill melanoma cells, either of parental or modified type. On the contrary, melanoma cells were not affected by the presence of spleen cells from mice injected with parental cells as well as with spleen cells from normal untreated mice (65).

These immune, humoral and cellular effector elements were also analyzed for their effects on the in vivo tumor development. In these in vivo assays, serum or spleen cells from mice vaccinated either with parental or modified, inhibited IGF-1 cells were injected together with melanoma cells to syngeneic hosts. Results obtained have shown that only spleen cells but not the immune serum from mice vaccinated with modified, IGF-1 inhibited B16 cells were able to control the tumor development in syngeneic hosts. No effect on tumor growth was observed with the spleen cells from mice vaccinated with parental cells or spleen cells from control untreated mice as well as their serum (65, 66). The discrepancy between the in vitro and in vivo, humoral and cellular results concerning the case of mice vaccinated with modified-inhibited IGF-1 cells could be explained by the cell surface movement or capping phenomenon which could mask the antibody to ADCC/complement fixing lysis. Another alternative could be relevant to the short half-life of antibody molecules compared to cellular effectors that would persist longer in the syngeneic host organisms.

Experiments were further performed for characterizing the active anti-tumor cell population(s) from spleen cells of mice vaccinated with modified, IGF-1 inhibited B16 cells. The above immune spleen cell suspension was thus submitted to negative selection by means of protein A - sepharose beads coated with specific antibody to CD4, CD8, NK (NK1.1), CD25, Ig (Immunoglobulin) and B220. It was shown that the anti-tumor activity was affected when spleen cell population was incubated with anti-CD8 antibody coated beads and removed from the cell suspension. The treatment of spleen cell suspension with other antibody-coated beads did not affect its anti-melanoma activity, indicating that spleen CD8+ T cells were the main immune effectors controlling in vivo melanoma development (66).

## 5. References

[1] Linos E, Swetter SM, Cockburn MG, Colditz MG, Clarke CA (2009) Increasing burden of melanoma in the United States. J Invest Dermatol 129:1666-74.

[2] Criscione VD, Weinstock MA (2010) Melanoma thickness trends in the Unites States, 1988-2006. J Invest Dermatol 130:793-797.

[3] Lipsker D, Engel F, Cribier B, Velten M, Hedelin G (2007) Trends in melanoma epidemiology suggest three different types of melanoma. Br J Dermatol 157:338-343.

[4] Tejera-Vaquerizo A, Mendiola-Fernandez M, Fernandez Orland A, Herrera-Ceballos E (2008) Thick melanoma: the problem continues. J Eur Acad Dermatol Venereol 22:575-579.

[5] Thompson JF, Scolyer RA, Kefford RF (2005) Cutaneous melanoma. Lancet 365:687-701.

[6] Curtin JA, Fridlyand J, Kageshita T, Patel HN, Busam KJ, et.al. (2005) Distinct sets of genetic alternatives in melanoma. N Engl J Med 353:2135-2147.

[7] Whiteman DC, Stickley M, Watt P, Hughes MC, Davis MB, Green AC (2006) Anatomic site, sun exposure, and risk of cutaneous melanoma. J Clin Oncol 24:3172-3177.

[8] Thomas NE, Edmiston SN, Alexander A, Millikan RC, et.al. (2007) Number of nevi and early-life ambient UV exposure are associated with BRAF-mutant melanoma. Cancer Epidemiol Biomarkers Prev 16:991-997.

[9] Hacker E, Hayward NK, Dumenil T, James MR and Whiteman DC (2010) The association between MC1R genotype and BRAF mutation status in cutaneous melanoma: findings from an Australian population. J Invest Dermatol 130:241-248.

[10] Davies H, Bignell GR, Cox C et.al. (2002) Mutations of the BRAF gene in human cancer. Nature 417:949-954.

[11] Omholt K, Karsberg S, Platz A et.al. (2002) Screening of N-ras codon 61 mutations in paired primary and metastatic cutaneous melanomas: mutations occur early and persist throughout tumor progression. Clin Cancer Res 8:3468-3474.

[12] Pollock PM, Harper UL, Hansen KS, Yudt LM, et.al. (2003) High frequency of BRAF mutations in nevi. Nat Genet 33:19-20.

[13] Gorden A, Osman I, Gay W et.al. (2003) Analysis of BRAF and N-RAS mutations in metastatic melanoma tissues. Cancer Res 63:3955-3957.

[14] De Snoo FA, Hayward NK (2005) Cutaneous melanoma susceptibility and progression genes. Cancer Lett 230:153-186.

[15] Landi MT, Bauer J, Pfeiffer RM, Elder DE et.al. (2006) MC1R germline variants confer risk for BRAF-mutant melanoma. Science 313:521-522.

[16] Shibata T, Kokubu A, Miyamoto M, Sasajima, Yamazaki N (2011) Mutant IDH1 confers an in vivo growth in a melanoma cell line with BRAF mutation. Am J Pathol 178:1395-1402.

[17] Baleh CM, Soong SJ, Gershenwald JE et.al. (2001) Pronostic factors analysis of 17,600 melanoma patients: validation of the American Joint Committee on Cancer melanoma staging system. J. Clin Oncol 19:3622-3634.

[18] Emanuel PO, Phelps RG, Mudgil A et.al. (2008) Immunohistochemical detection of XIAP in melanoma. J Cutan Pathol 35:292-297.

[19] Hiscutt E, Hill DS, Martin S, Kerr R et.al. (2010) Targeting X-linked inhibitor of apoptosis protein to increase the efficacity of endoplasmic reticulum stress-induced apoptosis for melanoma therapy. J Invest Dermatol 130:2250-2258.

[20] Bollag G, Hirth P, Tsai J, Zhang J et.al. (2010) Clinical efficacy of a RAF inhibitor needs broad target blockade in BRAF-mutant melanoma. Nature 467:596-599.

[21] Boon T, Gajewski TF, Coulie PG. (1995) From defined human tumor antigens to effective immunisation ? Immunol Today 16:334-336.

[22] Boon T, van der Bruggen. (1996) Human tumor antigens recognized by T lymphocytes. J Exp Med 183:725-729.

[23] De Plaen E, Lurkin C, Lethe B, van der Bruggen P et al. (1997) Identification of genes coding for tumor antigens recognized by cytotoxic T lymphocytes. Methods 12:125-142.

[24] Kawakami Y, Eliyahu S, Sakaguchi K, Robbins F et al. (1994) Identification of the immunodominant peptides of the MART-1 human melanoma antigen recognized by the majority of HLA-A2-restricted tumor infiltrating lymphocytes. J Exp Med 180: 347-352.

[25] Kawakami Y, Eliyahu S, Jennings C, et al. (1995) Recognition of multiple epitopes in the human melanoma antigen gp100 by tumor infiltrating T lymphocytes associated with in vivo tumor regression. J Immunol 154:3961-3968.

[26] Kawakami Y, Robbins PF, Wang X, Tupesis JP, et al. (1998) Identification of new melanoma epitopes on melanosomal proteins recognized by tumor infiltrating T lymphocytes restricted by HLA-A1, -A2 and –A3 alleles. J Immunol 161: 6985-6992.

[27] Kawakami Y. (2000) New cancer therapy by immunomanipulation : development of immunotherapy for human melanoma as a model system. Cornea 19: S2-6.

[28] Rosenberg SA, (1995) The devepment of new cancer therapies based on the molecular identification of cancer regression antigens. Cancer J Sci Am 1:90-100.

[29] Rammensee HG, Falk K, Rotzschke O. (1993) MHC molecules as peptide receptors. Curr Opin Immunol 5:35-44.

[30] Parkhurst MR, Salgaller ML, Southwood S, Robbins PF, et al. ( 1996) Improved induction of melanoma-reactive CTL with peptides from the melanoma antigen gp100 modified at HLA A 0201-binding residues. J Immunol 157: 2539-2548.

[31] Rosenberg SA, Yang JC, Schwartzentruber DJ, Hwu P, et al. (1998) Immunologic and therapeutic evaluation of a synthetic peptide vaccine for the treatment of patients with metastatic melanoma. Nat Med 4: 321-327.

[32] Aucouturier J, Dupuis L, Deville S, Ascarateil S, et al. (2002) Montanide ISA 720 and 51 : A new generation of water-in-oil emulsions adjuvants for humans vaccines. Expert Rev Vaccines 1:111-118.

[33] Hioe CE, Qui H, Chend PD, Bian Z, et al. (1996) Comparison of adjuvant formulations for cytotoxic T cell induction using synthetic peptides. Vaccines 14: 412-418.

[34] Walker EB, Haley D, Miller W, Floyd K et al. (2004) gp100 209-2M peptide immunization of human lymphocyte antigen-A2+ stage I-III melanoma patients induces significant increase in antigen-specific effector and long-term memory CD8+ T cells. Clin Cancer Res 10:668-680.

[35] Wang F, Bade E, Kuniyoshi C, Spears L, et al. (1999) Phase I trial of a MART-1 peptide vaccine with incomplete Freund's adjuvant for resected high-risk melanoma. Clin Cancer Res 5:2756-2765.

[36] Weber J, Sondak VK, Scotland R, Phillip R, et al. (2003) Granulocyte-macrophage-colony-stimulating factor added to a multiple vaccine for resected stage II melanoma. Cancer 97:186-200.

[37] Lee P, Wang F, Kuniyoshi J, et al. (2001) Effects of interleukin-12 on the immune response to a multiple vaccine for resected metastatic melanoma. J Clin Oncol 19:3836-3847.

[38] Yang S, Linette GP, Longerich S, Haluska G. (2002) Antimelanoma activity of CTL generated from peripheral blood mononuclear cells after stimulation with autologous dendritic cells pulsed with melanoma gp100 peptide G209-2M is correlated to TCR avidity. J Immunol 169:531-539.

[39] Rosenberg SA, Packard BS, Aebersold PM, Solomon D et.al. (1988) Use of infiltrating lymphocytes and interleukin-2 in the immunotherapy of patients with metastatic melanoma. A preliminary report. N Engl J Med 319:1676-1680.

[40] Topalian SL, Solomon D, Rosenberg SA (1989) Tumor-specific cytolysis by lymphocytes infiltrating human melanomas. J Immunol 142:3714-3725.

[41] Dudley ME, Wunderlich JR, Robbins PF, Yang JC et.al. (2002) Cancer regression and autoimmunity in patients after clonal repopulation with antitumor lymphocytes. Science 298:850-854.

[42] Hussein MR (2005) Tumour-infiltrating lymphocytes and melanoma tumorigenesis: an insight. Br J Dermatol 153:18-21

[43] Falo Jr LD, Kovacsovics-Bankowski M, Thompson K, Rock KL (1995) Targeting antigen into the phagocytic pathway in vivo induces protective tumour immunity. Nat Med 1:649- 653.

[44] Gorelik E, Peppoloni S, Overton R, Herberman R (1985) Increase in H-2 antigen expression and immunogenicity of BL6 melanoma cells treated with n-methyl-N'-nitro-N- nitrosoguanidine. Cancer Res 45:5341-5347.

[45] Pogador A, Feldman M, Eisenbach L (1989) H-2 Kb transfection of B16 melanoma cells results in reduced tumorigenicity and metastatic competence. J Immunogenet 16:291-303.

[46] Feldman M, Eisenbach L (1991) MHC class I genes controlling the metastatic phenotype of tumor cells. Semin Cancer Biol 2:337-346.

[47] Kim M, Duty L, Herberman R, Gorelik E (1994) Divergent effects of H-2k and H-2d genes on sensitivity of BL6 melanoma cells to NK cells or TNF-mediated cytotoxicity. Cell Immunol 155:358-371.

[48] Chiang EY, Henson M, Stroynowski I (2003) Correlation of defects responsible for impaired Qa-2 class I b MHC expression on melanoma cells protects mice from tumor growth. J Immunol 170:4515-4523.

[49] Fidler IJ. (1975) Biological behavior of malignant melanoma cells correlated to their survival in vivo. Cancer Res 35:218-24.

[50] Fidler IJ. (1973). The relationship of embolic homogeneity, number, size and viability to the incidence of experimental metastasis. Eur J cancer 9:223-227.

[51] Hart IR (1979). The selection and characterization of an invasive variant of the B16 melanoma. Am J Pathol 97:587-600.

[52] De Giovanni C, Palmieri G, Nicoletti G, Landuzzi L, Scotlandi K, Bontadini A (1991). Immunological and non-immunological influence of H-2Kb gene transfection on the metastatic ability of B16 melanoma cells. Int J Cancer 48:270-6.

[53] Herlyn M, Fukunaga-Kalabis M (2010) What is a good model for melanoma? J Invest Dermatol 130:911-912.

[54] Dankort D, Curley DP, Cartlidge RA et al. (2009) Braf (V600E) cooperates with Pten loss to induce metastatic melanoma. Nat Genet 41:544-552.

[55] Wang Y, Tan XH, DiGiovanna JJ et al. (2010) genetic diversity in melanoma metastases from a patient with xeroderma pigmentosum. J Invest Dermatol 130:1188-1191.

[56] Perego M, Tortoreto M, Tragni G et al. (2010) Heterogeneous phenotype of human melanoma cells with in vitro and in vivo features of tumor-initiating cells. J Invest Dermatol 130:1877-1886.

[57] Froesch ER, Schmid C, Schwander J, Zapf J (1985) Actions of insulin-like growth factors. Ann Rev Physiol 47:443-467.

[58] Humbel RE (1990) Insulin-like growth factors I and II. Eur J Biochem 190:445-462.

[59] Trojan J, Johnson TR, Rudin SD, Ilan J, Tylocinski ML (1993) Treatment and prevention of rat glioblastoma by immunogenic C6 cells expressing antisense insulin-like growth factor I RNA. Science 259:94-97.

[60] Lafarge-Frayssinet C, Duc HT, Frayssinet C, Sarasin A, Anthony D et al. (1997) Antisense insulin-like growth factor I transferred into a rat hepatoma cell line inhibits tumorigenesis by modulating major histocompatibility complex I cell surface expression. Cancer Gene Ther 4:276-285.

[61] Trojan J, Blossey BK, Johnson TR et al. (1992) Loss of tumorigenicity of rat glioblastoma directed by episome-based antisense cDNA transcription of insulin-like growth factor I. Proc Natl Acad Sci USA 89:4874-4879.

[62] Trabado S, Nguyen Van Binh P, Martin C et al. (2006) Modulated expression of cell surface molecules and in vivo outgrowth of modified melanoma cells. Biomed Pharmacother 60:693-697.

[63] Trojan J, Duc HT, Upegui-Gonzales LC, Hor F et al. (1996) Presence of MHC-I and B7 molecules in rat and human glioma cells expressing antisense IGF-1 mRNA. Neurosci Lett 212:9-12.

[64] Boucheix C, Huynh Thien Duc G, Jasmin C, Rubinstein E (2001) Tetraspanins and malignancy. Expert Reviews in molecular medicine.

[65] Trabado C, Nguyen Van Binh P, Martin C et al. (2007) Stimulation of anti-melanoma immune effectors via modified tumor cells exhibiting inhibited IGF-1 and low CD9. Biomed Pharmacother 61:494-498.

[66] Nguyen van Binh P, Trabado S, Lafarge-Frayssinet C et al] (2011) In Vitro and in vivo analyses of immune effectors stimulated by B16 melanoma cells exhibiting inhibited IGF-1 expression. Sumitted for publication.

# 9

# Melanin Hyperpigmentation Inhibitors from Natural Resources

Hideaki Matsuda, Kazuya Murata, Kimihisa Itoh,
Megumi Masuda and Shunsuke Naruto
*Faculty of Pharmacy, Kinki University*
*Japan*

## 1. Introduction

In Oriental countries, such as China, Korea and Japan, a female beauty criterion since ancient times has been a face with fair skin, and the admiration of women with young, healthy, bright and fair skin has created a whitening cosmetics market. The color of human skin and hair is determined by a number of factors. Biosynthesis of the melanin pigment, namely melanogenesis, is the most important factor. Melanogenesis is a multistage process involving melanin synthesis, melanin transport, and melanosome release. Tyrosinase is one of the key enzymes in the melanin biosynthetic pathway. Abnormal deposition of the melanin pigment causes hyperpigmentary disorders.

From natural sources, a number of ingredients with an inhibitory effect on melanin hyperpigmentation have been found, and some of them were developed as cosmetic agents and over the counter (OTC) drugs in Oriental countries. On the other hand, some medicinal chemists have recently paid a lot of attention to inhibitors of melanin production to prevent hyperpigmentary disorders such as melasma, freckles and age spots. To develop novel and useful cosmetic agents, supplements, functional foods and OTC drugs, we have continued to research regulators of melanin production from natural sources since 1980. We describe here our screening strategy and studies on targeted melanin hyperpigmentation inhibitors from natural plant sources, *e.g.* Umbelliferae, Ericaceae, Rubiaceae, Piperaceae and Rutaceae plants. Interesting findings originating from the screening results are also described.

## 2. The search for cosmetic whitening agents from Chinese herbal medicine

### 2.1 Literature search for cosmetic whitening agents in ancient Chinese herbal books

Recently, a retrospective search for cosmetic agents from traditional crude drugs including plants, animals, and inorganic compounds has become a global trend. Traditional application of herbs and biological components of animals to cosmetics and OTC drugs is based on long experience under the expectation that they exert the attributed physiological action. The historical application of Chinese crude drugs to cosmetics has been described in detail in many ancient Chinese herbal books and literature. Since some herbs used for cosmetics, such as flowers of *Carthamus tinctorius* (safflower) and the juice of *Aloe ferox* (aloe), have been used as crude drugs for thousands of years all over the world, knowledge and experience of these herbs have been accumulated.

The first strategy involves a literature search of ancient Chinese books of traditional Chinese herbal medicine to select target herbs which may have the desired biological activity. Herbs having an injury care effect, blood circulation improvement effect and anti-microbial activity could be applied to cosmetic agents with the expectation that they could exert the attributed activity. It was found that about 200 formulas for cosmetics which could be used to beautify a woman's face were listed in several ancient Chinese books of traditional Chinese herbal medicine about 1,500 years ago. A number of dosage delivery forms, such as creams, lotions, pastes, cologne water, suspensions, and emulations, as well some used in modern cosmetics, for external use are found in these 200 formulas. Several Chinese crude drugs, such as seeds of *Euphorbia lathyris* (caper spurge), flowers of *Prunus salicina* (Chinese plum), seeds of *Adenanthera pavonina* (red sandalwood tree), seeds of *Gleditsia japonica* (honey locust), rhizomes of *Kaempferia galangal* (galangale), and seeds of *Cuscuta japonica* were used as medicines for external use or cosmetics to prevent stains and freckles accompanied by hyperpigmentation. As a result of our literature search, Chinese herbs originating from Umbelliferae plants, *e.g.* roots of *Angelica dahurica* (angelica dahurica root), rhizomes of *Cnidium officinalis* (cnidium rhizome), roots of *Angelica acutiloba* (Japanese angelica root), roots and rhizomes of *Saposhnikovia divaricate* (saposhnikovia root), were most frequently listed for the prevention of hyperpigmentation in the 200 formulas for cosmetics described above. An example of the description of Umbelliferae plants which were used to beautify a woman's face in an ancient Chinese herbal book written in Chinese characters is illustrated in Fig. 1.

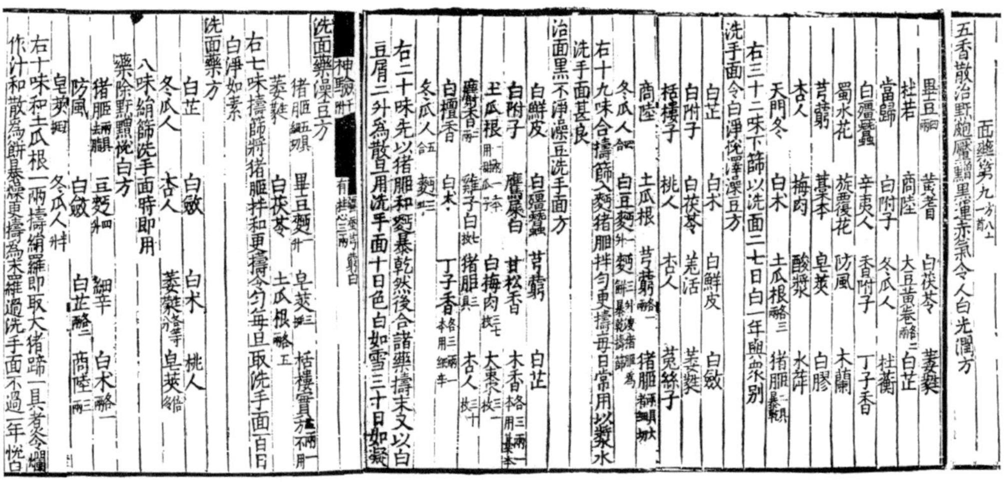

Fig. 1. Description of Umbelliferae plants used to beautify a woman's face in an ancient Chinese herbal book

## 2.2 Tyrosinase inhibitory activity of Umbelliferae plants

Tyrosinase catalyzes the oxidation of L-tyrosine to 3,4-dihydroxyphenyl-L-alanine (L-DOPA), followed by the oxidation of L-DOPA to dopaquinone, and oxidative polymerization of several dopaquinone derivatives produces melanin. Thus, the tyrosinase inhibitor is one of candidates for reducing melanogenesis.

In order to find novel ingredients for whitening cosmetics from natural resources, the effect of test samples on melanogenesis was assayed by using mushroom tyrosinase and/or cultured murine B16 melanoma cells (B16 melanoma cells) as the first screening (Mason & Peterson, 1965). On the basis of the first screening results of the selected herbs followed by pharmacological tests, we further examined whether the herbs and their active constituents could be used as cosmetic agents.

From 200 formulas for cosmetics which could be used to beautify a woman's face in the ancient Chinese books of the traditional Chinese herbal medicine, 22 crude drugs were selected as they were most frequently listed in the cosmetics formulas. We examined the tyrosinase inhibitory activity of 50% methanolic extract of the selected 22 crude drugs. Among them, 11 crude drugs originating from Umbelliferae plants exhibited relatively potent tyrosinase inhibitory activity compared to other crude drugs as shown in Table 1 (Masamoto et al., 1980). Although the inhibitory activity of the cited plants was not superior to that of the plants whose potent tyrosinase inhibitory activities have been reported, Umbelliferae plants are generally aromatic, and some of them improve blood circulation and have anti-inflammatory activity. Because of these characteristic physical and pharmacological properties, Umbelliferae plants seemed to be favorable for cosmetics, and were frequently used in the ancient cosmetics formula described in the ancient Chinese herbal books.

| Plant name | Parts | $IC_{50}$ (mg/ml)* |
|---|---|---|
| *Glebnia littoralis* | root | 1.2 |
| *Angelica acutiloba* var. *sugiyamae* | root | 1.8 |
| *Notopterygium forbesii* | rhizome | 3.0 |
| *Peucedanum praeruptorum* | root | 4.4 |
| *Angelica pubescens* | root | 5.1 |
| *Bupleurum falcatum* | root | 5.5 |
| *Ledebouriella seseloides* | root | 6.3 |
| *Ligusticum wallichii* | rhizome | 6.3 |
| *Ligusticum sinense* | rhizome and root | 7.0 |
| *Angelica acutiloba* | root | 7.0 |
| *Cnidium officinale* | rhizome | 9.6 |

Table 1. $IC_{50}$ values of tyrosinase inhibitory activities of 50% methanolic extract obtained from crude Umbelliferae drugs (*; $IC_{50}$ values are indicated as relevant to the concentration of dried crude drugs. *Ref.*; Masamoto et al., 1980)

## 3. The search for cosmetic whitening agents from Alpine plants

### 3.1 Tyrosinase inhibitory activity of Ericaceae plants

Considering the growing environment and characteristic constituents of plants provides another approach to look for novel tyrosinase inhibitors. The second strategy is based on the following consideration. Plants growing in high mountain regions or at the coast of islands in the South Pacific receive stronger solar ultraviolet (UV) radiation all year round than plants growing in other regions, and thus the former plants may have a specific biological self defense system against harmful UV radiation, such as anti-oxidative systems and biosynthesis of several pigments. It has been reported that superoxide dismutase (SOD) is one of the key factors that reduce melanin production caused by UV radiation. These facts

indicate that the anti-oxidative system may play an important role in the regulation of melanogenesis in humans, and that tyrosinase inhibitors with SOD-like activity and/or anti-oxidant activity may be useful ingredients in the field of whitening cosmetics (Tobin & Thody, 1994). Thus, anti-oxidative activity, *e.g.* the SOD-like activity, of some samples was assayed by various methods.
Ericaceae plants grow in arid zones of sub-high mountain regions rich in solar UV radiation. Bearberry (*Arctostaphylos uva-ursi*) was selected from the Ericaceae plants as a screening target because its leaves have historically been used as an anti-septic for the urinary tract in Europe and Japan. A 50% methanolic extract of bearberry leaves showed dose-dependent tyrosinase inhibitory activity. Activity-guided fractionation of the extract led to isolation of arbutin as an active component (Matsuda et al., 1992a). Arbutin (Fig. 2), a major constituent of bearberry, showed a weak tyrosinase inhibitory activity. The activity of the bearberry leaf extract was not fully explained by arbutin, so the extract may have contained other unidentified active components.

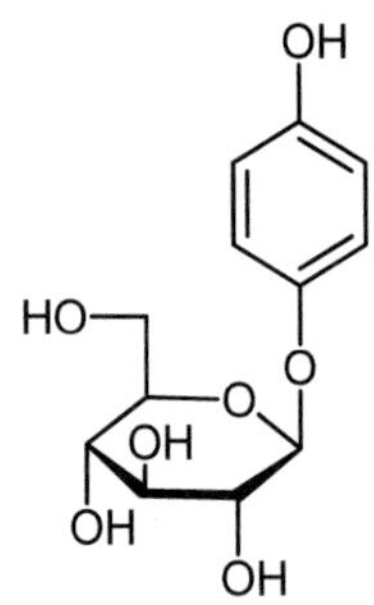


Fig. 2. Arbutin

In order to find a more potent tyrosinase inhibitor than bearberry leaf, the activity of 50% ethanolic leaf extracts obtained from five plants of the genus of *Arctostaphylos e.g. A. patula* (greenleaf manzanita), *A. viscida* (whiteleaf manzanita), *A. canescens* (hoary manzanita), *A. columbiana* (hairy manzanita), and *A. nevadensis* (pinemat manzanita), growing in a sub-high mountain region of North America was assayed (Matsuda et al., 1996). Simultaneously, the SOD-like activity of the five extracts was tested. All exhibited similar SOD-like activity, and the tyrosinase inhibitory activities of the extracts of *A. patula* and *A. viscida* were slightly more potent than that of *A. uva-ursi*, as shown in Table 2. These results indicated that the leaves of *A. uva-ursi*, *A. patula* and *A. viscida* may be useful agents for whitening cosmetics, and it is expected that further screening of Alpine plants may lead to more potent cosmetic whitening agents.

| Plants | Tyrosinase inhibitory activity ($IC_{50}$, μg/ml) | SOD-like activity ($IC_{50}$, μg/ml) |
|---|---|---|
| *A. patula* | 133 | 15.8 |
| *A. viscida* | 145 | 16.0 |
| *A. nevadensis* | 243 | 10.8 |
| *A. columbiana* | 246 | 11.5 |
| *A. canescens* | 226 | 15.3 |
| *A. uva-ursi* | 191 | 19.4 |

Table 2. $IC_{50}$ values of tyrosinase inhibitory and SOD-like activities of 50% methanolic extract from various Arctostaphylos plants (*Ref.*; Matsuda et al., 1996)

### 3.2 The application of cosmetic agents to OTC drugs

Adrenocortical steroids are externally used in the treatment of allergic and atopic dermatitis. These steroid drugs show excellent efficacy, but the long term external use of steroid drugs cause several adverse effects such as skin pigmentation. Although the pigmentation mechanism affected by steroids has not been fully elucidated, some agents with tyrosinase inhibitory and/or anti-oxidant activity may be useful in the prevention of pigmentation.

Bearberry leaf exhibited both tyrosinase inhibitory and anti-oxidative activities as described above. A Japanese lady who visited a Chinese medicinal pharmacy in Osaka told us that her allergic skin eruption caused by hair dye was improved by washing her face with an aqueous extract of bearberry leaf. This information prompted us to examine anti-allergic and anti-inflammatory activities of aqueous extract of bearberry leaf. We investigated the effect of external application of an ointment containing 1 and 2% of bearberry leaf extract to allergic and inflammatory model rodents in comparison with an ointment of 0.005% and 0.025% of dexamethazone, a steroid with potent anti-inflammatory activity (Matsuda et al., 1992b). Bearberry leaf extract did not show anti-allergic and anti-inflammatory activities. However, in the case of external application of a combination ointment of the bearberry extract and dexamethazone, the bearberry extract enhanced the anti-allergic and anti-inflammatory activities of dexamethazone via a synergistic effect without enhancement of adverse effects caused by the steroid. Based on these pharmacological results, Berrybear® ointment was launched on the Japanese OTC drug market after clinical trials by Daiichi Seiyaku Co. Ltd. (present affiliation: Daiichi Sankyo Co. Ltd.) in 2005.

## 4. The search for cosmetic whitening agents from plants in the South Pacific

It was thought that the plants growing at the coast of islands in the South Pacific may have a specific self-defense system against solar UV radiation. Therefore, we looked for cosmetic whitening agents from such plants. We collected a number of plants including tropical and folk medicinal plants at Palau island (The Republic of Palau), Fiji islands (The Republic of Fiji Islands), Tongatapu island (The Kingdom of Tonga), 'Eua island (The Kingdom of Tonga), and Tahiti (French Polynesia) under the approval of the respective governments. Tyrosinase inhibitory activity of the extracts obtained from the collected 150 plants was assayed. Among them, noni (*Morinda citrifolia*, Rubiaceae) was selected for further investigation to find novel cosmetic whitening agents. We simultaneously examined the effect of these extracts on melanogenesis in B16 melanoma cells. In the screening, the extract of kava (rhizome of *Piper methysticum*, Piperaceae) was found to stimulate melanogenesis in B16 melanoma cells, as described in the section 4.2.

### 4.1 *Morinda citrifolia* (Noni)

The fruit, roots, bark and leaves of a tropical tree, *Morinda citrifolia*, commonly known as "noni" in Hawaii and Tahiti, have long been used throughout Polynesia as a folk medicine in the treatment of many diseases, *e.g.* hypertension and diabetes. Recently, the juice of the noni fruit and tea made from noni leaves have been launched on the functional food market. Since noni fruit contains a lot of seeds in its flesh, these seeds are removed and discarded during the production process of noni fruit juice. Consequently, we focused on the utility value of noni seeds.

We examined the tyrosinase inhibitory activity and anti-oxidant activity of 50% ethanolic extracts of the fruit flesh, leaves, and seeds of noni, respectively (Masuda et al., 2009). As for anti-oxidant activity, 1,1-diphenyl-2-picrylhydrazyl (DPPH) radical scavenging activities of the extracts were tested. A 50% ethanolic extract from noni seeds (MCS-ext) showed more potent inhibition of tyrosinase and DPPH radical scavenging activities than extracts of noni leaves or flesh. Activity-guided fractionation followed by chromatography of MCS-ext led to the isolation of 3,3′-bisdemethylpinoresinol, americanin A, and quercetin as active constituents with both tyrosinase inhibitory and radical scavenging activities. Americanin A and quercetin also showed SOD-like activity (Table 3 and Fig. 3). In addition, MCS-ext exhibited potent *in vitro* inhibition of elastase, and ursolic acid was a major active constituent of MCS-ext. UV irradiation promotes photoaging of human skin. Chronic UV exposure denatures collagen and elastic fibers in the dermis and induces wrinkles in human skin. In the process of photoaging of human skin, neutrophils play an important role. They infiltrate the skin and release active enzymes such as human leukocyte elastase (HLE), which cleaves the helix structure of type I collagen and then degrades elastic fibers in human skin. Therefore, HLE inhibitors may be useful ingredients for prevention of skin wrinkles. MCS-ext was found to contain, tyrosinase inhibitory, anti-oxidant, and HLE inhibitory active constituents, namely 3,3′-bisdemethylpinoresinol, americanin A, quercetin and ursolic acid. These findings suggested that noni seeds could be a useful ingredient in cosmetics for whitening and/or wrinkle-prevention.

| Samples | Tyrosinase inhibitory activity (mM) | SOD-like activity (μM or U/ml) | Radical-scavenging activity (μM) |
|---|---|---|---|
| Americanin A | 2.7 | 170 μM | 11 |
| 3,3′-Bisdemethylpinoresinol | 0.3 | N.E. | 4 |
| Quercetin | 0.1 | 30 μM | 6 |
| Kojic acid | 0.03 | N.D. | N.D. |
| Arbutin | 83.3 | N.D. | N.D. |
| Superoxide dismutase (SOD) | N.D. | 0.3 U/ml | N.D. |
| L-Ascorbic acid | N.D. | N.D. | 23 |

Table 3. $IC_{50}$ values of tyrosinase inhibitory, SOD-like, and radical-scavenging activities of americanin A, 3,3′-bisdemethylpinoresinol, quercetin, kojic acid, arbutin, superoxide dismutase and L-ascorbic acid (N.D.; Not determined. N.E.; No effect. *Ref.*; Masuda et al., 2009)

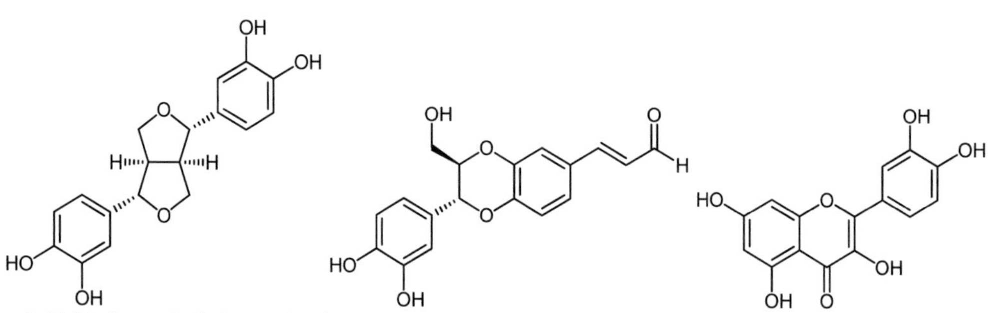


3,3′-bisdemethylpinoresinol americanin A quercetin

Fig. 3. 3,3′-Bisdemethylpinoresinol, americanin A and quercetin

### 4.2 Piperaceae plants

During the course of the first screening for the effects of plants collected from islands in the South Pacific on melanogenesis by using B16 melanoma cells, it was found that the extract of rhizome of *Piper methysticum* (Piperaceae) stimulated melanogenesis (Matsuda et al., 2006). The rhizomes are known as kava (kava-kava or kawa) in Oceania, and the South Pacific islanders have traditionally used the rhizome to prepare a psychoactive beverage for social and ceremonial events.

With the increase in the elderly population, many Asian people are develop gray hair. Thus, the cosmetic market for hair-dye and anti-gray hair agents is growing. Hair turning gray is caused by genetic predisposition, aging, reduced melanocytes caused by environmental stress, and reduced biosynthesis of melanin pigment, or melanogenesis. Hair-dye agents are used to treat gray hair, and many anti-gray hair agents are under development. However, there remain some problems with these agents, such as insufficient activity and side effects due to the dyes. Although anti-gray hair agents aim for the opposite effect of cosmetic whitening agents, there is a need for safer anti-gray hair agents that exhibit satisfactory melanogenesis activity and gray hair prevention. Therefore, we continued screening to look for ingredients with more potent melanogenesis stimulation activity among Piperaceae plants.

| Samples | Parts | Concentration (μg/ml) | Melanin content (μg/well) | Cell proliferation (%) |
|---|---|---|---|---|
| Control | | | 11.0 ± 0.8 | 100.0 ± 0.9 |
| *P. methysticum* | Leaf | 1 | 9.3 ± 0.1 | 101.8 ± 0.9 |
| | | 10 | 9.5 ± 0.5 | 106.9 ± 1.4* |
| | Stem | 1 | 10.7 ± 0.4 | 101.7 ± 2.0 |
| | | 10 | 12.8 ± 0.6* | 102.2 ± 1.3 |
| | Rhizome | 1 | 10.6 ± 0.8 | 102.4 ± 2.9 |
| | | 10 | 14.0 ± 0.6* | 108.6 ± 2.0* |
| *P. nigrum* | Leaf | 1 | 13.0 ± 0.3* | 99.9 ± 3.4 |
| | | 10 | 14.9 ± 0.2** | 104.0 ± 2.9 |
| | Stem | 1 | 11.7 ± 0.4 | 98.8 ± 1.0 |
| | | 10 | 11.8 ± 0.4 | 95.9 ± 1.5 |
| | Fruit | 1 | 11.2 ± 0.5 | 99.5 ± 0.6 |
| | | 10 | 15.5 ± 1.1** | 101.6 ± 0.4 |
| Theophylline | | 1 | 12.4 ± 0.3 | 99.1 ± 0.8 |
| | | 10 | 18.7 ± 0.5** | 96.9 ± 1.2 |

Table 4. Effects of 50% ethanolic extracts from Piperaceae plants and theophylline on melanin content in B16 melanoma cells (Each value represents the mean ± S.E. of triplicates. Statistical analysis was performed with a multiple comparison test using the Bonferroni/Dunn algorithm. Significantly different from the control group at *: $p<0.05$, **: $p<0.01$. *Ref.*; Matsuda et al., 2006)

Melanogenesis stimulation activity of 50% ethanolic extracts obtained from several different parts of six Piper species, namely *P. longum* (long pepper), *P. kadsura* (Japanese pepper), *P. methysticum*, *P. nigrum* (black pepper), *P. betle* (betel leaf), and *P. cubeba* (cubeb), were examined (Table 4). Among them, the extracts of kava and *P. nigrum* leaf showed a potent stimulatory effect on melanogenesis without any significant effect on cell proliferation, as shown in Table 4. Activity-guided fractionation of kava extract by using B16 melanoma cells led to the isolation of two active kavalactones, yangonin and (+)-7,8-epoxyyangonin (Fig. 4 and Table 5). (+)-7,8-Epoxyyangonin showed a significant stimulatory effect on melanogenesis in B16 melanoma cells. Yangonin exhibited a weak melanogenesis stimulation activity.

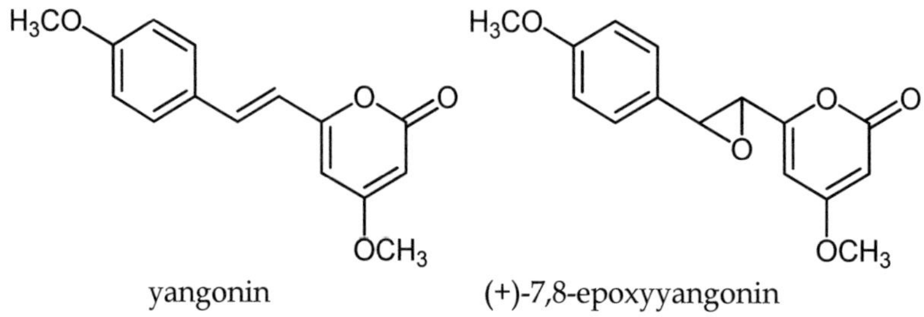


Fig. 4. Yangonin and (+)-7,8-epoxyyangonin

| Samples | Concentration (μg/ml) | Melanin content (μg/well) | Cell proliferation (%) |
|---|---|---|---|
| Control | | 10.6 ± 0.5 | 100.0 ± 1.6 |
| Yangonin | 1 | 13.4 ± 1.2** | 100.6 ± 2.3 |
| | 10 | 17.3 ± 0.5** | 108.2 ± 1.2* |
| (+)-7,8-Epoxyyangonin | 1 | 16.3 ± 1.1** | 107.9 ± 0.2** |
| | 10 | 25.4 ± 0.7** | 116.9 ± 2.8** |
| Theophylline | 1 | 10.2 ± 0.3 | 95.6 ± 1.2 |
| | 10 | 21.0 ± 0.2** | 94.6 ± 2.8 |

Table 5. Effects of yangonin, (+)-7,8-epoxyyangonin and theophylline on melanin content in B16 melanoma cells (Each value represents the mean ± S.E. of triplicates. Statistical analysis was performed with a multiple comparison test using the Bonferroni/Dunn algorithm. Significantly different from the control group at *: $p<0.05$, **: $p<0.01$. *Ref.*; Matsuda et al., 2006)

The *P. nigrum* leaf extract showed the most potent stimulation activity. Fruits of *P. nigrum* are widely used as a pungent spice. The use of Piper leaf has not yet been fully developed. Activity-guided fractionation followed by chromatography of the methanolic leaf extract led to the isolation of two active lignans, (-)-cubebin and (-)-3,4-dimethoxy-3,4-desmethylenedioxycubebin (Fig. 5) (Matsuda et al., 2004). Two lignans showed a significant melanogenesis stimulatory activity without any significant effects on cell proliferation, as shown in Table 6. Therefore, melanogenesis stimulation activity of the leaf extract was attributable to these two lignans. Especially, (-)-cubebin showed the most potent melanogenesis stimulation activity in B16 melanoma cells without any significant effects on cell proliferation. Since (-)-cubebin is a new melanogenesis stimulating substance, we tried to elucidate its melanogenesis stimulation mechanism by using B16 melanoma cells (Hirata et al., 2007). Tyrosinase activity was increased at 24 to 72 h after addition of (-)-cubebin to B16 melanoma cells, and then the intracellular melanin amount was increased at 48 to 96 h after the treatment. The expression levels of tyrosinase were time-dependently enhanced after the treatment with (-)-cubebin. The activation of microphthalmia-associated transcription factor (MITF), a transcription factor that regulates tyrosinase gene expression, is known to be a critical event during melanogenesis. (-)-Cubebin elevated the level of phosphorylation of p38 mitogen-activated protein kinase (p38 MAPK) of which the cascade activates MITF, whereas no effect was observed in the levels of phosphorylation of ERK 1/2 and p70 S6K1. SB203580, a selective inhibitor of p38 MAPK, completely blocked (-)-cubebin-induced expression of tyrosinase mRNA in B16 melanoma cells. These results suggest that one of the mechanisms for (-)-cubebin-induced melanogenesis in B16 melanoma cells is attributable to the increase in tyrosinase gene expression through a positive regulator, MITF, initiated by (-)-cubebin-induced activation of p38 MAPK, as shown in Fig. 6.

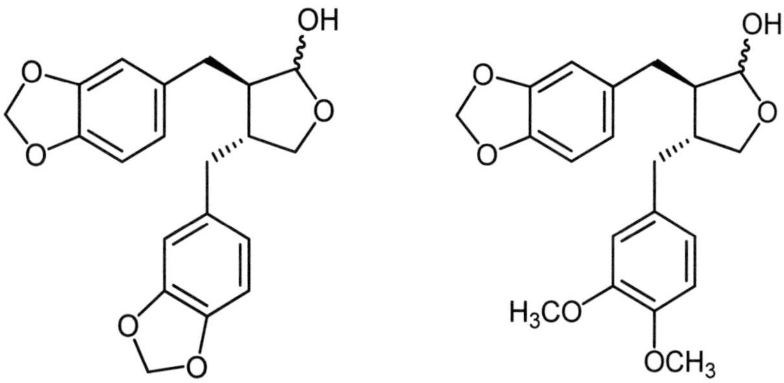


(-)-cubebin (-)-3,4-dimethoxy-3,4-desmethylenedioxycubebin

Fig. 5. (-)-Cubebin and (-)-3,4-dimethoxy-3,4- desmethylenedioxycubebin

| Samples | Concentration (μM) | Melanin content (μg/well) | Cell proliferation (%) |
|---|---|---|---|
| Control | | 7.1 ± 0.3 | 100.0 ± 2.6 |
| (-)-Cubebin | 0.3 | 8.6 ± 0.9 | 101.1 ± 2.5 |
| | 1.0 | 10.7 ± 0.2** | 102.5 ± 2.1 |
| | 3.0 | 11.8 ± 0.1** | 101.1 ± 0.9 |
| (-)-3,4-Dimethoxy-3,4-des-methylenedioxycubebin | 0.3 | 9.1 ± 0.3 | 98.9 ± 0.9 |
| | 1.0 | 10.7 ± 0.2* | 103.6 ± 1.4 |
| | 3.0 | 8.8 ± 0.3 | 109.9 ± 2.0* |
| Theophylline | 3.0 | 9.3 ± 1.0* | 105.5 ± 6.1 |
| | 10.0 | 8.3 ± 0.1 | 99.3 ± 1.1 |

Table 6. Effects of (-)-cubebin, (-)-3,4-dimethoxy-3,4-desmethylenedioxycubebin and theophylline on melanin content in B16 melanoma cells (Each value represents the mean ± S.E. of triplicates. Statistical analysis was performed with a multiple comparison test using the Bonferroni/Dunn algorithm. Significantly different from the control group at *: $p<0.05$, **: $p<0.01$. *Ref.*; Matsuda et al., 2004)

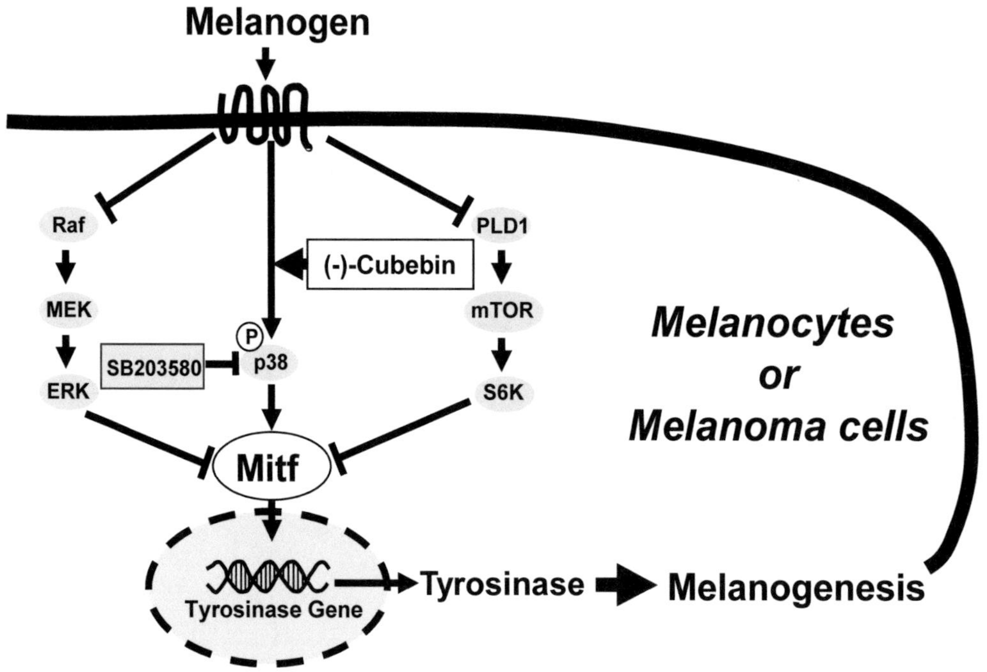


Fig. 6. Proposed scheme showing the activation mechanism of (-)-cubebin on the melanogenesis signaling pathway

Melanogenesis stimulating agents were found during the course of the screening using B16 melanoma cells for cosmetic ingredients with melanogenesis inhibitory activity. Some of the stimulation agents that originated in Piper plants may be useful as cosmetic ingredients for prevention of gray hair after further experimental studies, including clinical trials.

## 5. The search for cosmetic whitening agents from Citrus fruits

### 5.1 Citrus fruits are used as crude drugs throughout the world

Fruits of *Citrus*, *Fortunella*, and *Poncirus* genera (Rutaceae) are generally called Citrus fruits. Yellowish ripe fruits belonging to *Citrus* and *Fortunella* genera are popular, juicy and sour foods that are eaten all over the world. As for the historical medicinal use of Citrus fruits, the ancient Egyptians used them as an anti-bacterial mummification agent. The fruits were also used as insecticides and antidotes, and for the treatment of frostbite, external wounds and colds in the ancient Rome. It has been reported that the fruits were used as washing agents for hair and copper goods in the ancient India. Citrus fruits have been used as crude drugs from ancient times in China as well as other regions; for example, an illustration of Citrus-like fruit (Fig. 7) has been depicted in the oldest Chinese herbal book. In later years, unripe fruits of *C. aurantium* (bitter orange) and *C. natsudaidai* (natsudaidai), and the peals of the ripe fruits of *C. aurantium*, *C. natsudaidai*, and *C. unshiu* (satsuma mandarin) were described in several Chinese herbal books. All have historically been used as digestive medicines, cough remedies, and expectorants.

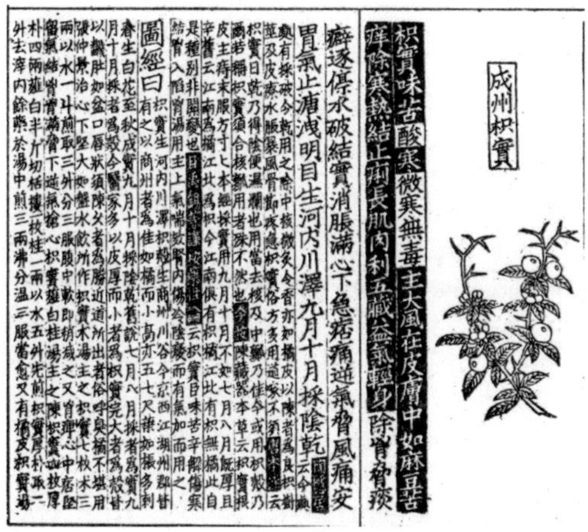


Fig. 7. Description on Citrus fruits in an ancient Chinese herbal book

### 5.2 Citrus plants

The anatomical taxonomy of Citrus plants is controversial because cultivated variations of Citrus plants for new entry into the fruit market increase year by year with recent improvements in breeding. On the other hand, chemotaxomomical classification of Citrus fruits based on our high performance liquid chromatography (HPLC) analysis (Kubo et al., 2004) of four flavanone glycosides (Fig. 8) in the fruits revealed that Citrus fruits could be classified into the following four groups; 1) a group in which the major flavanone glycosides are narirutin and hesperidin with a rutinoside moiety: 2) a group in which the major glycosides are naringin and neohesperidin with a neohesperidoside moiety: 3) a group in which the major glycoside is naringin: 4) a group in which none of the flavanone glycosides described above were detected. We reported that the content of the four flavanone glycosides cited above in unripe fruits was higher than that in ripe ones (Kubo et al., 2004), while the flavanone glycosides content in peel was higher than that in edible flesh.

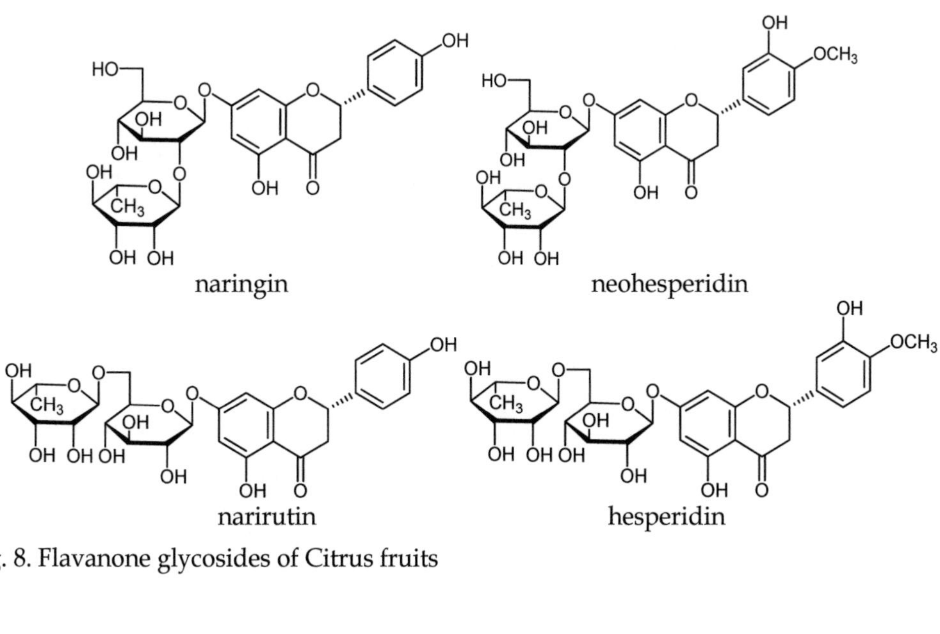


Fig. 8. Flavanone glycosides of Citrus fruits

Flavonoid compounds exhibit various biological activities, such as vasodilatory, anti-oxidative and radical scavenging activities. Since the peel of Citrus fruits is exposed to solar UV radiation, it was assumed that flavanone glycosides may exert an anti-photoaging effect by preventing sun damage. This assumption prompted us to examine the tyrosinase inhibitory activity of some Citrus fruits.

From the most popular Citrus fruits, *C. unshiu* fruit and *C. hassaku* (hassaku) fruit were selected as representatives of the group in which the major flavanone glycosides are narirutin and hesperidin and the group in which major glycosides are naringin and neohesperidin, respectively. Assay results for each 50% ethanolic extract, including seasonal variations in activity, are shown in Table 7 (Itoh et al., 2009). Tyrosinase inhibitory activity of unripe fruits was superior to that of ripe ones in accordance with the fact that the contents of four flavanone glycosides in unripe fruits were higher than those in ripe ones. Inhibitory activity of *C. hassaku* fruit was more potent than that of *C. unshiu* fruit. The 50% ethanolic extract (CH-ext) obtained from the unripe *C. hassaku* fruit collected in July exhibited significant tyrosinase inhibitory activity. Activity-guided fractionation and further examination revealed that the inhibitory activity of the CH-ext was attributable to two flavanone glycosides, naringin and neohesperidin. The tyrosinase inhibitory activities of naringin and neohesperidin are depicted in Table 8. Naringin showed the most potent activity. The SOD-like and anti-oxidant activities of CH-ext and its two flavanone glycosides were examined. As shown in Table 8, both CH-ext and neohesperidin showed potent SOD-like and DPPH radical-scavenging activities.

| Samples | Sampling month | $IC_{50}$ |
|---|---|---|
| CH-ext | July | 4.5 mg/ml |
| | August | 8.2 mg/ml |
| | September | >10 mg/ml |
| | October | >10 mg/ml |
| | November | >10 mg/ml |

Table 7. Seasonal variation in tyrosinase inhibitory activity ($IC_{50}$ value) of 50% ethanolic extract from *C. hassaku* fruits (*Ref.*; Itoh et al., 2009)

| Samples | Tyrosinase inhibitory activity | SOD-like activity | Radical-scavenging activity |
|---|---|---|---|
| CH-ext | 4.7 mg/ml | 0.5 mg/ml | 0.2 mg/ml |
| Naringin | 1.9 mM | >2000 μM | >4 mM |
| Neohesperidin | >5 mM | 26 μM | 0.6 mM |
| Narirutin | 2.0 mM | >2000 μM | >4 mM |
| Hesperidin | >5 mM | 268 μM | 3.2 mM |
| Arbutin | >10 mM | N.D. | N.D. |
| Kojic acid | 0.02 mM | N.D. | N.D. |
| Superoxide dismutase (SOD) | N.D. | 0.2 U/ml | N.D. |
| L-Ascorbic acid | N.D. | N.D. | 0.03 mM |

Table 8. $IC_{50}$ values of tyrosinase inhibitory, SOD-like, and radical-scavenging activities of 50% ethanolic extract from *C. hassaku* fruits (CH-ext), naringin, neohesperidin, narirutin, hesperidin, arbutin, kojic acid, superoxide dismutase, and L-ascorbic acid (N.D.: not determined. *Ref.*; Itoh et al., 2009)

The inhibitory effects of CH-ext on melanogenesis were evaluated (Itoh et al., 2009). The CH-ext showed significant inhibitory activity in a concentration-dependent manner without any significant effects on cell proliferation, as depicted in Table 9. Moreover, as for the pharmacological activity of CH-ext, we found anti-allergic, fibrinolytic, collagen-induced rabbit platelet aggregation inhibitory, and polybrene-induced rat erythrocyte aggregation inhibitory activities. These results imply that CH-ext can improve blood fluidity, which is related to skin problems such as infraorbital dark circles around the eyes and skin darkness resulting from unsmooth circulation or blood stagnation. Thus, CH-ext and its flavanone glycosides may be useful ingredients for whitening cosmetics.

| Samples | Concentration | Melanin content (μg/well) | Cell proliferation (%) |
|---|---|---|---|
| Control | | 13.3 ± 0.6 | 100.0 ± 5.9 |
| CH-ext | 100 μg/ml | 11.2 ± 0.6** | 113.3 ± 5.7 |
| | 250 μg/ml | 9.9 ± 0.5** | 122.2 ± 6.4 |
| | 500 μg/ml | 7.0 ± 0.2** | 101.8 ± 13.1 |
| Arbutin | 50 μM | 11.5 ± 0.1* | 84.6 ± 5.9 |
| | 100 μM | 11.6 ± 0.1* | 91.9 ± 7.6 |
| | 250 μM | 8.5 ± 0.2** | 103.3 ± 12.0 |
| | 500 μM | 6.5 ± 0.3** | 100.2 ± 8.8 |
| Kojic acid | 50 μM | 13.6 ± 1.0 | 100.9 ± 6.6 |
| | 100 μM | 13.2 ± 0.2 | 101.7 ± 11.1 |
| | 250 μM | 12.5 ± 0.6 | 116.4 ± 13.2 |
| | 500 μM | 10.6 ± 0.2** | 129.7 ± 10.1 |
| L-Ascorbic acid | 50 μM | 13.0 ± 0.4 | 120.7 ± 10.1 |
| | 100 μM | 15.4 ± 0.8** | 136.4 ± 15.2* |
| | 250 μM | 13.9 ± 0.8 | 134.1 ± 13.2 |
| | 500 μM | 14.9 ± 0.4* | 118.9 ± 15.1 |

Table 9. Effects of 50% ethanolic extract from unripe *C. hassaku* fruits (CH-ext) arbutin, kojic acid and L-ascorbic acid on melanin production in B16 melanoma cells (Each value represents the mean ± S.E. of triplicates. Statistical analysis was performed with a multiple comparison test using the Bonferroni/Dunn algorithm. Significantly different from the control group at *: $p<0.05$, **: $p<0.01$. *Ref.*; Itoh et al., 2009)

## 6. Conclusion

Research to find a novel inhibitor of melanin hyperpigmentation from natural resources was carried out based on our strategies. We found several seeds of melanogenesis regulators which exhibit various pharmacological actions. These seeds may become useful ingredients for cosmetics, supplements, functional foods and OTC-drugs.

Recent gradual destruction of the ozonosphere has raised solar UV exposure risk for all people. Solar UV radiation is a risk factor for photo-carcinogenesis, hyperpigmentation and photo-aging. Safer and more potent cosmetic whitening agents will be required to preserve beautiful and fair facial skin. We expect that superior melanin hyperpigmentation inhibitors with anti-aging effects and various anti-oxidative activities will be discovered from natural resources.

## 7. References


Itoh, K., Hirata, N., Masuda, M., Naruto, S., Murata, K., Wakabayashi, K. & Matsuda, H. (2009). Inhibitory Effects of *Citrus hassaku* Extract and its Flavanone Glycosides on Melanogenesis. *Biological & Pharmaceutical Bulletin*, Vol.32, No.3, (December 2008), pp. 410-415, ISSN 0918-6158

Hirata, N., Naruto, S., Ohguchi, K., Akao, Y., Nozawa, Y., Iinuma, M. & Matsuda, H. (2007). Mechanism of the Melanogenesis Stimulation Activity of (-)-Cubebin in Murine B16 Melanoma Cells. *Bioorganic & Medicinal Chemistry*, Vol.15, No.14, (July 2007 ), pp. 4897-4902, ISSN 0968-0896

Kubo, M., Fujita, T., Nishimura, S., Tokunaga, M., Matsuda, H., Gato, T., Tomohiro, N., Sasaki, K. & Utsunomiya, N. (2004). Seasonal Variation in Anti-Allergic Activity of Citrus Fruits and Flavanone Glycoside Content. *Natural Medicines*, Vol.58, No.6, (June 2004), pp. 284-294, ISSN 1349-9114

Mason, H.S. & Peterson, E.W. (1965). Melanoproteins. I. Reactions between Enzyme-Generated Quinones and Amino Acids. *Biochimica et Biophysica Acta*, Vol.111, No.1, (November 1965), pp. 134-146, ISSN 0304-4165

Masamoto, Y., Iida, S. & Kubo, M. (1980). Inhibitory Effect of Chinese Crude Drugs on Tyrosinase. *Planta Medica*, Vol.40, No.4, (December 1980), pp. 361-355, ISSN 0032-0943

Masuda, M., Murata, K., Fukuhama, A., Naruto, S., Fujita, T., Uwaya, A., Isami, F. & Matsuda, H. (2009). Inhibitory Effect of Constituents of *Morinda citrifolia* Seed on Elastase and Tyrosinase. *Journal of Natural Medicines*, Vol.63, No.3, (Mar 2009), pp. 267-273, ISSN 1340-3443

Matsuda, H., Higashino, M., Nakai, Y., Iinuma, M., Kubo, M. & Lang, F.A. (1996). Studies of Cuticle Drugs from Natural Sources. IV. Inhibitory Effects of Some *Arctostaphylos* Plants on Melanin Biosynthesis. *Biological & Pharmaceutical Bulletin*, Vol.19, No.1, (January 1996), pp. 153-156, ISSN 0918-6158

Matsuda, H., Hirata N., Kawaguchi, Y., Naruto, S., Takata, T., Oyama, M., Iinuma, M. & Kubo, M. (2006). Melanogenesis Stimulation in Murine B16 Melanoma Cells by Kava (*Piper methysticum*) Rhizome Extract and Kavalactones. *Biological & Pharmaceutical Bulletin*, Vol.29, No.4, (December 2005), pp. 834-837, ISSN 0918-6158

Matsuda, H., Kawaguchi, Y., Yamazaki, M., Hirata, N., Naruto, S., Asanuma, Y., Kaihatsu, T. & Kubo, M. (2004). Melanogenesis Stimulation in Murine B16 Melanoma Cells by *Piper nigrum* Leave Extract and Its Lignan Constituents. *Biological & Pharmaceutical Bulletin*, Vol.27, No.10, (July 2004), pp. 1611-1616, ISSN 0918-615

Matsuda, H., Nakamura, S., Shiomoto, H., Tanaka, T. & Kubo, M. (1992a). Pharmacological Studies on Leaf of *Arctostaphylos uva-ursi* (L.) SPRENG. IV. Effect of 50% Methanolic Extract from *Arctostaphylos uva-ursi* (L.) SPRENG. (Bearberry Leaf) on Melanin Synthesis. *Yakugaku Zasshi*, Vol.112, No.4, (April 1992), pp. 276-282, ISSN 0031-6903

Matsuda, M., Nakamura, S., Tanaka, T. & Kubo, M. (1992b). Pharmacological Studies on Leaf of *Arctostaphylos uva-ursi* (L.) SPRENG. V. Effect of Water Extract from *Arctostaphylos uva-ursi* (L.) SPRENG. (Bearberry Leaf) on the Anti-Allergic and Anti-Inflammatory Activities of Dexamethazone Ointment. *Yakugaku Zasshi*, Vol.112, No.9, (September 1992), pp. 673-677, ISSN 0031-6903

Tobin, D. & Thody, A.J. (1994). The Superoxide Anion May Mediate Short- but Not Long-term Effects of Ultraviolet Radiation on Melanogenesis. *Experimental Dermatology*, Vol.3, No.3, (June 1994), pp. 99-105, ISSN 0906-6705

# Part 4

# Advances in Melanoma Translational Research

# 10

# Caveolin-1 in Melanoma Progression

Lorena Lobos-González, Lorena Aguilar,
Gonzalo Fernández, Carlos Sanhueza and Andrew F.G Quest
*Centro de Estudios Moleculares de la Célula (CEMC),
Facultad de Medicina, Universidad de Chile,
Chile*

## 1. Introduction

Cancer is a leading cause of death world wide and mortality due to this group of diseases has doubled in the last 20 years. With an estimated 3 million cases, skin cancer is currently the third most common human malignancy and global incidence is rising at an alarming rate due to environmental changes. Within that category, melanomas represent the least common, but most dangerous form accounting for the majority of skin cancer-related deaths.

In general terms, cancer evolves as the consequence of a multi-factorial process that involves the loss of a cell's ability to respond in an appropriate fashion to cues provided by the microenvironment. The development of such aberrant, autonomous behavior is caused by both genetic mutations and epigenetic mechanisms. Particularly relevant in the context of melanoma are the Ras/Raf/MEK/Erk, PI3K/PTEN and NF-kB signaling pathways. The Wnt/β-catenin patway is also implicated, but it´s role still remains unclear. Depending on whether changes result in a "gain of function" or a "loss of function", the molecules involved are classified as either oncogenes or tumor suppressors, examples important in melanomas being NRas and B-Raf or PTEN, respectively. More recently, a new group of molecular participants has begun to emerge, which, depending on the cellular context, display the ability to either block tumor development or favor progression. Very little is still known about the underlying mechanisms that might explain such "ambiguous" behavior.

In this respect, work from our laboratory has focused on the study of a scaffolding protein called caveolin-1. This protein is implicated in a large number of cellular processes, including caveolae formation and vesicular transport, cholesterol transport and the regulation of signal transduction. With respect to tumor development, initial reports implicated caveolin-1 as a tumor suppressor. For instance, caveolin-1 expression is reduced in several human tumors including lung, mammary, colon, ovarian carcinoma and sarcomas, as wells as osteosarcomas and re-expression of the protein can reverse characteristics associated with the transformed phenotype. However, evidence to the contrary is also available showing that caveolin-1 promotes more aggressive traits in tumor cells, such as metastasis and multidrug resistance. Importantly, in human melanoma patients high levels of caveolin-1 are detected in exosomes found in the plasma and some data available associate caveolin-1 expression with increased metastatic potential in different human melanoma cell lines.

In this chapter, we summarize data available in the literature highlighting the ambiguity of caveolin-1 function in cancer development. Mechanisms that might explain one or the other type of behavior, as well as the possible relevance of caveolin-1 in the development of melanomas will be discussed. Finally, the potential of this understanding for developing therapies will be mentioned.

## 2. Cancer

Cancer is a leading cause of death worldwide that evolves as the consequence of genetic and epigenetic changes (Ponder 2001). This multifactorial process results in the loss of appropriate communication between cells and their microenviroment. During this transition, aberrant cells acquire specific molecular traits, including unlimited replicative potential, resistance to apoptosis, independence of growth factors and insensitivity to growth-inhibitory signals. Insipient tumors require then the formation *de novo* of blood vessels (angiogenesis) to grow beyond an initially limited size. Ultimately, tumor cells develop the ability to disseminate to distant sites and form new tumors (metastasis), which frequently are the cause of patient death. All these processes are thought to reflect the consequence of an inbalance in the activity of genes referred to as oncogenes and tumor suppressors, whereby mutations in both types of genes (genetic regulation), in addition to changes in the levels of expression (epigenetic regulation), contribute to such abnormal development (Weinberg 1989; Hanahan and Weinberg 2000; Hanahan and Weinberg 2011).

Skin cancer is a common disease and the high incidence has generated global concern. Although many of these cancers are not aggressive, some, like melanoma, are extremely lethal. As indicated, aberrant cellular signaling underlies the development of essentially all tumors. Not surprisingly, therefore, in the transition from melanocytes to melanomas, many signaling pathways become constitutively activated, as will be discussed later and promote the acquisition of molecular traits associated with melanoma development. (Figure 1).

Malignant melanomas are a serious public health problem in many countries; however, data from less developed countries is often either not available or not reliable. The data available in developed countries reveals that mortality associated with melanomas has increased gradually in the past 40 years. Perhaps more problematic in this context is the fact that the incidence rate is increasing faster in younger people, an aspect which tends to amplify the impact of this deadly cancer. Malignant melanoma is known to initially develop in melanocytes located at the interphase between epidermis and dermis. These peripherally located, proliferative cells suffer damage upon excessive UV exposure that can translate ultimately into cell transformation and invasion of deeper structures of the skin. While still at an early stage of development, equivalent to less than 4 mm of vertical penetration and the absence of distant spread, surgical resection represents an appropriate treatment for melanomas. However, in more advanced cases, the success of surgical and therapeutical procedures is severely limited by tumor recurrence, metastasis and relatively rapid patient death. Hence, in order to develop more effective treatments, it is important to understand better the mechanisms leading to melanocyte damage and, particularly, to identify those responsible for the alterations in signaling that initiate and propagate the transformation process. In recent years, a large body of evidence has accumulated identifying sun exposure as a mayor risk factor in developing this disease. However, simply eliminating this risk by protective measures is not an option, since sun exposure is necessary for a number of reasons, including being required for vitamin D synthesis. Hence, it is important to define when precisely sun exposure becomes deleterious, in order to identify groups of the population at risk and thereby improve early diagnosis and treatment.

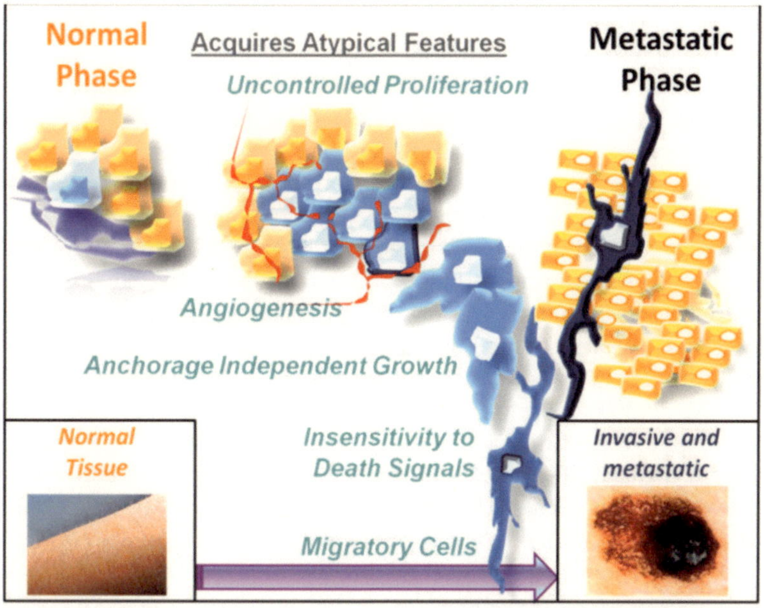


Fig. 1. Atypical characteristics acquired by melanocytes in the transition to malignant melanomas

Melanocytes are intimately associated with keratinocytes in the intermediate cell layer between dermis and epidermis. The acquisition of atypical features, such as uncontrolled proliferation, angiogenesis, anchorage-independent growth and insensitivity to death-inducing signals are depicted. Additionally, the cells eventually begin to migrate, become invasive and metastatic. These cells invade both the dermis and epidermis layers, thereby increasing the size of the primary tumor before disseminating via the blood stream to other tissues.

## 3. Melanoma incidence

The International Agency for Research on cancer publishes a document entitled "Cancer Incidence in Five Continents", which permits comparisons between countries. In general terms, countries with white/Kaukasian-populations have the highest incidence rates (above 2/100.000) in the world, while asians, africans and indigenous americans are much less at risk (1-0.1/100.000). The highest registered incidence for melanomas in the world is found in Australia, whereby a latitude gradient exists, such that rates are highest in the northern part of the country (over 50/100.000 in men, and 40/100.000 for women). Also in New Zealand the incidence of 30/100.000 is well above the global average and higher to the north. Given that in both these countries the predominantly white population is homogeneously distributed, differences is incidence rates can be largely explained by the latitude gradient in sun exposure. Amongst european countries, Scandinavia and Switzerland have the highest incidence rates, being in the latter case 16/100.000 for men and 19/100.000 for women. For Scandinavian countries, there is no straightforward explanation, although the population is extremely fair, because sun exposure is low. In Switzerland, ozone depletion may be a relevant factor. Interestingly, Italy also has latitude a gradient which is inverted compared to the one in Australia, such that for residents of northern regions (less sun exposure) incidence rates are higher than in southern regions with increased exposure. The question arising here is whether a "skin gradient" exists within the Italian population. Also in the USA incidence rates are quite high, but only in non-hispanic, white populations (19/100.000 men, 16/100.000 women). Relevant factors are again the ethnic background and sun exposure. However, no latitude gradient has been described in the USA. For the rest of the world, the incidence appears low. However, data is frequently either not available or not reliable, in the latter case mainly due to confusion with non-melanoma skin cancer.

A this point, we wish to dwell briefly on the problem of malignant melanoma in Chile. This narrow and extremely long country (approx. 200 by 5000 km) extends from 18°S to 55°S and covers, therefore, geographical zones particularly in the center and to the north with intense sun exposure. Moreover, UV irradiation has also increased dramatically in the southern-most region (ie: XII region) close to the Antarctic, due to ozone depletion that has become evident since the 1970s. Consistent with this development, epidemiological data accumulated over the last 30-40 years indicate a notable increment in the incidence of melanomas also in these areas. The genetic background of the population is fairly homogeneous, being predominantly a mixture between the indigenous population of asian origin and europeans, whereby interracial mixing has occurred over the last 500 years. The population is homogeneously distributed, such that this factor does not contribute to the latitude gradient. In any case, available epidemiological studies do not segregate data according to ethnic background.

Malignant melanoma is a relevant public health problem given the prevalence throughout the country and the relatively high mortality rate associated with this disease (slightly above 1:100.000 deaths/year). Currently, melanomas are the 9$^{th}$ most frequent cause of cancer death in Chile. Unfortunately, as mentioned previously, for a large number of countries in the world, no useful incidence data is available due to registration problems and confusion with non-melanoma skin cancer. The mortality rate within the country ranges from about 3.0/100.000 inhabitants (in the northern-most region of Chile) down to 1.2/100000 in the southern region (XI region). However, in the region furthest south in Chile (XII), death rates are again higher and reach values of approximately 2.1/100.000. For malignant melanoma, certain differences in body distribution are observed for Chile in comparison to melanomas in Europe, North America, Australia and New Zealand. In Chile the most frequent cases are of the acral-lentiginous type, that are observed in non sun-exposed regions of the skin, such as hand palms, foot soles and under the nails. For the other countries mentioned, in most cases the body, face and arms are affected, suggesting sun exposure as an important causing factor. Treatments for malignant melanoma in Chile are similar to those employed in the other countries. Generally, surgical resection of large areas, with or without removal of sentinel lymph nodes, remains the procedure of choice.

## 4. Melanoma biology

Melanoma is a highly complex disease that involves activation of oncogenes, such as BRAF, NRAS, the Wnt pathway and loss or mutation of tumor suppressors, such as p53 or PTEN. For the subsequent discussion, we will focus in this chapter on the possible contribution of the Wnt/β-catenin pathway to melanoma development. Excellent reviews concerning the other alterations mentioned can be found elsewhere (Straume and Akslen 1997; Larue and Delmas 2006; Gray-Schopfer, Wellbrock et al. 2007).

## 5. The Wnt/β-catenin pathway

The canonical Wnt pathway is involved in the control of a large variety of processes, including cell proliferation, cell migration and differentiation, all key events in the initiation and progression of cancer. A crucial component of this pathway is β-catenin (Bienz and Clevers 2000; Polakis 2000; Widelitz 2005) (Klaus and Birchmeier 2008).

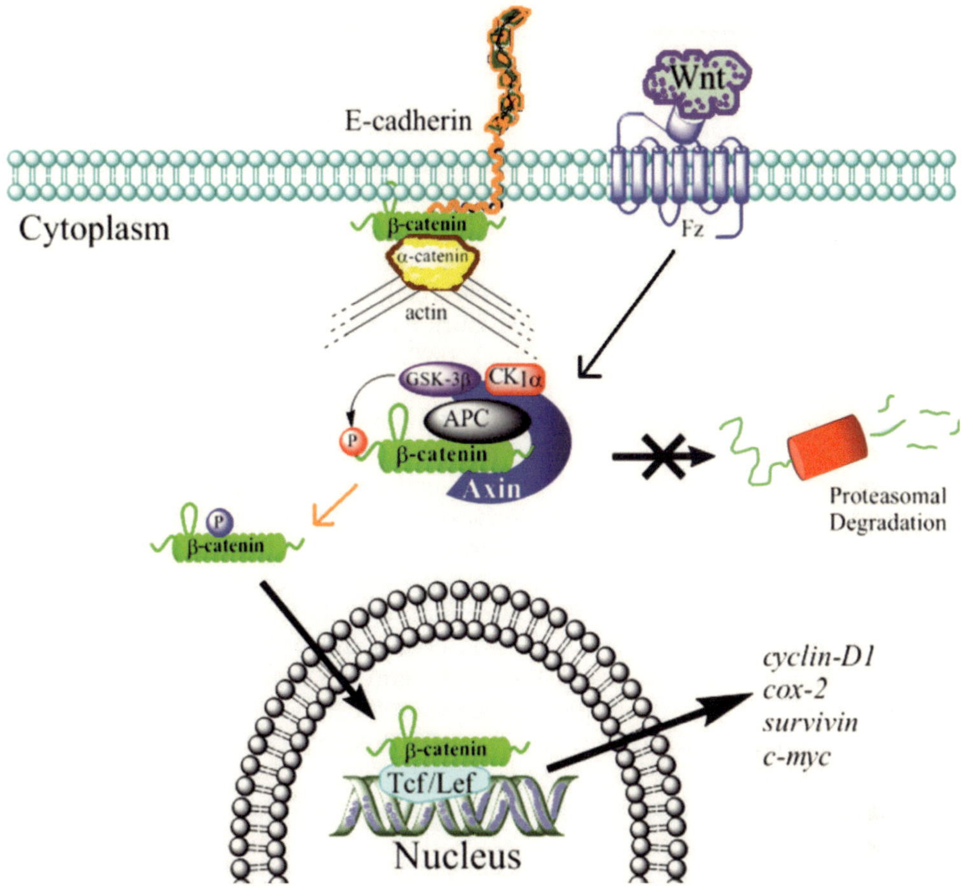


Fig. 2. Wnt/β-catenin pathway.

Schematic showing some of the relevant components of the pathway and highlighting three key locations of β-catenin in the cell. On the one hand, β-catenin is found at the plasma membrane in a multiprotein complex with E-cadherin important for cell-cell interactions. Additionally, β-catenin is present in the cytosol, generally associated with another multi-protein complex that includes adenomatous polyposis coli (APC), axin and GSK-3β and is responsible for promoting degradation via the proteasome pathway. Finally, β-catenin is also present within the nucleus, where it acts as a cofactor that promotes transcription by Tcf/Lef family members of a large number of genes including *survivin, cox-2, cyclin D1 and c-myc.*

In non-stimulated cells, cytoplasmic free β-catenin is associated within a multiprotein complex containing Axin/Conductin, glycogen synthase kinase 3β (GSK3β/Shaggy) and the tumor suppressor APC (Bienz and Clevers 2000; Polakis 2000; Henderson and Fagotto 2002; Nathke 2004; Heeg-Truesdell and LaBonne 2006). In this complex, Axin/Conductin acts as a scaffolding protein that binds APC, GSK3β and β-catenin, thereby promoting the phosphorylation of APC and β-catenin. Axin also associates with the protein kinase CK1, which phosphorylates β-catenin prior to GSK3β engagement and thereby promotes subsequent GSK3β-dependent phosphorylation, in a process referred to as hierarchical phosphorylation (Heeg-Truesdell and LaBonne 2006). Subsequent phosphorylation of β-catenin by GSK3β drives β-catenin ubiquitination by the SCF complex, thus promoting proteasome-mediated degradation of β-catenin (Kimelman and Xu 2006).

Following Wnt stimulation of Frizzled receptors, Dishevelled is recruited to the receptor. Dishevelled binding serves to help maintain the Axin/APC/GSK3β protein complex in the vicinity of the Frizzled receptor. Additionally, this interaction favors release of β-catenin from the degradative Axin/APC/GSK3β protein complex, hence preventing proteasomal-mediated degradation of β-catenin (Logan and Nusse 2004; Huang and He 2008). Then, β-catenin translocates and accumulates in the nucleus, where it forms a protein complex with T-cell factor/ lymphoid enhancer factor (Tcf/Lef) transcription factors and thereby promotes transcription of Wnt target genes, such as *cyclin D1, survivin, cox-2, c-myc* (He, Sparks et al. 1998; Shtutman, Zhurinsky et al. 1999; Haertel-Wiesmann, Liang et al. 2000; Kim, Plescia et al. 2003).

As indicated (Figure 2), another pool of β-catenin is present in adhesion junctions, where β-catenin forms a protein complex with E-cadherin, α-catenin and actin. This protein complex has been suggested to mediate cell adhesion and confer mechanical stability to cells (Gottardi, Wong et al. 2001; Brembeck, Rosario et al. 2006; Jeanes, Gottardi et al. 2008; Schmalhofer, Brabletz et al. 2009). By sequestering β-catenin within the plasma membrane, E-cadherin reduces β-catenin-Tcf/Lef-dependent transcription in a manner that is independent of its function as a cell-cell adhesion molecule (Gottardi, Wong et al. 2001). Consistent with this view, loss or inactivation of E-cadherin increase responses to Wnt-Ligands (Jeanes, Gottardi et al. 2008). Thus, E-cadherin is a negative regulator of the Wnt pathway and a strong inhibitor of cancer progression (Ma, Young et al. ; Berx, Nollet et al. 1998; Gottardi, Wong et al. 2001; Hajra and Fearon 2002; Margineanu, Cotrutz et al. 2008).

## 6. Alterations in the Wnt/β-catenin pathway in melanoma

The contribution of the Wnt/β-catenin pathway to melanoma development is highly controversial. Some authors suggest that Wnt/β-catenin activation promotes melanoma development (Rimm, Caca et al. 1999; Larue and Delmas 2006; Larue, Luciani et al. 2009). This view is supported by the observation that alterations in the Wnt/β-catenin pathway are detectable in 70-80% of melanomas. Specifically, mutations in β-catenin have been detected in both melanoma biopsies and melanoma cell lines (Larue and Delmas 2006). These findings are reinforced by immuno-histochemical studies showing that β-catenin staining is frequently observed in primary melanomas, but is less abundant in metastatic melanomas (Pecina-Slaus, Zigmund et al. 2007; De Panfilis, Ferrari et al. 2009) and appears to be inversely correlated with the Clark stage (Pecina-Slaus, Zigmund et al. 2007). In both cases, β-catenin is observed predominantly at the cell membrane and in the cytoplasm (Pecina-Slaus, Zigmund et al. 2007; Tucci, Lucarini et al. 2007; De Panfilis, Ferrari et al. 2009). Furthermore, β-catenin has been detected in the nucleus in 30% of the melanomas analyzed (Rimm, Caca et al. 1999). It is important to note, that APC alterations are not frequently observed in melanomas in comparison to colon cancer (Lucero, Dawson et al. ; Larue and Delmas 2006). However, based on such evidence it remains poorly understood how aberrant β-catenin function may be related to melanoma progression. Possibly, its function in this sense is dependent on direct association of β-catenin with the promoter of Microphthalmia-associated transcription factor (MITF), which is frequently amplified in melanoma cell lines (Garraway, Widlund et al. 2005) and is required for Wnt/β-catenin to induce melanoma growth (Widlund, Horstmann et al. 2002). Interestingly, MITF has been proposed to contribute to melanoma development, by promoting expression of target genes, such as cdk2 that favors cell-cycle progression, anti-apoptotic *bcl2,* and *c-met* that enhances cell motility (Cheli, Ohanna et al. ; Levy, Khaled et al. 2006). Consistent with this view, reduction in MITF levels sensitizes melanoma cells to chemotherapy-induced cell death (Garraway, Widlund et al. 2005).

Alternatively, other groups propose that β-catenin prevents melanoma progression (Lucero, Dawson et al. ; Kageshita, Hamby et al. 2001; Maelandsmo, Holm et al. 2003; Bachmann, Straume et al. 2005; Chien, Moore et al. 2009). This view is supported by clinical data associating more aggressive melanomas and melanoma progression with loss of β-catenin (Kageshita, Hamby et al. 2001). Consistent with this view, loss of cytoplasmic β-catenin correlates with increased thickness of lesions and reduced disease-free patient survival (Maelandsmo, Holm et al. 2003). Additionally, loss of nuclear β-catenin is associated with a reduction in patient life span (Bachmann, Straume et al. 2005). Alternatively, activation of β-catenin is associated with reduced tumor cell proliferation (Chien, Moore et al. 2009). Taken together, these observations favor the notion that β-catenin plays a protective role in melanoma development. To date, however, neither how β-catenin develops such a role nor the mechanisms that lead to loss of β-catenin are fully understood.

A possible explanation for these striking differences in comparison to colon cancer may be related to the type of Wnt ligand present. Analysis of melanocytic tumors reveals that levels of the Wnt ligands 3A and 5A are increased (Larue and Delmas 2006). However, these two Wnt ligands are thought to have opposite functions. *In vitro* assays show that Wnt 3A reduces cell proliferation in association with activation of the β-catenin pathway. Microarray analysis of 350 melanoma samples showed that high levels of β-catenin correlated with better patient prognosis, suggesting that activation of β-catenin pathway by Wnt 3A reduces melanoma cell proliferation (Chien, Moore et al. 2009). How activation of the Wnt/ β-catenin pathway causes such effects in melanoma cells remains unclear, particularly since the opposite is seen in other cell types (Giles, van Es et al. 2003; Logan and Nusse 2004; Khan, Bradstock et al. 2007).

Alternatively, Wnt 5A expression in melanomas correlates with tumor progression and metastasis (McDonald and Silver 2009), and Wnt 5A has been shown to increase melanoma cell migration (Dissanayake, Wade et al. 2007). Interestingly, these effects of Wnt 5A have been described both in *in vitro* and *in vivo* melanoma models (Dissanayake, Olkhanud et al. 2008). In general, Wnt 5A enhances-melanoma cell migration but does so in a manner independent of the canonical Wnt/β-catenin pathway (Dissanayake, Wade et al. 2007; Dissanayake, Olkhanud et al. 2008; O'Connell and Weeraratna 2009).

Another important factor that contributes to changes in the Wnt/β-catenin pathway is the tumor suppressor E-cadherin (Margineanu, Cotrutz et al. 2008; Wu, Lin et al. 2008). Mutations or loss of this cell-cell adhesion protein are associated with increases in β-catenin Tcf/Lef-dependent transcription and cell proliferation (Berx, Nollet et al. 1998). Thus, loss of E-cadherin generally correlates with poor patient prognosis. Moreover, changes in the expression pattern of Cadherins are relevant. For instance, replacement of E-cadherin by N-cadherin is linked to the epithelial-mesenquimal transition and acquisition of a more malignant cell phenotype (Gray-Schopfer, Wellbrock et al. 2007; Kreizenbeck, Berger et al. 2008)

## 7. Caveolin-1

Caveolins are a family of membrane-associated scaffolding proteins implicated in variety of functions in cells, including vesicle trafficking, cholesterol transport and regulation of signal transduction (Anderson 1998; Okamoto, Schlegel et al. 1998; Quest, Leyton et al. 2004). To date three major isoforms have been described in mammals, namely caveolin-1, -2 and -3 (18-24 kDa). All three isoforms are encoded by distinct genes (Williams and Lisanti 2004). While caveolin-1 and -2 are fairly generically expressed, caveolin-3 presence is limited to muscle and glial cells (Okamoto, Schlegel et al. 1998; Razani, Schlegel et al. 2000; Williams and Lisanti 2004). Different variants have been described for caveolin-1 and -2 (Razani, Woodman et al. 2002; van Deurs, Roepstorff et al. 2003).

Since caveolin-1 is the best characterized isoform, the discussion here will focus on this protein. Two variants referred to as caveolin-1α and-1β have been described that are generated by alternative initiation or splicing (Scherer, Tang et al. 1995; Kogo and Fujimoto 2000; Kogo, Aiba et al. 2004). Caveolin-1β lacks the first 31 amino acids present in caveolin-1α. This region contains the amino acid tyrosine 14, which is phosphorylated by src family kinases (Cao, Courchesne et al. 2002; Labrecque, Nyalendo et al. 2004). Caveolin-1 assumes an unusual topology, whereby a central hydrophobic domain (residues 102-134) is thought to form a hairpin structure within the membrane (Figure 3). As a consequence, both the N-terminal (residues 1-101) and C-terminal domain (residues 135-178) face the cytoplasm. A 41-amino acid region in the N-terminal domain, as well as COOH-terminal elements are required for the formation of caveolin-1 homo-oligomers. In the C-terminal segment, three palmitoylation sites are present at positions 133, 143 and 156 (Figure 3).

Caveolin-1 is phosphorylated on tyrosine-14 in response to growth factors like insulin (Mastick, Brady et al. 1995; Mastick and Saltiel 1997; Lee, Volonte et al. 2000; Kimura, Mora et al. 2002) or EGF (Lee, Volonte et al. 2000; Orlichenko, Huang et al. 2006) and by extracellular stimuli including, UV, oxidative stress or hyperosmolarity (Li, Seitz et al. 1996; Volonte, Galbiati et al. 2001; Sanguinetti and Mastick 2003; Cao, Sanguinetti et al. 2004). These observations have implicated caveolin-1 and particularly phosphorylation on tyrosine 14 in cellular stress responses. Consistent with this notion, caveolin-1 knockout mice have a reduced lifespan and are less resistant to partial hepatectomy (Park, Cohen et al. 2003; Fernandez, Albor et al. 2006).

Caveolin-1 and phosphorylated caveolin-1 are also implicated in cell migration. A specific aminoacid sequence (aminoacids 46-55) is required for localization of the protein to the rear of migrating cells (Sun, Flynn et al. 2007; Sun, Liu et al. 2009) and such polarized distribution of caveolin-1 and associated cell signaling elements is considered important for directional migration of some cell types (Isshiki, Ando et al. 2002; Parat, Anand-Apte et al. 2003; Beardsley, Fang et al. 2005). Although phosphorylation of caveolin-1 on tyrosine 14 has been shown to favor migration via a process involving recruitment of the adaptor protein Grb7 (Lee, Volonte et al. 2000), the precise role of caveolin-1 in these events remains an issue of controversy. In part this is attributable to technical problems associated with the precise identification of phospho-caveolin-1 localization in migrating cells (Hill, Scherbakov et al. 2007).

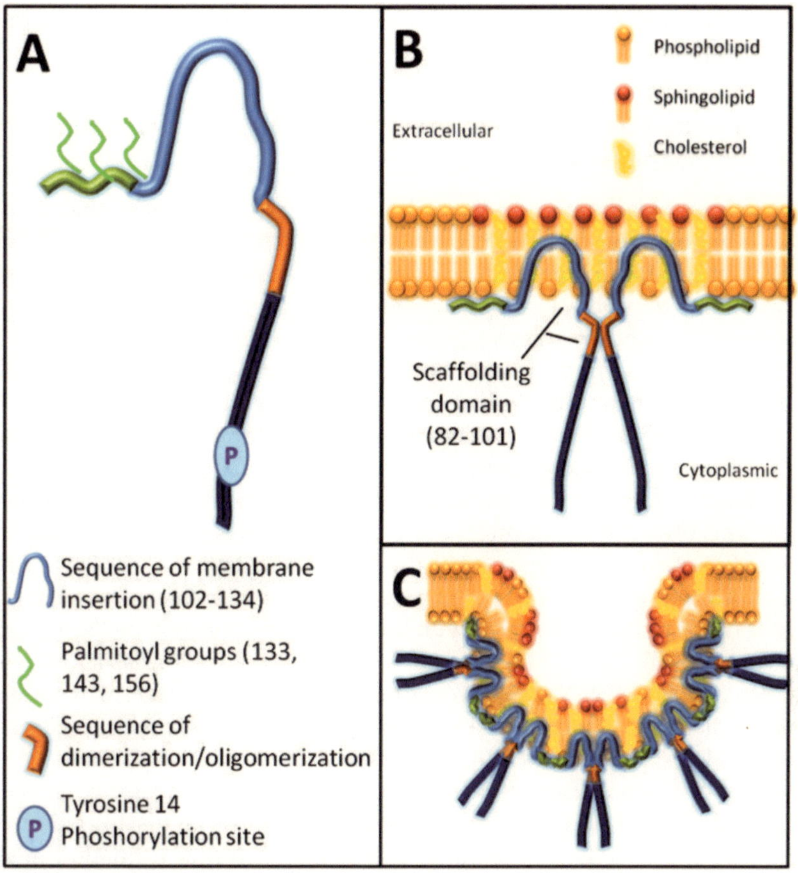


Fig. 3. Caveolin-1 structure and caveolae morphology.

A) Schematic showing the different domains present in caveolin-1 that permit interaction with other proteins and membranes. B) Caveolin-1 anchorage via the membrane insertion domain into regions enriched in sphingolipids and cholesterol. C) Caveolin-1 oligomerizes to generate the proteinaceous coat of caveolae, small invaginations (50-100 nm) of the plasma membrane. Additional proteins called cavins are also essential for the formation of these structures (not shown).

Despite these issues, a large body of literature is available linking the expression of caveolin-1 not only to enhanced migration but also metastasis of cancer cells. Likewise, caveolin-1 is implicated in development of the multi-drug resistant phenotype of aggressive cancer cells. All three characteristics of caveolin-1 mentioned, namely its participation in cellular stress responses and regeneration, migration and metastasis, as well as multi-drug resistance tend to favor the interpretation that caveolin-1 represents a protein whose presence is associated with tumor progression. Such evidence, however, has generated an intense discussion concerning the precise role of caveolin-1 in cancer, since also a large body of data is available suggesting that caveolin-1 functions as a tumor suppressor (see subsequent sections). A key objective in the remaining section of this chapter will be to highlight important aspects of this ongoing discussion and attempt to reconcile these different and opposing functions of caveolin-1 in a working model (see Figure 4). In doing so, we will focus our attention mostly on studies dealing with the role of caveolin-1 in modulating the Wnt/β-catenin pathway.

## 8. Role of caveolin-1 as tumor suppressor: Inhibition of β-catenin-Tcf/Lef-dependent gene expression

Over the last 15 years, a large amount of data has become available associating the presence of caveolin-1 with tumor suppression. However, as will be discussed, the ability of caveolin-1 to act in this fashion depends on the cellular context. Thus, caveolin-1 should be considered a "conditional" tumor suppressor. In initial studies, oncogene-mediated transformation of NIH3T3 fibroblasts was shown to correlate with reduced caveolin-1 mRNA and protein levels, and re-expression of the protein was sufficient to revert cell transformation (Koleske, Baltimore et al. 1995; Engelman, Wykoff et al. 1997). Likewise selective loss of caveolin-1 expression using an siRNA approach was sufficient to transform NIH3T3 fibroblasts (Galbiati, Volonte et al. 1998). Furthermore, caveolin-1 expression is reduced in a number of human tumors, including lung, mammary, colon and ovarian carcinomas, as well as osteosarcomas (Lee, Reimer et al. 1998; Racine, Belanger et al. 1999; Bender, Reymond et al. 2000; Wiechen, Diatchenko et al. 2001; Wiechen, Sers et al. 2001; Bender, Montoya et al. 2002; Ho, Huang et al. 2002; Cantiani, Manara et al. 2007). Here too, re-expression of caveolin-1 frequently, but not always, reverts characteristics associated with the transformed phenotype (Yang, Truong et al. 1998; Li, Yang et al. 2001; Tahir, Yang et al. 2001; Karam, Lotan et al. 2007; Yang, Addai et al. 2007; Bartz, Zhou et al. 2008). More recently, decreased caveolin-1 levels have been reported for lymph node metastases from head and neck squamous cell carcinoma and restoration of caveolin-1 expression suppresses growth and metastasis (Zhang, Su et al. 2008).

Despite the fact that caveolin-1 depletion in knockout mice does not lead to drastic changes in viability, it is now clear that caveolin-1 absence favors lung and mammary hyperplasia, angiogenesis, as well as carcinogen induced tumor formation in skin tissue (Drab, Verkade et al. 2001; Razani, Engelman et al. 2001; Capozza, Williams et al. 2003; Williams, Cheung et al. 2003). Also, increased mammary and intestinal stem cell proliferation is observed in caveolin-1 knockout mice and caveolin-1 was also shown to control neural stem cell proliferation (Jasmin, Yang et al. 2009). Finally, stromal expression of caveolin-1 in breast cancer predicts outcome, recurrence and survival, further highlighting its relevance as a potential therapeutic target (Sloan, Ciocca et al. 2009; Witkiewicz, Dasgupta et al. 2009). Indeed, caveolin-1 mutation of P132L, which was previously linked to breast cancer (Hayashi, Matsuda et al. 2001), was recently demonstrated to predict recurrence and metastasis in an orthotopic mouse model (Bonuccelli, Casimiro et al. 2009). Taken together, these reports demonstrate that caveolin-1 displays traits consistent with a role of the protein as a tumor suppressor. This ability of caveolin-1 has often been linked to inhibition of signalling events associated with cell survival and proliferation. However, it is important to note that alternative mechanisms have also been proposed. For a more detailed discussion of literature related to the tumor suppressor hypothesis, the interested reader is referred to additional reviews (Williams and Lisanti 2005; Quest, Gutierrez-Pajares et al. 2008).

Initially, our entrance to the caveolin-1 field came with the demonstration that caveolin-1 protein levels are reduced both in tumors from patients with colon cancer, as well as in colon adenocarcinoma cells and that caveolin-1 functions as a tumor suppressor *in vivo* upon re-expression in different colon adenocarcinoma cells (Bender, Reymond et al. 2000; Bender,

Montoya et al. 2002). Despite the ever-increasing abundance of signaling molecules available in the literature for regulation by caveolin-1, at the time relatively few were linked to specific transcriptional events. Thus, as one approach, we set out to compare, by microarray analysis, colon cancer cell lines expressing or not caveolin-1. Rather intriguingly, those studies identified in an initial screen the IAP protein survivin as one of the most strongly down-regulated targets at the transcriptional level (Torres, Tapia et al. 2006). This protein is of tremendous interest, since it is abundantly expressed in a variety of human tumors including lung, colon, breast, prostate, pancreatic, and gastric carcinoma, but is essentially absent in most normal tissues. Importantly, survivin expression in cancer cells is linked to tumor survival. These characteristics define survivin as a tumor specific antigen (Li, Ambrosini et al. 1998; Reed 2001; Altieri 2003).

The mayor challenge then was identifying a mechanism that permitted connecting events thought to occur at the plasma membrane with transcription in the nucleus. Given the importance of canonical Wnt signaling in colon cancer, this pathway became an attractive potential caveolin-1 target. This possibility was further substantiated by reports showing on the one hand that caveolin-1 expression prevented transcription of cyclinD1 by sequestering β-catenin (Hulit, Bash et al. 2000) and on the other that survivin is a β-catenin/Tcf/lef target gene (Kolligs, Bommer et al. 2002). With this in mind, we then established that caveolin-1 controled survivin expression by sequestering β-catenin to the plasma membrane (Torres, Tapia et al. 2006) and subsequently that this ability required the expression of E-cadherin in both colon cancer and melanoma cell lines (Torres, Tapia et al. 2007). Finally, evidence was obtained showing that caveolin-1 regulates in a similar fashion also the expression of cyclooxygenase-2 (COX2; (Rodriguez, Tapia et al. 2009).

Since loss of E-cadherin is frequently observed in human epithelial tumors (Cavallaro and Christofori 2004), our studies suggest that the combined loss of caveolin-1 and E-cadherin in epithelial cells is likely to promote increased expression of genes relevant to epithelial-mesenchymal transition, loss of cell-cell contacts and cell transformation. Perhaps even more importantly, they provide mechanistic insight to how caveolin-1-specific suppression of genes associated with its role as a tumor suppressor becomes "conditional", that is dependent on the cellular context (Torres, Tapia et al. 2007; Quest, Gutierrez-Pajares et al. 2008). Interestingly, this ability of caveolin-1 is not only limited by the proteins present within cells expressing caveolin-1, but also by factors present in the cellular medium. In particular, caveolin-1 expression was shown to limit $PGE_2$ accumulation in the culture media of HEK293T, DLD-1 and HT29 cells. Alternatively, supplementation of media with $PGE_2$ disrupted caveolin-1 complexes responsible for sequestration of β-catenin to the plasma membrane (Rodriguez, Tapia et al. 2009).

Despite the abundance of evidence summarized previously indicating that caveolin-1 functions as a tumor suppressor, there is also evidence suggesting a radically different, even opposite role for caveolin-1. Specifically, caveolin-1 is known to promote tumor formation and presence is correlated with poor prognosis and survival in prostate cancer. Indeed, the expression of caveolin-1 reportedly increases in primary tumors from prostate (Yang, Truong et al. 1998) and certain leukemia derived cell lines (Hatanaka, Maeda et al. 1998). Also, in prostate cancer cells caveolin-1 presence increases tumor growth and the incidence of metastasis (Li, Yang et al. 2001; Tahir, Yang et al. 2001; Karam, Lotan et al. 2007; Bartz, Zhou et al. 2008). Increased caveolin-1 expression in tumor samples is not restricted to cases, like the prostate, where normal tissues have low relative caveolin-1 levels, since increased expression was also reported in tumor models where initial caveolin-1 loss is observed, such as colon (Bender, Reymond et al. 2000) and breast cancer (Fiucci, Ravid et al. 2002; Garcia, Dales et al. 2007; Savage, Lambros et al. 2007).

In most of these cases, the available data argue for a strong positive correlation between expression of caveolin-1, metastasis and multidrug resistance (Lavie, Fiucci et al. 1998; Lavie and Liscovitch 2000; Garcia, Dales et al. 2007). Moreover, studies in samples derived from esophageal squamous cell carcinoma (Ando, Ishiguro et al. 2007), small cell lung carcinomas (Ho, Huang et al. 2002), colon cancer cells with elevated metastatic potential ((Bender, Reymond et al. 2000), see below) and gastric cancer (Burgermeister, Tencer et al. 2003), revealed that caveolin-1 expression correlates with poor patient prognosis. Furthermore, caveolin-1 is also overexpressed in nasopharyngeal carcinoma and protein levels correlate there with poor prognosis, enhanced tumor cell migration and metastasis (Du, Hu et al. 2009). Finally, caveolin-1 was recently associated with tumor progression in a panel of melanoma cell lines, since increased expression correlated with enhanced proliferation, cell migration and tumorigenicity (Felicetti, Parolini et al. 2009).

## 9. Caveolin-1 function as a promoter of metastasis: The role of phosphorylation on tyrosine-14

A variety of potential mechanisms have been invoked to explain how caveolin-1 presence may favor tumor progression. For example, in prostate cancer cells, increased caveolin-1 levels were found to favor growth factor release and regulation by a positive feedback loop that enhances tumor cell invasiveness (Li, Ren et al. 2009) and VEGF-associated pro-angiogenic signaling (Tahir, Park et al. 2009). Futhermore, Caveolin-1 is located on prostasomes secreted by prostate cancer cells (Llorente, de Marco et al. 2004) and the presence of antibodies against caveolin-1 in blood plasma decreased prostate cancer cell metastasis in animal models (Watanabe, Yang et al. 2009). In breast cancer cells, caveolin-1 was recently shown to associate with type 1 matrix metalloproteinase and thereby promote invadopodia formation, as well as matrix degradation, both of which favor invasiveness (Yamaguchi, Takeo et al. 2009). Also, caveolin-1 enhanced hepatocellular carcinoma cell motility and invasiveness is associated with augmented metalloproteinase expression and secretion, together with down-regulation of E-cadherin (Cokakli, Erdal et al. 2009). Alternatively, re-expression of caveolin-1 in lung adenocarcinoma cells is sufficient to promote filopodia formation, cell migration and metastatic potential of these cells (Ho, Huang et al. 2002). Thus, as so often, the alterations observed due to the presence of caveolin-1 depend on the model under study. However, all the aforementioned observations have in common that caveolin-1 promotes traits associated with increased malignancy of cancer cells.

Successful tumor cell metastasis to distant sites requires the acquisition of multiple traits, including the ability to migrate. Interestingly, caveolin-1 is required for cell polarization and migration in two and three dimensions (Parat, Anand-Apte et al. 2003; Beardsley, Fang et al. 2005; Santilman, Baran et al. 2007; Yamaguchi, Takeo et al. 2009). Additionally, caveolin-1 regulates the small GTPases Rho and Rac, which are required for actin dynamics, cell polarization and directional migration (del Pozo, Balasubramanian et al. 2005; Grande-Garcia, Echarri et al. 2007; Grande-Garcia and del Pozo 2008). Furthermore, phosphorylation of caveolin-1 on tyrosine-14 favors cell migration (Grande-Garcia, Echarri et al. 2007) and anchorage-independent growth via the adaptor protein Grb7 (Lee, Volonte et al. 2000). Thus, in addition to its role as a tumor suppressor, caveolin-1 clearly also displays characteristics of a protein that promotes cell migration and metastasis.

Many explanations for such variations in function exist. One possibility is that the role of caveolin-1 depends on the cellular environment and that tumor suppressor activity is developed in systems where negative signalling occurs downstream of caveolin-1. Alternatively, when presence of the protein is associated with more aggressive tumor behavior, positive caveolin-1 mediated signalling is likely to be more important (reviewed in (Quest, Leyton et al. 2004; Quest, Gutierrez-Pajares et al. 2008)). A fundamental problem here is that direct comparisons are difficult, since these distinct characteristics were observed in different experimental settings and cell models. Ideally, to begin to test the aforementioned working hypothesis and identify molecular features of caveolin-1 that contribute to one or the other behavioral pattern, an approach that permits evaluation of these two characteristics in the same cell/animal model would be required. In this respect, some recent results from our laboratory suggest that melanomas may represent an interesting model.

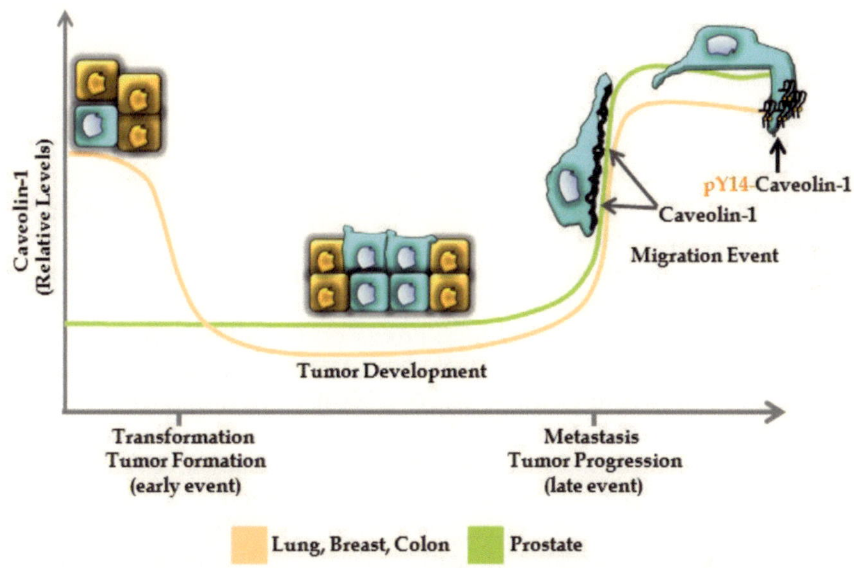


| | Caveolin-1 expression | | | | | |
|---|---|---|---|---|---|---|
| Tissue | Normal | Cancer | Late Phase | knock-out mice* | Cell transfection** | Repression** |
| Lung | High | Low | Metastasis | Hyperplasia | Cell polarization and migration | ? |
| Breast | High | Low | Metastasis | Increased susceptibility to tumors | Resistance to anoikis, sensitization to Gefitinib | High sensitivity to chemotherapy, invadopodia |
| Colon | High | Low | Multidrug resistance, Metastasis | Increased susceptibility to tumors | ? | ? |
| Prostate | Low | High | Metastasis | ? | ? | ? |
| Melanoma | ? | ? | Metastasis | ? | ? | ? |

* *in vivo* model
** *in vitro* model

Fig. 4. Dual role of caveolin-1 in cancer: Representative profiles of caveolin-1 expression in different types of human cancer cells.

Two profiles of caveolin-1 expression appear to prevail in human cancer (Figure 4). In the first case, caveolin-1 expression is as follows: i) caveolin-1 is expressed in normal tissue. ii) During the development of cancer, caveolin-1 levels decline. iii) In later stages caveolin-1 re-expression occurs. Examples here include lung, colon and breast cancer. The second possibility is: i) Essentially, caveolin-1 is not expressed in normal tissue. ii) Caveolin-1 expression increases with tumor progression. The typical example here is prostate cancer. As, indicated, in many cancer cell types expression of caveolin-1 is associated with enhanced migratory capacity and multidrug resistance. How changes in caveolin-1 expression relate to melanoma development remain unclear. These characteristics are summarized again in the table (Figure 4). Additionally, the effects of loss of caveolin-1 expression in different tissues of knock-out mice are mentioned, as well as the consequences of either over-expressing or down-regulating caveolin-1 in tumor cells.

## 10. Caveolin-1 in melanoma

Relatively little information is available concerning the role of caveolin-1 in melanomas. Early reports focussed on studying the relationship between this protein and glycosphingolipids, which are important constituents of membrane microdomains referred to as "glycolipid-enriched membranes", "detergent-insoluble microdomains" (DIMs) or simply "membrane rafts" because of their flotation behaviour on sucrose gradients following centrifugation. Depending on whether or not caveolin-1 is associated with such membrane rafts, these may become detectable as 50-100 nm invaginations of the membrane called caveolae. Both membrane rafts and caveolae have received considerable attention due to their participation in a variety of cellular processes, including endocytosis, cholesterol transport, micro-organism infection and signal transduction. A detailed discussion of these aspects can be found elsewhere (Quest et al., 2004; 2008). Here, they are relevant because of their reported role in the regulation of signals associated with the development of malignant properties in cancer cells. For instance, in B16 mouse melanoma cells, a GM3-enriched membrane subdomain implicated in adhesion and migration was found to contain a number of relevant signaling molecules, including c-Src, FAK, and RhoA. This GM3 enriched "glycosphingolipid signaling domain" however does not contain caveolin-1 and appears to represent a functionally distinct identity from caveolin-1 and cholesterol-enriched microdomains in these cells (Iwabuchi et al 1998).
Acidic glycosphingolipids also play an important role in tumor biology and particularly GD3 expression is increased in almost all malignant melanomas and melanoma cell lines. In human melanoma cells, GD3 presence is associated with enhanced tyrosine phosphorylation of the two adaptor molecules p130Cas and paxillin. In SK-MEL-28 human melanoma cells, GD3 accumulates at the leading edge together with the aforementioned adaptor molecules and is thought to promote migration. In cells expressing caveolin-1, GD3 becomes homogeneously distributed in the membrane, rather than concentrated in specific regions. Hence, caveolin-1 is suggested to function as a tumor suppressor in melanoma cells by disrupting GD3-mediated malignant signaling (Nakashima, Hamamura et al. 2007).
Alternatively, for a non-cutaneous, retinal melanoma, increased caveolin-1 expression was associated with enhanced malignancy. Previous reports had documented low levels of caveolin-1 expression in different cell types of normal murine retinal tissue. Essentially this was corroborated in human tissue and, additionally, the level of expression of caveolin-1

was shown to increase in retinal melanoma cells (Berta, Kiss et al. 2007). An even more recent study identified exosomes in the plasma of melanoma patients, with high levels of caveolin-1. Exosomes are small vesicle secreted by both normal and tumoral cells. In this particular case, they were attributed immunosuppressive effects and associated with malignant tumor progression (Logozzi, De Milito et al. 2009). This study suggests that mechanisms similar to those already mentioned for prostate cancer may be relevant to caveolin-1 function in melanoma metastasis.

The notion that caveolin-1 presence may favor metastasis is supported by additional studies. Felicetti and co-workers proposed that caveolin-1 expression is associated with increased metastatic potential in different human melanoma cell lines. Specifically, caveolin-1 expression was increased using retroviral vectors in human melanoma cell lines. For the WM983A melanoma cell line, caveolin-1 increased cell proliferation, anchorage-independent growth, migration and invasion. Also, caveolin-1 down-regulation in metastatic caveolin-1-expressing melanomas reduces their proliferation, as well as their tumorigenicity (Felicetti, Parolini et al. 2009). Rather surprisingly, another recent report indicates that caveolin-1 blocks metastasis of malignant melanomas in a murine model (Trimmer, Whitaker-Menezes et al. 2010). Caveolin-1 has previously been shown to down-regulate survivin expression by sequestering β-catenin to the plasma membrane and reducing β-catenin-Tcf/Lef dependent transcription (Torres, Tapia et al. 2006). To do so, cells must express E-cadherin. However, E-cadherin is frequently silenced in melanomas and downregulation of this protein is considered one of the possible causes of melanoma progression and metastasis. Indeed, B16F10 cells do not express E-cadherin. Accordingly, E-cadherin re-expression in B16F10 murine melanoma cell line restored the ability of caveolin-1 to reduce cell proliferation and increase apoptosis by repressing survivin (Torres, Tapia et al. 2007).

Once again these findings highlight the apparent ambiguity of caveolin-1 function in melanomas and clearly more studies are warranted. As mentioned previously, an ideal experimental system would permit observing the role of caveolin-1 as a tumor suppressor and promoter of metastasis in the same cell/animal model.

## 11. Tumor formation assays in mouse melanoma models

Currently available models for the study of melanomas include: i) Xeno-transplantation models using genetically modified animals. One frequently employed possibility here are immunosuppressed animals that can be challenged with cells of another species. (ii) Syngeneic transplantation models. In this case, melanoma cells are derived from the same host so that immunological responses are avoided. Some examples here include Harding-Passey melanoma in BALB/c x DBA/2F1 mice, the Cloudman S91 melanoma in DBA/2 mice and the B16 melanoma in C57BL/6 mice. (iii) Genetically modified animals that develop spontaneous melanomas. Examples here include mouse lines expressing known oncogenes, such as Ret or mutant forms of Ras and Raf under the control of ubiquitous or tissue-specific promoters. Such mice develop melanocytic hyperplasia, retinal pigmented epithelial tumors and melanomas (Becker, Houben et al. 2010).

### 11.1 Syngeneic B16-F10 murine melanoma model

In our laboratory, the effects of caveolin-1 have been evaluated using two *in vivo* model systems, a xeno-transplantation model for HT29 and DLD-1 human colon adenocarcinoma cell lines in nude mice (Bender, Reymond et al. 2000) and the syngeneic B16 murine melanoma model in C57BL6 mice (Nicolson, Brunson et al. 1978). Both models serve well to assess the ability of a protein like caveolin-1 to function as a tumor suppressor or promoter upon subcutaneous injection of the tumor cells. However, a major advantage of the latter model is that the behaviour of cells injected into the tail vein can also be readily evaluated. Since these cells are pigmented, dissemination throughout the body or specifically to the lung can be quantified for cells independent of whether they have been selected for homing or not (B16F10 versus B16F0 cells). Additionally, this model is closer to the situation in human patients because the tumors develop from cells in syngeneic mice with a fully functional immune system.

The schematic below (Figure 5) summarizes the origin of B16F0 cells (poorly metastatic) and how B16F10 cells (highly metastatic) were obtained by repetitive cycles of injection into the tail vein and recovery from the lung. Moreover, the figure highlights how the behaviour of such cells can be evaluated in tumor formation and metastasis assays.

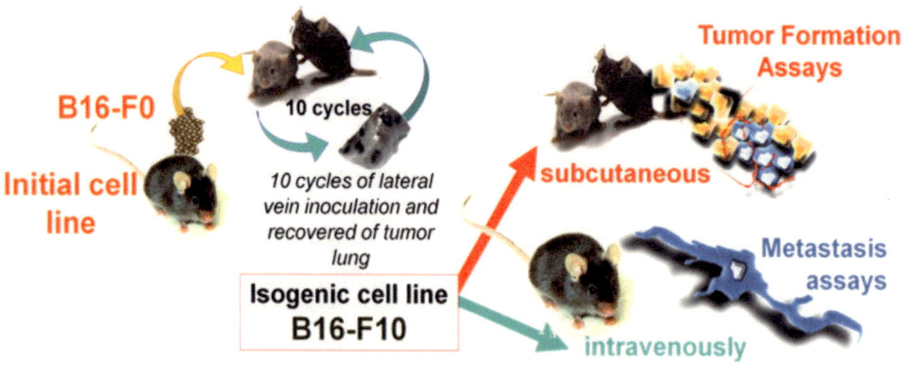


Fig. 5. Generation of B16F0 and B16-F10 cells (Nicolson, Brunson et al. 1978).

The parent tumor cell population of B16-F0 cells was isolated from a spontaneous melanoma in C57BL6 mice. These cells were then selected for their ability to colonize the lung following intravenous injection. To that end, B16-F0 cells were injected into the tail vein of C57BL/6 mice. Cells that formed tumors in the lung were expanded in culture and then injected again into the tail vein. This process was repeated ten times and the resulting population is referred to as B16-F10 cells. These cells behave very differently depending on the microenvironment. When B16-F10 cells are injected sub-cutaneously they form defined, palpable tumors. Alternatively, when injected intravenously these cells colonize the lung to form well defined black melanocytic nodules. See also figures 6 and 7, respectively.

### 11.2 Tumour formation in the B16F10 melanoma model

To study the ambiguity of caveolin-1 function, B16-F10 cells transfected or not with a plasmid (placIOP) permitting IPTG-inducible expression of caveolin-1 (plaIOP(cav-1)) were employed. These cells have been described previously (Torres, Tapia et al. 2007). The *in vivo* effect of the caveolin-1 expression in B16-F10 melanoma cells was evaluated by subcutaneous injection into of the flanks of mice. Appearance of tumors was monitored by palpitation and in initial experiments confirmed by histopathological analysis (Figure 6). Histological sections revealed that the tumors were composed entirely of proliferating melanoma cells, whereas extracellular matrix, blood vessels and the stroma were largely confined to the tumor perifery. Hence, the tumors observed in this model system are rather soft and gelatinous, making manipulation for immunohistochemical analysis more difficult (Figure 6). Mice were monitored for 7 to 30 days after the challenge with tumor cells. As shown, our preliminary results using this syngeneic murine melanoma model indicated that caveolin-1 was able to suppress tumor formation *in vivo* (see Fig. 6A and 6B).

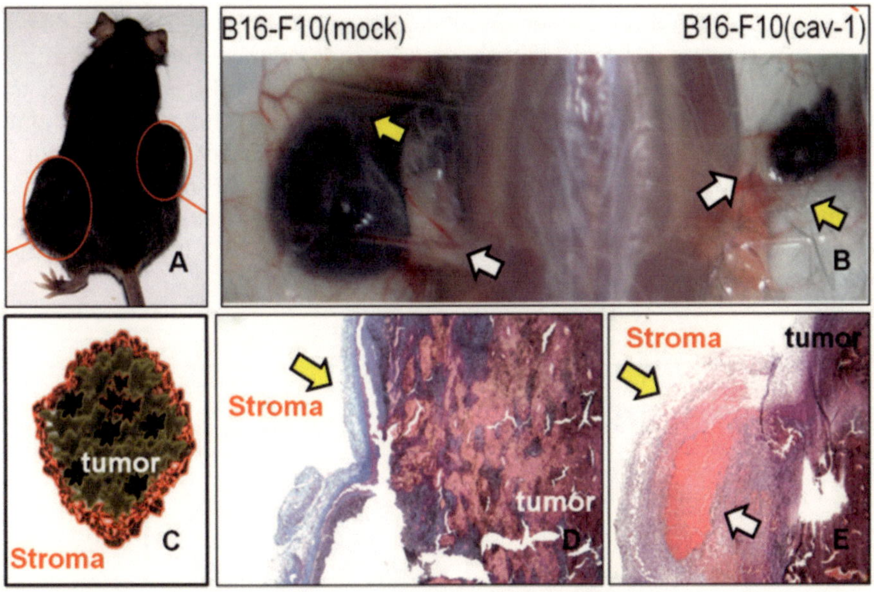


Fig. 6. Characterization of subcutaneous tumors.

C57BL/6 mice were inoculated with B16-F10 (mock) and B16-F10 (cav-1) cells on the left and right side of the animal, respectively. When the tumors of B16-F10(mock) cells reached the bioethically permitted limit the animals were sacrificed and the tumors were fixed in paraformaldehyde, embedded in paraffin, sectioned and stained with hematoxylin and eosin for histological analysis. A) Mouse inoculated with B16-F10(mock) and B16-F10(cav-1) cells injected into the left and right flank, respectively. B) Dissected tumors from mouse injected with cells as indicated in A. White arrows indicate external blood vessels. Yellow arrows highlight the tumor overlying serous tissue. C) Scheme showing how stroma support tissue surrounds the tumor. D) Histological section of a subcutaneous melanoma tumor, where the stroma and blood vessels surround the homogeneous tumor mass. E) Histological section of another subcutaneous tumor. White arrow: blood vessel located outside of the tumor; yellow arrow: stromal tissue.

## 12. Metastasis assays

To date, studies that employ the B16F10 model of lung metastasis generally quantify the metastastic nodules that are apparent at the lung surface (Figure 7). However, evidence in the literature indicates that this mode of quantification probably sub-estimates the actual extent of metastasis. Specifically, for B16F10 cells it is known that the cell adhesion molecule Lu-ECAM-1 plays a fundamental role in retention of these cells in the lung. This molecule is present to some extent in venes of the parenchyma, but is strongly expressed particularly in sub-pleural and pleural venes, as well as in large venes of the lung and venes of the mesenchyma (Zhu, Cheng et al. 1991). The sites of expression Lu-ECAM-1 are entirely consistent with the distribution of melanomas we observed upon dissection of the lung. Moreover, the extent of lung metastasis observed by freezing the lungs of experimental animals, separating melanoma from normal tissue and then weighing both yielded results that were distinct from those obtained by simply counting nodules at the surface, as was reported (Trimmer, Whitaker-Menezes et al. 2010). In our hands, preliminary experiments indicated that the approach of actually quantifying lung tumor mass was far superior in detecting lung metastasis for B16 F10 cells expressing caveolin-1. Results obtained in this manner with B16-F10 cells clearly indicate that augmented caveolin-1 expression levels enhanced the metastatic potential of these melanoma cells when injected intravenously into animals. Taken together, the results discussed here suggest that the B16F10/C57BL6 model represents an ideal experimental system to identify molecular traits in caveolin-1 associated with its role as a tumor suppressor and promoter of metastasis.

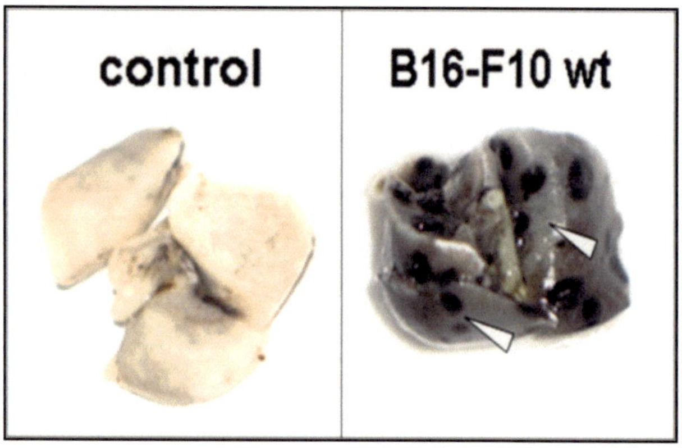


Fig. 7. Lung metastases.

B16-F10 cells were cultured in 100 mm plates for 48 h. Control mice were inoculated intravenously with saline solution (left panel) and the other group of mice were inoculated with 200,000 B16-F10 cells in 500 µl of saline solution (right panel). On day 21 post-injection, the animals were sacrificed, organs were removed and necropsied to identify melanocytic nodules. The lungs shown were fixed in Feketes buffer for 48 h. Arrowheads indicate nodules.

## 13. The caveolin-1 dilema: Summary and outlook

The data summarized here reinforce the notion that caveolin-1 potentially plays a dual role in melanoma development, as has been described for other cancers (reviewed in (Quest, Leyton et al. 2004; Quest, Gutierrez-Pajares et al. 2008)). The ambiguity of caveolin-1 function is perhaps best reconciled by the view portrayed in Figure 4. Colon cancer is an example where initial loss of caveolin-1 is followed by re-expression at later stages. If caveolin-1 is re-expressed at early stages, it develops traits consistent with a role as a tumor suppressor. Regulation of the Wnt signaling pathway is one possibly relevant mechanism discussed here, although several more are likely to exist. During tumor progression, the cellular context changes, since expression of a large number of proteins is altered. One such possibility we eluded to is the loss of E-cadherin. However, extracellular components, such as $PGE_2$ are also relevant. Hence, both "intracellular" and also "extracellular" changes define caveolin-1 function in a cell. When then later in tumor progression caveolin-1 expression is triggered by as yet poorly defined mechanisms, the protein no longer encounters conditions that permit function as a tumor suppressor, and for instance suppression of β-catenin-dependent transcription. Instead, characteristics associated with malignant cell behavior, including increased cell migration, may prevail. For prostate cancer, the situation is different because caveolin-1 is not expressed in normal tissue. At this point, it is still not clear which of these examples is closest to the situation in melanomas. However, particularly the studies by Felicetti and co-workers (Felicetti, Parolini et al. 2009) indicate that prostate may represent a more appropriate comparison. However, it should be noted that loss of E-cadherin represents a crucial step towards metastasis in the development of melanomas. Bearing this in mind, one may suspect that augmented expression of caveolin-1 in later stages of melanoma development will promote the acquisition of a more malignant phenotype in these cells. The availability of an experimental model where both characteristics of the protein can be detected and analyzed *in vivo*, now permit defining the molecular traits associated with tumor suppression and enhanced metastasis. With such insight at hand, we may anticipate the design and use of successful caveolin-1-based strategies in the treatment of melanoma.

## 14. Acknowledgements

The work was supported by the FONDECYT-FONDAP grant #15010006, FONDECYT grant #1090071 (to A.F.G.Q).

## 15. Abbreviations

AA, arachidonic acid; APC, adenomatous polyposis coli; CSD, caveolin scaffolding domain; GSK3β, glycogen synthase kinase; IAP, inhibitor of apoptosis; MDR, multidrug resistance; NSAIDs, non-steroidal anti-inflammatory drugs; PCP, planar cell polarity; $PGE_2$, prostaglandin E2; $PGH_2$, prostaglandin H2; Tcf/Lef, T cell factor/lymphoid enhancer binding factor; SCF, Skp1-Cul1-F-box-protein.

## 16. References

Altieri, D. C. (2003). Validating survivin as a cancer therapeutic target. *Nat Rev Cancer* 3(1): 46-54.

Anderson, R. G. (1998). The caveolae membrane system. *Annu Rev Biochem* 67: 199-225.

Ando, T., H. Ishiguro, et al. (2007). The overexpression of caveolin-1 and caveolin-2 correlates with a poor prognosis and tumor progression in esophageal squamous cell carcinoma. *Oncol Rep* 18(3): 601-609.

Bachmann, I. M., O. Straume, et al. (2005). Importance of P-cadherin, beta-catenin, and Wnt5a/frizzled for progression of melanocytic tumors and prognosis in cutaneous melanoma. *Clin Cancer Res* 11(24 Pt 1): 8606-8614.

Bartz, R., J. Zhou, et al. (2008). Caveolin-1 secreting LNCaP cells induce tumor growth of caveolin-1 negative LNCaP cells in vivo. *Int J Cancer* 122(3): 520-525.

Beardsley, A., K. Fang, et al. (2005). Loss of caveolin-1 polarity impedes endothelial cell polarization and directional movement. *J Biol Chem* 280(5): 3541-3547.

Becker, J. C., R. Houben, et al. (2010). Mouse models for melanoma: a personal perspective. *Exp Dermatol* 19(2): 157-164.

Bender, F., M. Montoya, et al. (2002). Caveolae and caveolae-like membrane domains in cellular signaling and disease: identification of downstream targets for the tumor suppressor protein caveolin-1. *Biol Res* 35(2): 151-167.

Bender, F. C., M. A. Reymond, et al. (2000). Caveolin-1 levels are down-regulated in human colon tumors, and ectopic expression of caveolin-1 in colon carcinoma cell lines reduces cell tumorigenicity. *Cancer Res* 60(20): 5870-5878.

Berta, A. I., A. L. Kiss, et al. (2007). Different caveolin isoforms in the retina of melanoma malignum affected human eye. *Mol Vis* 13: 881-886.

Berx, G., F. Nollet, et al. (1998). Dysregulation of the E-cadherin/catenin complex by irreversible mutations in human carcinomas. *Cell Adhes Commun* 6(2-3): 171-184.

Bienz, M. and H. Clevers (2000). Linking colorectal cancer to Wnt signaling. Cell 103(2): 311-320.

Bonuccelli, G., M. C. Casimiro, et al. (2009). Caveolin-1 (P132L), a common breast cancer mutation, confers mammary cell invasiveness and defines a novel stem cell/metastasis-associated gene signature. *Am J Pathol* 174(5): 1650-1662.

Brembeck, F. H., M. Rosario, et al. (2006). Balancing cell adhesion and Wnt signaling, the key role of beta-catenin. *Curr Opin Genet Dev* 16(1): 51-59.

Burgermeister, E., L. Tencer, et al. (2003). Peroxisome proliferator-activated receptor-gamma upregulates caveolin-1 and caveolin-2 expression in human carcinoma cells. *Oncogene* 22(25): 3888-3900.

Cantiani, L., M. C. Manara, et al. (2007). Caveolin-1 reduces osteosarcoma metastases by inhibiting c-Src activity and met signaling. *Cancer Res* 67(16): 7675-7685.

Cao, H., W. E. Courchesne, et al. (2002). A phosphotyrosine-dependent protein interaction screen reveals a role for phosphorylation of caveolin-1 on tyrosine 14: recruitment of C-terminal Src kinase. *J Biol Chem* 277(11): 8771-8774.

Cao, H., A. R. Sanguinetti, et al. (2004). Oxidative stress activates both Src-kinases and their negative regulator Csk and induces phosphorylation of two targeting proteins for Csk: caveolin-1 and paxillin. *Exp Cell Res* 294(1): 159-171.

Capozza, F., T. M. Williams, et al. (2003). Absence of caveolin-1 sensitizes mouse skin to carcinogen-induced epidermal hyperplasia and tumor formation. *Am J Pathol* 162(6): 2029-2039.

Cavallaro, U. and G. Christofori (2004). Cell adhesion and signalling by cadherins and Ig-CAMs in cancer. *Nat Rev Cancer* 4(2): 118-132.

Cokakli, M., E. Erdal, et al. (2009). Differential expression of Caveolin-1 in hepatocellular carcinoma: correlation with differentiation state, motility and invasion. *BMC Cancer* 9: 65.

Cheli, Y., M. Ohanna, et al. Fifteen-year quest for microphthalmia-associated transcription factor target genes. *Pigment Cell Melanoma Res* 23(1): 27-40.

Chien, A. J., E. C. Moore, et al. (2009). Activated Wnt/beta-catenin signaling in melanoma is associated with decreased proliferation in patient tumors and a murine melanoma model. *Proc Natl Acad Sci U S A* 106(4): 1193-1198.

De Panfilis, G., D. Ferrari, et al. (2009). Cytoplasmic beta-catenin is lacking in a subset of melanoma-associated naevi, but is detectable in naevus-associated melanomas: potential implications for melanoma tumorigenesis? *Br J Dermatol* 160(3): 600-608.

del Pozo, M. A., N. Balasubramanian, et al. (2005). Phospho-caveolin-1 mediates integrin-regulated membrane domain internalization. *Nat Cell Biol* 7(9): 901-908.

Dissanayake, S. K., P. B. Olkhanud, et al. (2008). Wnt5A regulates expression of tumor-associated antigens in melanoma via changes in signal transducers and activators of transcription 3 phosphorylation. *Cancer Res* 68(24): 10205-10214.

Dissanayake, S. K., M. Wade, et al. (2007). The Wnt5A/protein kinase C pathway mediates motility in melanoma cells via the inhibition of metastasis suppressors and initiation of an epithelial to mesenchymal transition. *J Biol Chem* 282(23): 17259-17271.

Drab, M., P. Verkade, et al. (2001). Loss of caveolae, vascular dysfunction, and pulmonary defects in caveolin-1 gene-disrupted mice. *Science* 293(5539): 2449-2452.

Du, Z. M., C. F. Hu, et al. (2009). Upregulation of caveolin-1 and CD147 expression in nasopharyngeal carcinoma enhanced tumor cell migration and correlated with poor prognosis of the patients. *Int J Cancer* 125(8): 1832-1841.

Engelman, J. A., C. C. Wykoff, et al. (1997). Recombinant expression of caveolin-1 in oncogenically transformed cells abrogates anchorage-independent growth. *J Biol Chem* 272(26): 16374-16381.

Felicetti, F., I. Parolini, et al. (2009). Caveolin-1 tumor-promoting role in human melanoma. *Int J Cancer* 125(7): 1514-1522.

Fernandez, M. A., C. Albor, et al. (2006). Caveolin-1 is essential for liver regeneration. *Science* 313(5793): 1628-1632.

Fiucci, G., D. Ravid, et al. (2002). Caveolin-1 inhibits anchorage-independent growth, anoikis and invasiveness in MCF-7 human breast cancer cells. *Oncogene* 21(15): 2365-2375.

Galbiati, F., D. Volonte, et al. (1998). Targeted downregulation of caveolin-1 is sufficient to drive cell transformation and hyperactivate the p42/44 MAP kinase cascade. *Embo J* 17(22): 6633-6648.

Garcia, S., J. P. Dales, et al. (2007). Poor prognosis in breast carcinomas correlates with increased expression of targetable CD146 and c-Met and with proteomic basal-like phenotype. *Hum Pathol* 38(6): 830-841.

Garraway, L. A., H. R. Widlund, et al. (2005). Integrative genomic analyses identify MITF as a lineage survival oncogene amplified in malignant melanoma. *Nature* 436(7047): 117-122.

Giles, R. H., J. H. van Es, et al. (2003). Caught up in a Wnt storm: Wnt signaling in cancer. *Biochim Biophys Acta* 1653(1): 1-24.

Gottardi, C. J., E. Wong, et al. (2001). E-cadherin suppresses cellular transformation by inhibiting beta-catenin signaling in an adhesion-independent manner. *J Cell Biol* 153(5): 1049-1060.

Grande-Garcia, A. and M. A. del Pozo (2008). Caveolin-1 in cell polarization and directional migration. *Eur J Cell Biol* 87(8-9): 641-647.

Grande-Garcia, A., A. Echarri, et al. (2007). Caveolin-1 regulates cell polarization and directional migration through Src kinase and Rho GTPases. *J Cell Biol* 177(4): 683-694.

Gray-Schopfer, V., C. Wellbrock, et al. (2007). Melanoma biology and new targeted therapy. *Nature* 445(7130): 851-857.

Haertel-Wiesmann, M., Y. Liang, et al. (2000). Regulation of cyclooxygenase-2 and periostin by Wnt-3 in mouse mammary epithelial cells. *J Biol Chem* 275(41): 32046-32051.

Hajra, K. M. and E. R. Fearon (2002). Cadherin and catenin alterations in human cancer. *Genes Chromosomes Cancer* 34(3): 255-268.

Hanahan, D. and R. A. Weinberg (2000). The hallmarks of cancer. *Cell* 100(1): 57-70.

Hanahan, D. and R. A. Weinberg (2011). Hallmarks of cancer: the next generation. *Cell* 144(5): 646-674.

Hatanaka, M., T. Maeda, et al. (1998). Expression of caveolin-1 in human T cell leukemia cell lines. *Biochem Biophys Res Commun* 253(2): 382-387.

Hayashi, K., S. Matsuda, et al. (2001). Invasion activating caveolin-1 mutation in human scirrhous breast cancers. *Cancer Res* 61(6): 2361-2364.

He, T. C., A. B. Sparks, et al. (1998). Identification of c-MYC as a target of the APC pathway. *Science* 281(5382): 1509-1512.

Heeg-Truesdell, E. and C. LaBonne (2006). Wnt signaling: a shaggy dogma tale. *Curr Biol* 16(2): R62-64.

Henderson, B. R. and F. Fagotto (2002). The ins and outs of APC and beta-catenin nuclear transport. *EMBO Rep* 3(9): 834-839.

Hill, M. M., N. Scherbakov, et al. (2007). Reassessing the role of phosphocaveolin-1 in cell adhesion and migration. *Traffic* 8(12): 1695-1705.

Ho, C. C., P. H. Huang, et al. (2002). Up-regulated caveolin-1 accentuates the metastasis capability of lung adenocarcinoma by inducing filopodia formation. *Am J Pathol* 161(5): 1647-1656.



Ho, C. C., P. H. Huang, et al. (2002). Up-regulated caveolin-1 accentuates the metastasis capability of lung adenocarcinoma by inducing filopodia formation. *Am J Pathol* 161(5): 1647-1656.



Huang, H. and X. He (2008). Wnt/beta-catenin signaling: new (and old) players and new insights. *Curr Opin Cell Biol* 20(2): 119-125.

Hulit, J., T. Bash, et al. (2000). The cyclin D1 gene is transcriptionally repressed by caveolin-1. *J Biol Chem* 275(28): 21203-21209.

Isshiki, M., J. Ando, et al. (2002). Sites of Ca(2+) wave initiation move with caveolae to the trailing edge of migrating cells. *J Cell Sci* 115(Pt 3): 475-484.

Jasmin, J. F., M. Yang, et al. (2009). Genetic ablation of caveolin-1 increases neural stem cell proliferation in the subventricular zone (SVZ) of the adult mouse brain. *Cell Cycle* 8(23): 3978-3983.

Jeanes, A., C. J. Gottardi, et al. (2008). Cadherins and cancer: how does cadherin dysfunction promote tumor progression? *Oncogene* 27(55): 6920-6929.

Kageshita, T., C. V. Hamby, et al. (2001). Loss of beta-catenin expression associated with disease progression in malignant melanoma. *Br J Dermatol* 145(2): 210-216.

Karam, J. A., Y. Lotan, et al. (2007). Caveolin-1 overexpression is associated with aggressive prostate cancer recurrence. *Prostate* 67(6): 614-622.

Khan, N. I., K. F. Bradstock, et al. (2007). Activation of Wnt/beta-catenin pathway mediates growth and survival in B-cell progenitor acute lymphoblastic leukaemia. *Br J Haematol* 138(3): 338-348.

Kim, P. J., J. Plescia, et al. (2003). Survivin and molecular pathogenesis of colorectal cancer. *Lancet* 362(9379): 205-209.

Kimelman, D. and W. Xu (2006). beta-catenin destruction complex: insights and questions from a structural perspective. *Oncogene* 25(57): 7482-7491.

Kimura, A., S. Mora, et al. (2002). The insulin receptor catalyzes the tyrosine phosphorylation of caveolin-1. *J Biol Chem* 277(33): 30153-30158.

Klaus, A. and W. Birchmeier (2008). Wnt signalling and its impact on development and cancer. *Nat Rev Cancer* 8(5): 387-398.

Kogo, H., T. Aiba, et al. (2004). Cell type-specific occurrence of caveolin-1alpha and -1beta in the lung caused by expression of distinct mRNAs. *J Biol Chem* 279(24): 25574-25581.

Kogo, H. and T. Fujimoto (2000). Caveolin-1 isoforms are encoded by distinct mRNAs. Identification of mouse caveolin-1 mRNA variants caused by alternative transcription initiation and splicing. *FEBS Lett* 465(2-3): 119-123.

Koleske, A. J., D. Baltimore, et al. (1995). Reduction of caveolin and caveolae in oncogenically transformed cells. *Proc Natl Acad Sci U S A* 92(5): 1381-1385.

Kolligs, F. T., G. Bommer, et al. (2002). Wnt/beta-catenin/tcf signaling: a critical pathway in gastrointestinal tumorigenesis. *Digestion* 66(3): 131-144.

Kreizenbeck, G. M., A. J. Berger, et al. (2008). Prognostic significance of cadherin-based adhesion molecules in cutaneous malignant melanoma. *Cancer Epidemiol Biomarkers Prev* 17(4): 949-958.

Labrecque, L., C. Nyalendo, et al. (2004). Src-mediated tyrosine phosphorylation of caveolin-1 induces its association with membrane type 1 matrix metalloproteinase. *J Biol Chem* 279(50): 52132-52140.

Larue, L. and V. Delmas (2006). The WNT/Beta-catenin pathway in melanoma. Front Biosci 11: 733-742.

Larue, L., F. Luciani, et al. (2009). Bypassing melanocyte senescence by beta-catenin: a novel way to promote melanoma. *Pathol Biol* (Paris) 57(7-8): 543-547.

Lavie, Y., G. Fiucci, et al. (1998). Up-regulation of caveolae and caveolar constituents in multidrug-resistant cancer cells. *J Biol Chem* 273(49): 32380-32383.

Lavie, Y. and M. Liscovitch (2000). Changes in lipid and protein constituents of rafts and caveolae in multidrug resistant cancer cells and their functional consequences. *Glycoconj J* 17(3 -4): 253-259.

Lee, H., D. Volonte, et al. (2000). Constitutive and growth factor-regulated phosphorylation of caveolin-1 occurs at the same site (Tyr-14) in vivo: identification of a c-Src/Cav-1/Grb7 signaling cassette. *Mol Endocrinol* 14(11): 1750-1775.

Lee, S. W., C. L. Reimer, et al. (1998). Tumor cell growth inhibition by caveolin re-expression in human breast cancer cells. *Oncogene* 16(11): 1391-1397.

Levy, C., M. Khaled, et al. (2006). MITF: master regulator of melanocyte development and melanoma oncogene. *Trends Mol Med* 12(9): 406-414.

Li, F., G. Ambrosini, et al. (1998). Control of apoptosis and mitotic spindle checkpoint by survivin. *Nature* 396(6711): 580-584.

Li, L., C. Ren, et al. (2009). Caveolin-1 promotes autoregulatory, Akt-mediated induction of cancer-promoting growth factors in prostate cancer cells. *Mol Cancer Res* 7(11): 1781-1791.

Li, L., G. Yang, et al. (2001). Caveolin-1 mediates testosterone-stimulated survival/clonal growth and promotes metastatic activities in prostate cancer cells. *Cancer Res* 61(11): 4386-4392.

Li, S., R. Seitz, et al. (1996). Phosphorylation of caveolin by src tyrosine kinases. The alpha-isoform of caveolin is selectively phosphorylated by v-Src in vivo. *J Biol Chem* 271(7): 3863-3868.

Logan, C. Y. and R. Nusse (2004). The Wnt signaling pathway in development and disease. *Annu Rev Cell Dev Biol* 20: 781-810.

Logozzi, M., A. De Milito, et al. (2009). High levels of exosomes expressing CD63 and caveolin-1 in plasma of melanoma patients. *PLoS One* 4(4): e5219.

Lucero, O. M., D. W. Dawson, et al. A re-evaluation of the oncogenic nature of Wnt/beta-catenin signaling in melanoma and other cancers. *Curr Oncol Rep* 12(5): 314-318.

Llorente, A., M. C. de Marco, et al. (2004). Caveolin-1 and MAL are located on prostasomes secreted by the prostate cancer PC-3 cell line. *J Cell Sci* 117(Pt 22): 5343-5351.

Ma, L., J. Young, et al. miR-9, a MYC/MYCN-activated microRNA, regulates E-cadherin and cancer metastasis. *Nat Cell Biol* 12(3): 247-256.

Maelandsmo, G. M., R. Holm, et al. (2003). Reduced beta-catenin expression in the cytoplasm of advanced-stage superficial spreading malignant melanoma. *Clin Cancer Res* 9(9): 3383-3388.

Margineanu, E., C. E. Cotrutz, et al. (2008). Correlation between E-cadherin abnormal expressions in different types of cancer and the process of metastasis. *Rev Med Chir Soc Med Nat Iasi* 112(2): 432-436.

Mastick, C. C., M. J. Brady, et al. (1995). Insulin stimulates the tyrosine phosphorylation of caveolin. *J Cell Biol* 129(6): 1523-1531.

Mastick, C. C. and A. R. Saltiel (1997). Insulin-stimulated tyrosine phosphorylation of caveolin is specific for the differentiated adipocyte phenotype in 3T3-L1 cells. *J Biol Chem* 272(33): 20706-20714.

McDonald, S. L. and A. Silver (2009). The opposing roles of Wnt-5a in cancer. *Br J Cancer* 101(2): 209-214.

Nakashima, H., K. Hamamura, et al. (2007). Overexpression of caveolin-1 in a human melanoma cell line results in dispersion of ganglioside GD3 from lipid rafts and alteration of leading edges, leading to attenuation of malignant properties. *Cancer Sci* 98(4): 512-520.

Nathke, I. S. (2004). The adenomatous polyposis coli protein: the Achilles heel of the gut epithelium. *Annu Rev Cell Dev Biol* 20: 337-366.

Nicolson, G. L., K. W. Brunson, et al. (1978). Specificity of arrest, survival, and growth of selected metastatic variant cell lines. *Cancer Res* 38(11 Pt 2): 4105-4111.

O'Connell, M. P. and A. T. Weeraratna (2009). Hear the Wnt Ror: how melanoma cells adjust to changes in Wnt. *Pigment Cell Melanoma Res 22*(6): 724-739.

Okamoto, T., A. Schlegel, et al. (1998). Caveolins, a family of scaffolding proteins for organizing preassembled signaling complexes at the plasma membrane. *J Biol Chem* 273(10): 5419-5422.

Orlichenko, L., B. Huang, et al. (2006). Epithelial growth factor-induced phosphorylation of caveolin 1 at tyrosine 14 stimulates caveolae formation in epithelial cells. *J Biol Chem* 281(8): 4570-4579.

Parat, M. O., B. Anand-Apte, et al. (2003). Differential caveolin-1 polarization in endothelial cells during migration in two and three dimensions. *Mol Biol Cell* 14(8): 3156-3168.

Park, D. S., A. W. Cohen, et al. (2003). Caveolin-1 null (-/-) mice show dramatic reductions in life span. *Biochemistry* 42(51): 15124-15131.

Pecina-Slaus, N., M. Zigmund, et al. (2007). E-cadherin and beta-catenin expression patterns in malignant melanoma assessed by image analysis. *J Cutan Pathol* 34(3): 239-246.

Polakis, P. (2000). Wnt signaling and cancer. *Genes Dev* 14(15): 1837-1851.

Ponder, B. A. (2001). Cancer genetics. *Nature* 411(6835): 336-341.

Quest, A. F., J. L. Gutierrez-Pajares, et al. (2008). Caveolin-1: an ambiguous partner in cell signalling and cancer. *J Cell Mol Med* 12(4): 1130-1150.

Quest, A. F., L. Leyton, et al. (2004). Caveolins, caveolae, and lipid rafts in cellular transport, signaling, and disease. *Biochem Cell Biol* 82(1): 129-144.

Racine, C., M. Belanger, et al. (1999). Reduction of caveolin 1 gene expression in lung carcinoma cell lines. *Biochem Biophys Res Commun* 255(3): 580-586.

Razani, B., J. A. Engelman, et al. (2001). Caveolin-1 null mice are viable but show evidence of hyperproliferative and vascular abnormalities. *J Biol Chem* 276(41): 38121-38138.

Razani, B., A. Schlegel, et al. (2000). Caveolin proteins in signaling, oncogenic transformation and muscular dystrophy. *J Cell Sci* 113 ( Pt 12): 2103-2109.

Razani, B., S. E. Woodman, et al. (2002). Caveolae: from cell biology to animal physiology. *Pharmacol Rev* 54(3): 431-467.

Reed, J. C. (2001). The Survivin saga goes in vivo. *J Clin Invest* 108(7): 965-969.

Rimm, D. L., K. Caca, et al. (1999). Frequent nuclear/cytoplasmic localization of beta-catenin without exon 3 mutations in malignant melanoma. *Am J Pathol* 154(2): 325-329.

Rodriguez, D. A., J. C. Tapia, et al. (2009). Caveolin-1-mediated suppression of cyclooxygenase-2 via a beta-catenin-Tcf/Lef-dependent transcriptional mechanism reduced prostaglandin E2 production and survivin expression. *Mol Biol Cell* 20(8): 2297-2310.

Sanguinetti, A. R. and C. C. Mastick (2003). c-Abl is required for oxidative stress-induced phosphorylation of caveolin-1 on tyrosine 14. *Cell Signal* 15(3): 289-298.

Santilman, V., J. Baran, et al. (2007). Caveolin-1 polarization in transmigrating endothelial cells requires binding to intermediate filaments. *Angiogenesis* 10(4): 297-305.

Savage, K., M. B. Lambros, et al. (2007). Caveolin 1 is overexpressed and amplified in a subset of basal-like and metaplastic breast carcinomas: a morphologic, ultrastructural, immunohistochemical, and in situ hybridization analysis. *Clin Cancer Res* 13(1): 90-101.

Scherer, P. E., Z. Tang, et al. (1995). Caveolin isoforms differ in their N-terminal protein sequence and subcellular distribution. Identification and epitope mapping of an isoform-specific monoclonal antibody probe. *J Biol Chem* 270(27): 16395-16401.

Schmalhofer, O., S. Brabletz, et al. (2009). E-cadherin, beta-catenin, and ZEB1 in malignant progression of cancer. *Cancer Metastasis Rev* 28(1-2): 151-166.

Shtutman, M., J. Zhurinsky, et al. (1999). The cyclin D1 gene is a target of the beta-catenin/LEF-1 pathway. *Proc Natl Acad Sci U S A* 96(10): 5522-5527.

Sloan, E. K., D. R. Ciocca, et al. (2009). Stromal cell expression of caveolin-1 predicts outcome in breast cancer. *Am J Pathol* 174(6): 2035-2043.

Straume, O. and L. A. Akslen (1997). Alterations and prognostic significance of p16 and p53 protein expression in subgroups of cutaneous melanoma. *Int J Cancer* 74(5): 535-539.

Sun, X. H., D. C. Flynn, et al. (2007). Identification of a novel domain at the N terminus of caveolin-1 that controls rear polarization of the protein and caveolae formation. *J Biol Chem* 282(10): 7232-7241.

Sun, X. H., Z. Y. Liu, et al. (2009). A conserved sequence in caveolin-1 is both necessary and sufficient for caveolin polarity and cell directional migration. *FEBS Lett* 583(22): 3681-3689.

Tahir, S. A., S. Park, et al. (2009). Caveolin-1 regulates VEGF-stimulated angiogenic activities in prostate cancer and endothelial cells. *Cancer Biol Ther* 8(23): 2286-2296

Tahir, S. A., G. Yang, et al. (2001). Secreted caveolin-1 stimulates cell survival/clonal growth and contributes to metastasis in androgen-insensitive prostate cancer. *Cancer Res* 61(10): 3882-3885.

Torres, V. A., J. C. Tapia, et al. (2007). E-cadherin is required for caveolin-1-mediated down-regulation of the inhibitor of apoptosis protein survivin via reduced beta-catenin-Tcf/Lef-dependent transcription. *Mol Cell Biol* 27(21): 7703-7717.

Torres, V. A., J. C. Tapia, et al. (2006). Caveolin-1 controls cell proliferation and cell death by suppressing expression of the inhibitor of apoptosis protein survivin. *J Cell Sci* 119(Pt 9): 1812-1823.

Trimmer, C., D. Whitaker-Menezes, et al. (2010). CAV1 inhibits metastatic potential in melanomas through suppression of the integrin/Src/FAK signaling pathway. *Cancer Res* 70(19): 7489-7499.

Tucci, M. G., G. Lucarini, et al. (2007). Involvement of E-cadherin, beta-catenin, Cdc42 and CXCR4 in the progression and prognosis of cutaneous melanoma. *Br J Dermatol* 157(6): 1212-1216.

van Deurs, B., K. Roepstorff, et al. (2003). Caveolae: anchored, multifunctional platforms in the lipid ocean. *Trends Cell Biol* 13(2): 92-100.

Volonte, D., F. Galbiati, et al. (2001). Cellular stress induces the tyrosine phosphorylation of caveolin-1 (Tyr(14)) via activation of p38 mitogen-activated protein kinase and c-Src kinase. Evidence for caveolae, the actin cytoskeleton, and focal adhesions as mechanical sensors of osmotic stress. *J Biol Chem* 276(11): 8094-8103.

Watanabe, M., G. Yang, et al. (2009). Functional analysis of secreted caveolin-1 in mouse models of prostate cancer progression. *Mol Cancer Res* 7(9): 1446-1455.

Weinberg, R. A. (1989). Oncogenes, antioncogenes, and the molecular bases of multistep carcinogenesis. *Cancer Res* 49(14): 3713-3721.

Widelitz, R. (2005). Wnt signaling through canonical and non-canonical pathways: recent progress. *Growth Factors* 23(2): 111-116.

Widlund, H. R., M. A. Horstmann, et al. (2002). Beta-catenin-induced melanoma growth requires the downstream target Microphthalmia-associated transcription factor. *J Cell Biol* 158(6): 1079-1087.

Wiechen, K., L. Diatchenko, et al. (2001). Caveolin-1 is down-regulated in human ovarian carcinoma and acts as a candidate tumor suppressor gene. *Am J Pathol* 159(5): 1635-1643.

Wiechen, K., C. Sers, et al. (2001). Down-regulation of caveolin-1, a candidate tumor suppressor gene, in sarcomas. *Am J Pathol* 158(3): 833-839.

Williams, T. M., M. W. Cheung, et al. (2003). Loss of caveolin-1 gene expression accelerates the development of dysplastic mammary lesions in tumor-prone transgenic mice. *Mol Biol Cell* 14(3): 1027-1042.

Williams, T. M. and M. P. Lisanti (2004). The caveolin proteins. *Genome Biol* 5(3): 214.

Williams, T. M. and M. P. Lisanti (2005). Caveolin-1 in oncogenic transformation, cancer, and metastasis. *Am J Physiol Cell Physiol* 288(3): C494-506.

Witkiewicz, A. K., A. Dasgupta, et al. (2009). An absence of stromal caveolin-1 expression predicts early tumor recurrence and poor clinical outcome in human breast cancers. *Am J Pathol* 174(6): 2023-2034.

Wu, Y., Y. Lin, et al. (2008). Inhibition of invasion and up-regulation of E-cadherin expression in human malignant melanoma cell line A375 by (-)-epigallocatechin-3-gallate. J Huazhong Univ Sci Technolog *Med Sci* 28(3): 356-359.

Yamaguchi, H., Y. Takeo, et al. (2009). Lipid rafts and caveolin-1 are required for invadopodia formation and extracellular matrix degradation by human breast cancer cells. *Cancer Res* 69(22): 8594-8602.

Yang, G., J. Addai, et al. (2007). Correlative evidence that prostate cancer cell-derived caveolin-1 mediates angiogenesis. *Hum Pathol* 38(11): 1688-1695.

Yang, G., L. D. Truong, et al. (1998). Elevated expression of caveolin is associated with prostate and breast cancer. *Clin Cancer Res* 4(8): 1873-1880.

Zhang, H., L. Su, et al. (2008). Restoration of caveolin-1 expression suppresses growth and metastasis of head and neck squamous cell carcinoma. *Br J Cancer* 99(10): 1684-1694.

Zhu, D. Z., C. F. Cheng, et al. (1991). Mediation of lung metastasis of murine melanomas by a lung-specific endothelial cell adhesion molecule. *Proc Natl Acad Sci U S A* 88(21): 9568-9572.

# 11

# IMP3 and Malignant Melanoma

Mark J. Mentrikoski[1] and Haodong Xu[2]
[1]*Department of Pathology, University of Virginia Health System, Charlottesville, Virginia,*
[2]*Department of Pathology and Laboratory Medicine, University of Rochester Medical Center, Rochester, New York, USA*

## 1. Introduction

Malignant melanoma is the deadliest form of skin cancer arising from the abnormal proliferation of epidermal melanocytes. With the incidence and mortality from this disease rising, accurate histopathologic diagnosis is crucial. Most cases of melanoma can be appropriately diagnosed based on morphologic criteria, but a subset of lesions including Spitz and dysplastic nevi, can be difficult to distinguish from malignant proliferations. In addition, even though current immunohistochemical stains tend to be rather sensitive and specific for most types of malignant melanoma (S-100, Melan-A/MART-1, HMB-45 and tyrosinase), they are unable to distinguish malignant from benign melanocytes--a potential pitfall in architecturally and cytologically borderline cases, which can lead to inadequate treatment or surveillance. Also, the distinction between intranodal nevi and metastatic melanoma in sentinel lymph nodes is not morphologically straightforward in certain cases; however, the confirmative status of these lymph nodes is very important for clinical outcome and guiding treatment. Thus, finding a method to precisely distinguish melanoma from its benign mimickers is needed. Despite advances in melanoma investigation and research, no reliable diagnostic biomarkers have yet been identified.

Another challenge in melanoma treatment is to determine patients' prognosis. Currently, depth of invasion, tumor ulceration, and status of sentinel lymph node are three common objective measures of prognosis; with invasion greater than 1 mm, ulceration, and lymph node metastases portending a worse outcome. Other features, such as assignment of radial versus vertical growth phase, tumor infiltrating lymphocytes, and Clark's levels, are also useful for prognosis, but tend to be more subjective. Thus, an immunohistochemical marker predictive of disease progression and poorer prognosis would be useful, to identify melanomas with a more aggressive phenotype.

### 1.1 IMP3

Insulin-like growth factor-II (IGF-II) messenger RNA (mRNA)-binding protein-3 (IMP3), also known as K homology domain-containing protein overexpressed in cancer (KOC) and L523S, is an mRNA-binding protein which has been considered to play a dual role in both embryogenesis and tumor proliferation (Nielsen, Christiansen et al. 1999; Yaniv and Yisraeli 2002). IMP3 is a 580 amino-acid protein encoded by a 4350-bp mRNA transcript produced by a gene located on chromosome 7p11.5 (Mueller-Pillasch, Lacher et al. 1997). As a member of the IGF-II mRNA-binding protein (IMP) family, IMP3 is expressed in first trimester human embryos and term placenta (Yaniv and Yisraeli 2002). By binding downstream transcripts of IGF-II, IMP3 plays a role in early cell growth and proliferation through RNA trafficking and stabilization (Mueller-Pillasch, Pohl et al. 1999; Nielsen, Nielsen et al. 2001). After embryogenesis and development, IMP3 expression is detectable in occasional adult tissues, including the internal root sheath of hair follicles, germinal centers of lymph nodes (Figure 1B), patchy gastrointestinal tract and bronchiolar epithelium (Righi, Zhang et al.; Mueller-Pillasch, Pohl et al. 1999; Nielsen, Christiansen et al. 1999; Hammer, Hansen et al. 2005; Simon, Bourne et al. 2007; Xu, Bourne et al. 2007; Mentrikoski, Ma et al. 2009).

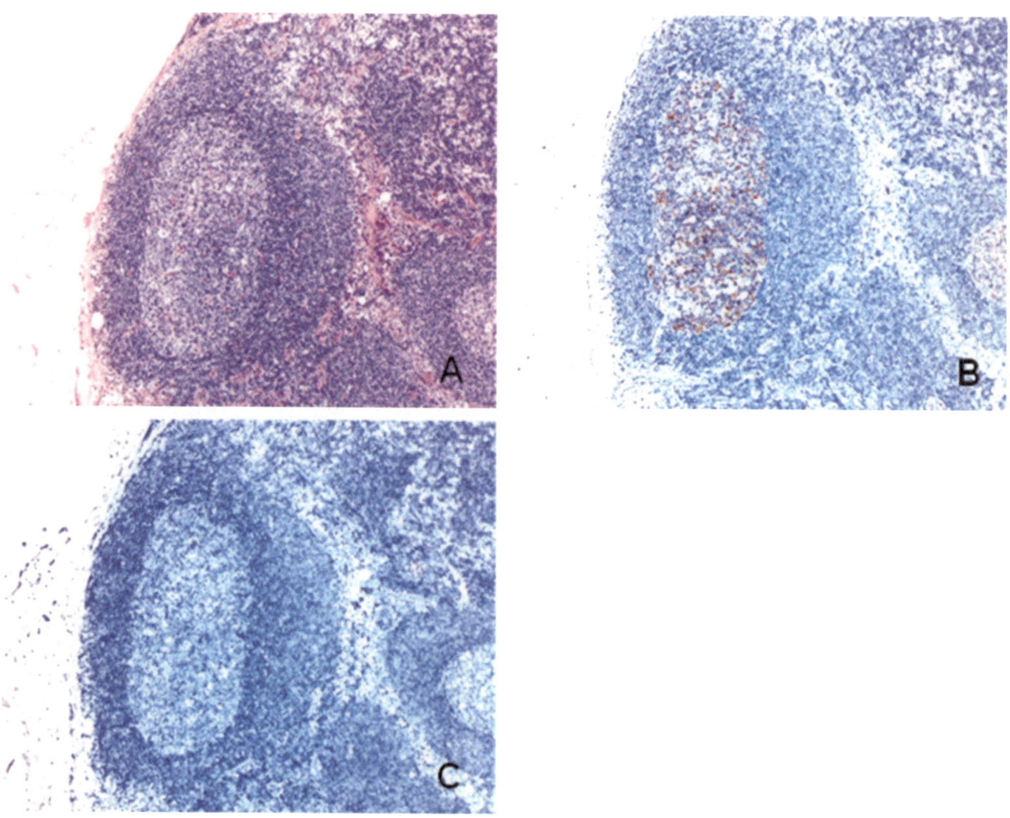


Fig. 1. IMP3 expression in lymph node germinal centers. A: Hematoxylin and Eosin stain shows normal lymph node with germinal center. B: IMP3 staining shows positivity in germinal center lymphocytes. C: Melan-A staining does not highlight any nodal elements. Original magnification is 100x for A, B and C.

In addition to its expression in fetal development, IMP3 has been detected in numerous malignancies including germ cell carcinomas, renal cell carcinoma, small and non-small cell lung carcinomas, urothelial carcinoma, endometrial serous and cervical carcinomas, Merkel cell carcinoma, extrapulmonary small cell carcinoma, various lymphomas, thyroid carcinoma, mammary breast carcinoma, colonic, gastric and esophageal adenocarcinomas, and osteogenic sarcoma (Asioli, Erickson et al. ; Findeis-Hosey, Yang et al. ; Jin, Seys et al. ; Righi, Zhang et al. ; Wang, Fan et al. 2003; Hammer, Hansen et al. 2005; Jiang 2007; Li, Rock et al. 2007; Simon, Bourne et al. 2007; Do, Kim et al. 2008; Li, Xu et al. 2008; Pryor, Bourne et al. 2008; Zheng, Yi et al. 2008; Jeng, Wang et al. 2009; King, Pasha et al. 2009; Li, Yan et al. 2009; Li, Huang et al. 2009; Lu, Vohra et al. 2009; Mentrikoski, Ma et al. 2009; Pryor, Simon et al. 2009; Slosar, Vohra et al. 2009; Walter, Prasad et al. 2009; Yuan, Wang et al. 2009). Moreover, IMP3 expression has been shown to be a marker of poorer prognosis with decreased overall survival in several tumors including renal cell carcinoma, mammary breast carcinoma, non-small cell lung carcinoma, and numerous gastrointestinal malignancies (Findeis-Hosey, Yang et al. ; Jiang, Chu et al. 2006; Hoffmann, Sheinin et al. 2008; Kobel, Xu et al. 2009; Walter, Prasad et al. 2009). Furthermore, another member of the IMP family of proteins, IMP1, was found to be expressed in primary melanomas, and melanoma cell lines suggesting that these proteins may also play a role in melanoma oncogenesis (Thomas and Erickson 2008).

Although IMP3's precise role in malignant transformation is as yet unknown, it has been shown to promote proper extra-cellular matrix formation, cell adhesion, and tumor invasion (Vikesaa, Hansen et al. 2006; Jeng, Chang et al. 2008), in various cell lines *in vitro*. These study results, combined with clinicopathologic evidence of a poorer prognosis in tumors with IMP3 overexpression, indicate that regardless of IMP3's exact role in primary oncogenesis, its expression in tumors indicates a more aggressive phenotype. Below we review the identification of IMP3 in cutaneous melanocytic lesions, including malignant melanoma, and discuss its role in the diagnosis and potential prognosis of these lesions.

## 2. IMP3 expression in cutaneous melanocytic lesions

Given IMP3's expression in a plethora of different malignancies, our group hypothesized that IMP3 may be of value in segregating malignant melanoma from benign melanocytic lesions. This was proven to be the case in the original paper by Pryor et al. (Pryor, Bourne et al. 2008). In this study, 56 melanocytic neoplasms, including 11 benign nevi, 8 dysplastic nevi, 10 Spitz nevi, 17 primary melanomas, and 10 metastatic melanomas, were evaluated for IMP3 expression through immunohistochemistry. The results revealed that 23 of 27 melanomas (85%) showed moderate-to-strong staining for IMP3, while no benign or dysplastic nevi expressed IMP3. These findings were statistically significant ($P$=0.0003). Spitz nevi showed weak staining in 30% of lesions, which was also significantly less than melanoma ($P$=0.0215) (Pryor, Bourne et al. 2008). Interestingly, when the primary melanomas were subdivided by tumor thickness, IMP3 overexpression was noted to be stronger and more prevalent in tumors with >1 mm of invasion, which suggests that IMP3 may be a marker of melanoma progression. In addition, the results also showed that IMP3 is expressed in metastatic melanoma (Figure 2B) significantly more than in thin melanomas. Whether these findings of IMP3 expression are suggestive of a poorer prognosis, is currently being evaluated using long-term outcomes and survival data.

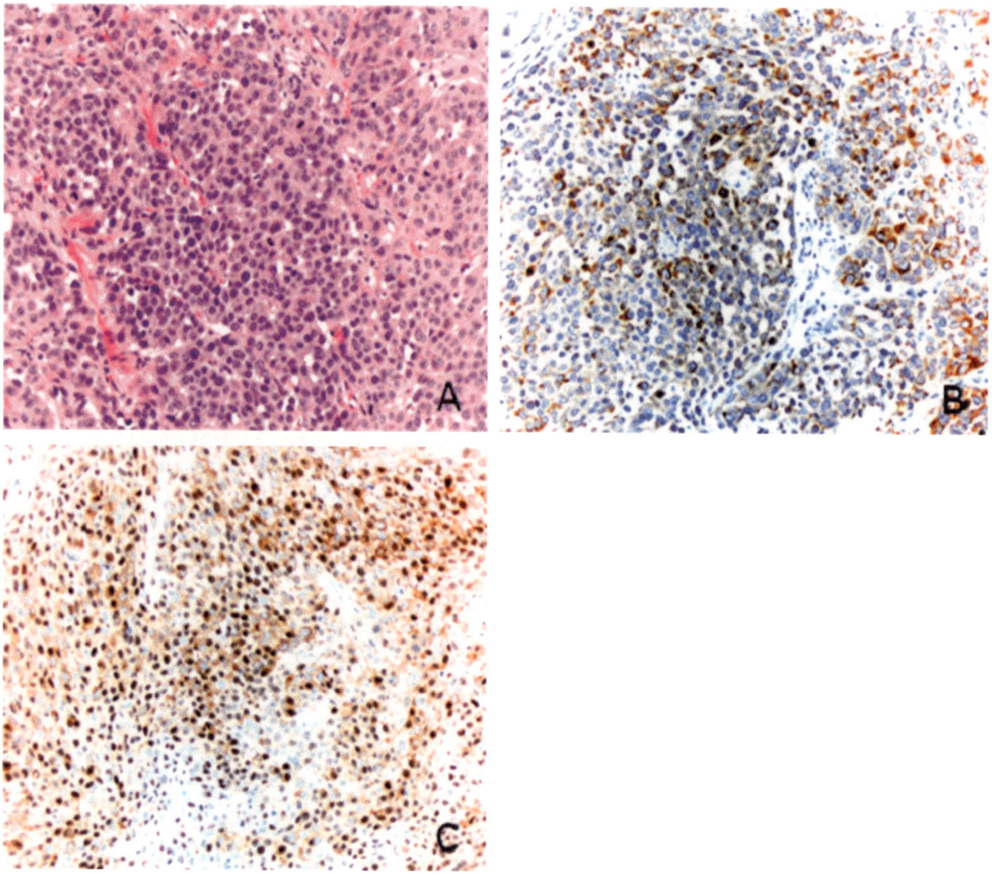


Fig. 2. Metastatic malignant melanoma in soft tissue is strongly and diffusely positive for IMP3. A: Hematoxylin and eosin staining shows metastatic malignant melanoma. B: Strong IMP3 positivity in melanoma cells. C: Strong nuclear immunohistochemical staining for S-100 in malignant melanoma. Original magnification is 200x for A, B and C.

A second study examining IMP3 and malignant melanoma was performed by Yu et al., and investigated its expression in atypical Spitz tumors, melanoma *in situ* (MIS), and desmoplastic melanoma (Yu, Xu et al.). The group confirmed the lack of staining in benign and dysplastic nevi, and only occasional, scattered staining in Spitz nevi. Atypical Spitz nevi showed weak to moderate staining in 7 of 10 cases. Desmoplastic melanoma showed overexpression in 4 of 23 (17%) of cases, similar to results obtained with other melanocytic markers (Busam 2005). In MIS, IMP3 staining was noted as isolated, single cells in 40% of cases; a similar percentage was observed in superficially invasive melanomas (<1 mm), but the positive cells had a more prominent, linear arrangement. Although the specificity of IMP3 detection in non-desmoplastic melanomas was less than the original study (50% vs. 85%, see above), there was nonetheless a significant difference between expression in melanoma compared to benign nevi ($P$=0.0251). As in the original study, the trend was for deeper non-desmoplastic melanomas to show stronger and more diffuse positivity than those with <1 mm of invasion.

### 2.1 IMP3 expression pattern in metastatic melanoma and intranodal nevi

Depending on the Breslow depth of a primary melanoma, sentinel lymph node biopsy is often performed for clinical staging and prognosis. In pathology departments and dermatopathology practice groups, it is not uncommon to stain sections of these sentinel nodes with various melanocytic markers in order to pick up metastatic melanoma cells. When benign, intranodal nevi occur in these specimens, the melanocytic markers will pick them up and can make diagnosis difficult if only a few cells are present. Although the clinical applicability of detecting these so-called micrometastases is debatable, accurate diagnosis is critical. As such, another study by our group was performed to see if IMP3 retained its ability to distinguish melanoma from benign nevi; and this time metastatic melanoma was compared to intranodal nevi (Mentrikoski, Ma et al. 2009).

A total 43 sentinel lymph node specimens were examined, including 30 with metastatic melanoma and 13 with intranodal nevi. The benign nevi were located both in the capsule (n=11) and trabeculae (n=2) (Figure 3). Melan-A was used as a general melanocytic marker, and both intranodal nevi and metastatic melanoma showed Melan-A diffuse and strong positivity (Figure 3C and 4C).

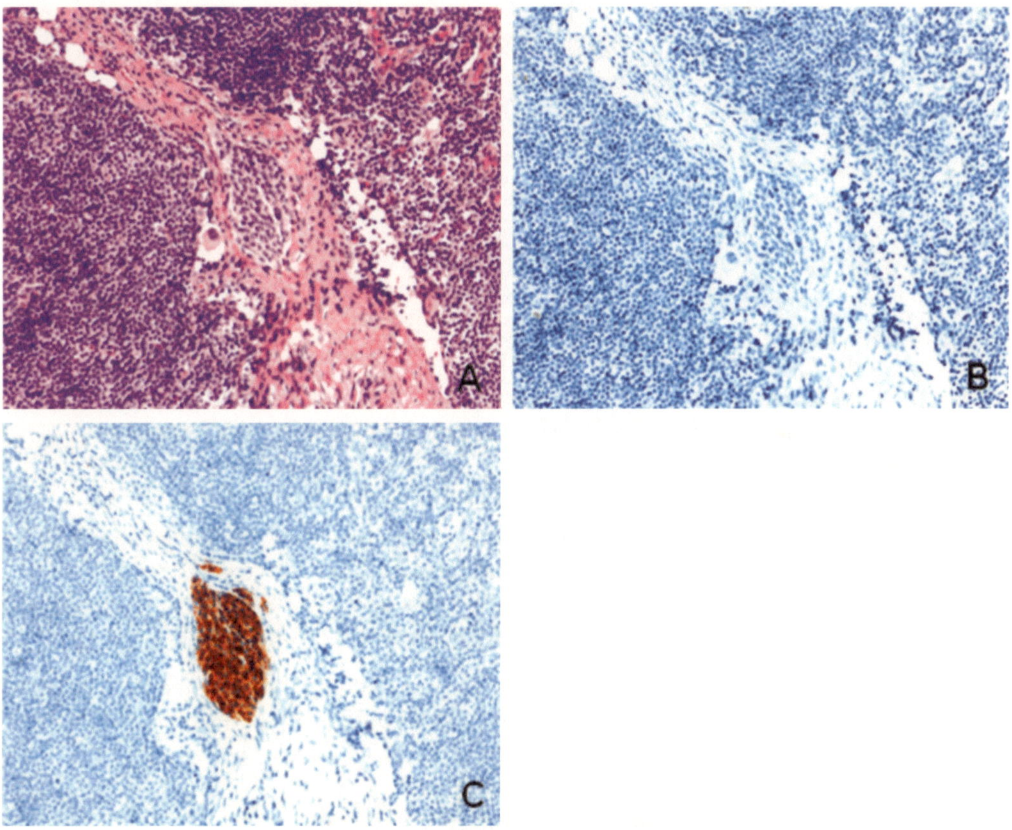


Fig. 3. Intranodal nevus is negative for IMP3. A: Hematoxylin and eosin staining shows a collection of small nevus in the trabeculae in the lymph node. B: IMP3 staining is negative in the benign nevi. C: The intranodal nevus is highlighted by Melan-A staining. Original magnification is 400x for A, B and C.

A diagnosis of melanoma was then made based on usual cytologic features. Examination of the same lymph nodes with immunohistochemistry for IMP3 revealed expression in 21 of 30 metastatic foci (70%) (Figure 4B) while no intranodal nevi showed positive staining (Figure 3B).

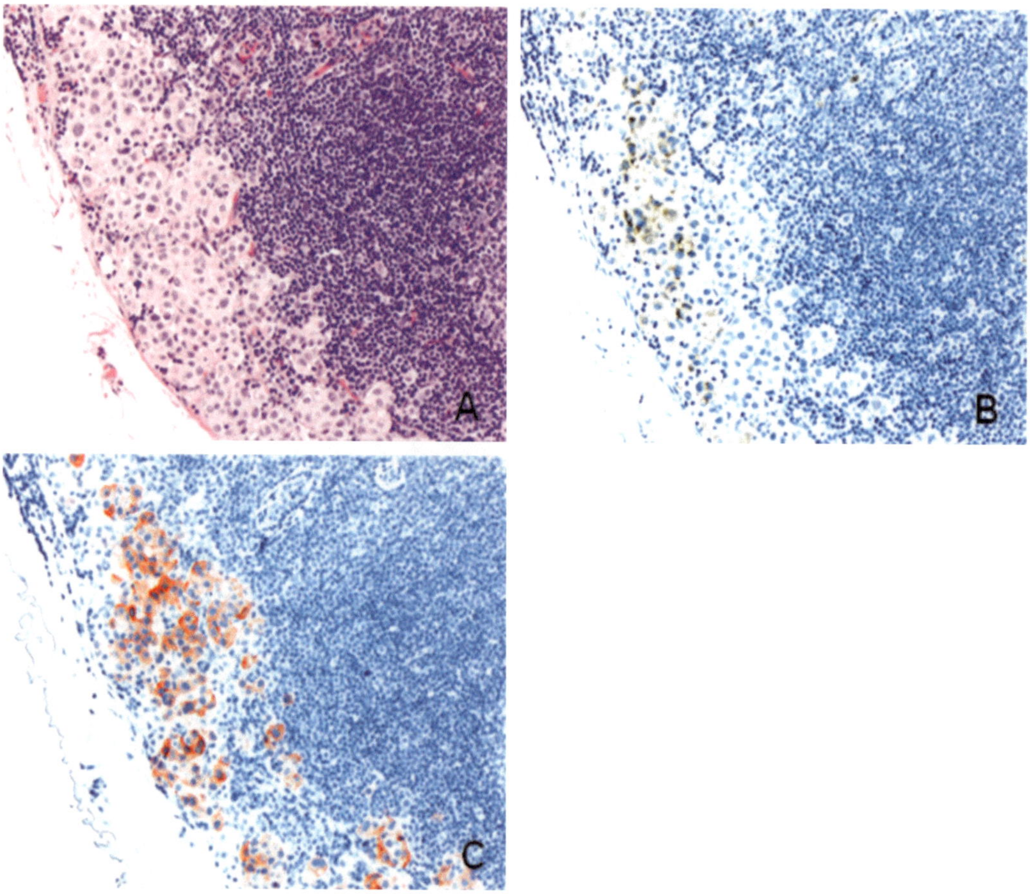


Fig. 4. Subcapsular deposit of metastatic melanoma is positive for IMP3. A: Hematoxylin and eosin staining shows a collection of malignant melanocytes within subcapsular area of the lymph node. B: Metastatic melanoma is positive for IMP3. C: Metastatic melanoma is highlighted by Melan-A staining. Original magnification are 400x for A, B and C.

The overall specificity and sensitivity in this study was comparable to the two previous cutaneous studies, and suggests that IMP3 has diagnostic utility in segregating benign nodal nevi from metastatic melanoma.

### 2.2 Comparing IMP3 to other common melanocytic markers

In general, the diagnosis of both cutaneous and metastatic melanoma can often be done on hematoxylin & eosin stained sections alone. However, there are many times when special and immunohistochemical stains are needed to aid in proper classification; IMP3 is just one of numerous such stains that can be used.

Although particular preference often varies amongst pathologists, and can be institutional-dependent, the immunohistochemical stains commonly used in the evaluation of questionable cases include S-100, HMB-45, and/or Melan-A. S-100 is considered the most sensitive marker (Nakajima, Watanabe et al. 1982; Ohsie, Sarantopoulos et al. 2008), but it is rather nonspecific; showing positivity in benign melanocytes, melanin-laden macrophages, dendritic cells, nerves, and adipose tissue. Both Melan-A (as used in our studies) and HMB-45 show increased specificities for melanocytes when compared to S-100, but with a loss of sensitivity in melanoma cases (Ohsie, Sarantopoulos et al. 2008). With regard to lymph node metastases, one study showed HMB-45 may be more helpful than S-100 or Melan-A, as it was typically negative in most benign nevic cell rests within sentinel lymph nodes (Lohmann, Iversen et al. 2002); yet, it should be noted that HMB-45 can still be positive in up to 16% of these cases, potentially leading to false positive results. (Abrahamsen, Hamilton-Dutoit et al. 2004).

Overall, it is evident that while there is not an exceedingly high sensitivity with IMP3, the specificity is such that it is able to discriminate between benign nevi and malignant melanocytes, in both cutaneous and metastatic lesions. Like some of the other immunohistochemical stains, specifically Melan-A and HMB-45, IMP3 is hurt by its low sensitivity. Therefore, although positive immunohistochemical staining with IMP3 can increase a pathologist's confidence in the proper diagnosis of malignant melanoma, one needs to be aware of false negative results. The sensitivity and specificity of IMP3 immunohistochemical staining in malignant melanoma are summarized in table 1.

| Study | Sensitivity | Specificity |
|---|---|---|
| Pryor J. G. et al. | 85% | 100% |
| Yu L. et al. | 50%[1] | 100%[2] |
| Mentrikoski M. J. et al. | 70%[3] | 100%[3] |

Note: [1]Percentage includes only non-desmoplastic melanoma; [2]percentage does not include staining in both Spitz or so-called atypical Spitz nevi; [3]percentage includes metastatic melanoma in lymph nodes.

Table 1. Combined sensitivity and specificity of IMP3 immunohistochemical staining for the diagnosis of malignant melanoma versus benign or dysplastic nevi.

## 3. Conclusions

Although the histopathologic diagnosis of malignant melanoma can be straightforward, many borderline cases exist where objective means to determine the proper diagnosis are largely suspected. To date, no biomarker has been found with high specificity and sensitivity for distinguishing benign from malignant melanocytic proliferations. IMP3 immunohistochemical staining has been shown to have a high specificity for identifying malignant melanoma, and with its overall sensitivity of 70%, a positive immunohistochemical result can give the pathologist confidence when making a diagnosis of malignancy. In addition, IMP3 can also aid in sentinel lymph node biopsy interpretation when the differential is melanoma micrometastasis versus intranodal nevus. Future studies utilizing long-term clinical data will be needed to see if the trend of stronger IMP3 staining in deeper, more advanced lesions correlates with poorer patient prognosis; and ultimately a more aggressive tumor phenotype.

## 4. References


Abrahamsen, H. N., S. J. Hamilton-Dutoit, et al. (2004). "Sentinel lymph nodes in malignant melanoma: extended histopathologic evaluation improves diagnostic precision." Cancer 100(8): 1683-91.

Asioli, S., L. A. Erickson, et al. "Poorly differentiated carcinoma of the thyroid: validation of the Turin proposal and analysis of IMP3 expression." Mod Pathol 23(9): 1269-78.

Busam, K. J. (2005). "Cutaneous desmoplastic melanoma." Adv Anat Pathol 12(2): 92-102.

Do, S. I., Y. W. Kim, et al. (2008). "Expression of insulin-like growth factor-II mRNA binding protein 3 (IMP3) in osteosarcoma." Oncol Res 17(6): 269-72.

Findeis-Hosey, J. J., Q. Yang, et al. "IMP3 expression is correlated with histologic grade of lung adenocarcinoma." Hum Pathol 41(4): 477-84.

Hammer, N. A., T. O. Hansen, et al. (2005). "Expression of IGF-II mRNA-binding proteins (IMPs) in gonads and testicular cancer." Reproduction 130(2): 203-12.

Hoffmann, N. E., Y. Sheinin, et al. (2008). "External validation of IMP3 expression as an independent prognostic marker for metastatic progression and death for patients with clear cell renal cell carcinoma." Cancer 112(7): 1471-9.

Jeng, Y. M., C. C. Chang, et al. (2008). "RNA-binding protein insulin-like growth factor II mRNA-binding protein 3 expression promotes tumor invasion and predicts early recurrence and poor prognosis in hepatocellular carcinoma." Hepatology 48(4): 1118-27.

Jeng, Y. M., T. H. Wang, et al. (2009). "Prognostic significance of insulin-like growth factor II mRNA-binding protein 3 expression in gastric adenocarcinoma." Br J Surg 96(1): 66-73.

Jiang, Z. (2007). "Prognostic biomarkers in renal cell carcinoma." Expert Rev Mol Diagn 7(3): 293-307.

Jiang, Z., P. G. Chu, et al. (2006). "Analysis of RNA-binding protein IMP3 to predict metastasis and prognosis of renal-cell carcinoma: a retrospective study." Lancet Oncol 7(7): 556-64.

Jin, L., A. R. Seys, et al. "Diagnostic utility of IMP3 expression in thyroid neoplasms: a quantitative RT-PCR study." Diagn Mol Pathol 19(2): 63-9.

King, R. L., T. Pasha, et al. (2009). "IMP-3 is differentially expressed in normal and neoplastic lymphoid tissue." Hum Pathol 40(12): 1699-705.

Kobel, M., H. Xu, et al. (2009). "IGF2BP3 (IMP3) expression is a marker of unfavorable prognosis in ovarian carcinoma of clear cell subtype." Mod Pathol 22(3): 469-75.

Li, C., K. L. Rock, et al. (2007). "IMP3 is a novel biomarker for adenocarcinoma in situ of the uterine cervix: an immunohistochemical study in comparison with p16(INK4a) expression." Mod Pathol 20(2): 242-7.

Li, D., D. Yan, et al. (2009). "IMP3 is a novel prognostic marker that correlates with colon cancer progression and pathogenesis." Ann Surg Oncol 16(12): 3499-506.

Li, K. H., Y. P. Huang, et al. (2009). "[Expression of IMP3 in osteosarcoma and its clinical significance]." Xi Bao Yu Fen Zi Mian Yi Xue Za Zhi 25(5): 426-7.

Li, L., H. Xu, et al. (2008). "Expression of RNA-binding protein IMP3 (KOC) in benign urothelium and urothelial tumors." Hum Pathol 39(8): 1205-11.

Lohmann, C. M., K. Iversen, et al. (2002). "Expression of melanocyte differentiation antigens and ki-67 in nodal nevi and comparison of ki-67 expression with metastatic melanoma." Am J Surg Pathol 26(10): 1351-7.

Lu, D., P. Vohra, et al. (2009). "An oncofetal protein IMP3: a new molecular marker for the detection of esophageal adenocarcinoma and high-grade dysplasia." Am J Surg Pathol 33(4): 521-5.

Mentrikoski, M. J., L. Ma, et al. (2009). "Diagnostic utility of IMP3 in segregating metastatic melanoma from benign nevi in lymph nodes." Mod Pathol 22(12): 1582-7.

Mueller-Pillasch, F., U. Lacher, et al. (1997). "Cloning of a gene highly overexpressed in cancer coding for a novel KH-domain containing protein." Oncogene 14(22): 2729-33.

Mueller-Pillasch, F., B. Pohl, et al. (1999). "Expression of the highly conserved RNA binding protein KOC in embryogenesis." Mech Dev 88(1): 95-9.

Nakajima, T., S. Watanabe, et al. (1982). "Immunohistochemical demonstration of S100 protein in malignant melanoma and pigmented nevus, and its diagnostic application." Cancer 50(5): 912-8.

Nielsen, F. C., J. Nielsen, et al. (2001). "A family of IGF-II mRNA binding proteins (IMP) involved in RNA trafficking." Scand J Clin Lab Invest Suppl 234: 93-9.

Nielsen, J., J. Christiansen, et al. (1999). "A family of insulin-like growth factor II mRNA-binding proteins represses translation in late development." Mol Cell Biol 19(2): 1262-70.

Ohsie, S. J., G. P. Sarantopoulos, et al. (2008). "Immunohistochemical characteristics of melanoma." J Cutan Pathol 35(5): 433-44.

Pryor, J. G., P. A. Bourne, et al. (2008). "IMP-3 is a novel progression marker in malignant melanoma." Mod Pathol 21(4): 431-7.

Pryor, J. G., R. A. Simon, et al. (2009). "Merkel cell carcinoma expresses K homology domain-containing protein overexpressed in cancer similar to other high-grade neuroendocrine carcinomas." Hum Pathol 40(2): 238-43.

Righi, A., S. Zhang, et al. "Analysis of IMP3 expression in normal and neoplastic human pituitary tissues." Endocr Pathol 21(1): 25-31.

Simon, R., P. A. Bourne, et al. (2007). "Extrapulmonary small cell carcinomas express K homology domain containing protein overexpressed in cancer, but carcinoid tumors do not." Hum Pathol 38(8): 1178-83.

Slosar, M., P. Vohra, et al. (2009). "Insulin-like growth factor mRNA binding protein 3 (IMP3) is differentially expressed in benign and malignant follicular patterned thyroid tumors." Endocr Pathol 20(3): 149-57.

Thomas, A. J. and C. A. Erickson (2008). "The making of a melanocyte: the specification of melanoblasts from the neural crest." Pigment Cell Melanoma Res 21(6): 598-610.

Vikesaa, J., T. V. Hansen, et al. (2006). "RNA-binding IMPs promote cell adhesion and invadopodia formation." EMBO J 25(7): 1456-68.

Walter, O., M. Prasad, et al. (2009). "IMP3 is a novel biomarker for triple negative invasive mammary carcinoma associated with a more aggressive phenotype." Hum Pathol 40(11): 1528-33.

Wang, T., L. Fan, et al. (2003). "L523S, an RNA-binding protein as a potential therapeutic target for lung cancer." Br J Cancer 88(6): 887-94.

Xu, H., P. A. Bourne, et al. (2007). "High-grade neuroendocrine carcinomas of the lung express K homology domain containing protein overexpressed in cancer but carcinoid tumors do not." Hum Pathol 38(4): 555-63.

Yaniv, K. and J. K. Yisraeli (2002). "The involvement of a conserved family of RNA binding proteins in embryonic development and carcinogenesis." Gene 287(1-2): 49-54.

Yu, L., H. Xu, et al. "IMP-3 expression in melanocytic lesions." J Cutan Pathol 37(3): 316-22.

Yuan, R. H., C. C. Wang, et al. (2009). "Diffuse expression of RNA-binding protein IMP3 predicts high-stage lymph node metastasis and poor prognosis in colorectal adenocarcinoma." Ann Surg Oncol 16(6): 1711-9.

Zheng, W., X. Yi, et al. (2008). "The oncofetal protein IMP3: a novel biomarker for endometrial serous carcinoma." Am J Surg Pathol 32(2): 304-15.

# 12

# Effects of Social Stress on Immunomodulation and Tumor Development

Oscar Vegas, Larraitz Garmendia,
Amaia Arregi and Arantza Azpiroz
*Basque Country University*
*Spain*

## 1. Introduction

Over the last 30 years, much interesting research has been carried out in the field of psychoneuroimmunology which has shown, with scientific rigor, that psychological states, including those generated by exposure to stress-inducing agents, may alter the immune balance and influence both health and illness. Psychoneuroimmunology is the convergence of various different disciplines (behavioral science, endocrinology, neuroscience and immunology) which studies the immune changes associated with behavioral change and the behavioral changes associated with immunological changes, as well as the mechanisms involved in this relationship. It is based on the reciprocal relationships which exist between the Central Nervous System (CNS) and the Immune System (IS), the two most complex systems involved in the maintenance of homeostasis. Communications between the CNS and the IS are bidirectional and involve neurotransmitters, neurohormones, neuropeptides and cytokines, which together form a complex network that is still being explored today.

Four general research areas have found evidence of the existence of afferent and efferent communication channels between the two systems. These areas are:

- Studies focusing on lesions to or stimulations of certain regions of the brain which alter the immune response (Rassnick et al., 1994).
- Studies which have revealed the extensive presence of sympathetic nervous system fibers, mainly noradrenergic in nature, innervating both the primary and secondary lymphoid organs. These nervous fibers innervate the vascular and parenchymal zones of lymphoid organs, thus providing a close anatomical link between the two systems (D. L. Felten et al., 1985).
- Studies focusing on the influence of numerous CNS neurohormones, mainly hypothalamic-pituitary in nature, which have a strong regulatory effect on the IS, as well as on the expression of numerous receptors which the immune cells have for them (Blalock et al., 1985).
- Finally, other studies have shown that products of immune cells, such as cytokines, have a neuroendocrine activity which is capable of influencing diverse brain functions, as well as providing information to the neuroendocrine system, activating inhibitory feedback circuits to ensure their own regulation (Dantzer et al., 2001).

These discoveries have given rise to a new approach to the IS. This new model, known as the "danger model", was first proposed by Polly Matzinger in 1994. The key idea of this model is that the main function of the immune system is to recognize and protect the organism from any potentially dangerous threat. According to the model, "danger" is anything capable of harming or destroying the cell or tissue. Polly Matzinger argues that in order to carry out this function, the IS has to communicate with the organism's other systems (Matzinger, 2002).

This way of conceiving the IS function has opened up a whole new field of study in diverse models in which the activation/modification of the immune response cannot be explained solely by pathogens from outside the organism. Rather, other variables are also involved, including the effect of situations of psychological stress on the development of infectious diseases, autoimmune diseases and cancer. In this chapter we aim to highlight the importance of social stress and the effects of the hormones released during stressful situations in the study of tumor development, particularly in relation to melanoma tumor progression. To this end, the chapter first outlines the basic physiological aspects of neuroimmunomodulation, which underpin the effects that stress may have on immunity and tumor development. Next, we will examine the studies carried out in relation to melanoma tumor development, and the possible therapeutic benefits of psychosocial intervention.

## 2. Communication pathways between the Central Nervous System and the Immune System

The recognition and integration of internal and external sensorial stimuli by the CNS triggers changes in the synthesis and release of neurotransmitters, hormones and neuropeptides. These substances reach the organs and lymphoid cells through two main descending communication pathways, which enable the CNS to control the activity of peripheral organs, including the organs of the immune system.

On the one hand, the neurovegetative communication pathway, through automatic innervation and the subsequent secretion of norepinephrine from nerve endings and epinephrine from the adrenal medulla, enables the CNS to control the activity of immune organs such as the spleen, the thymus and the lymph nodes, among others. And on the other, the neuroendocrine communication pathway refers to the synthesis and release of secretion factors by certain cells to the pituitary gland's pituitary portal system. This stimulation causes the pituitary gland to synthesize and release diverse hormones into the bloodstream, and in turn, these trigger the synthesis and secretion of new hormones capable of influencing diverse organs and peripheral cells (Fig. 1).

The activation of these two neurochemical communication pathways and the subsequent secretion of hormones and neurotransmitters may have a major effect on the immune system function. By means of receptor-ligand interaction, these endogenous substances affect diverse processes of the immune response, such as cell development and differentiation, lymphocyte activation and proliferation, cell migration, the production and release of cytokines and the expression of cytokine receptors.

Receptors for monoamines (norepinephrine, epinephrine, dopamine and serotonin), cholecystokinin, adrenocorticotropic hormone (ACTH), methionine-enkephalin, leucine-enkephalin, β-endorphin, neurotensin, substance P, vasoactive intestinal peptide (VIP), prolactin (PRL), growth hormone, thyroid-stimulating hormone (TSH), melatonin, dynorphin, corticotropin-releasing hormone (CRH), cortisol, somatostatin and gonadal hormones have all been found in IS cells (Weigent & Blalock, 1987; Yada et al., 2004). The activation of these receptors by selective agonists triggers well-defined changes in the working of these cells, both *in vivo* and *in vitro*.

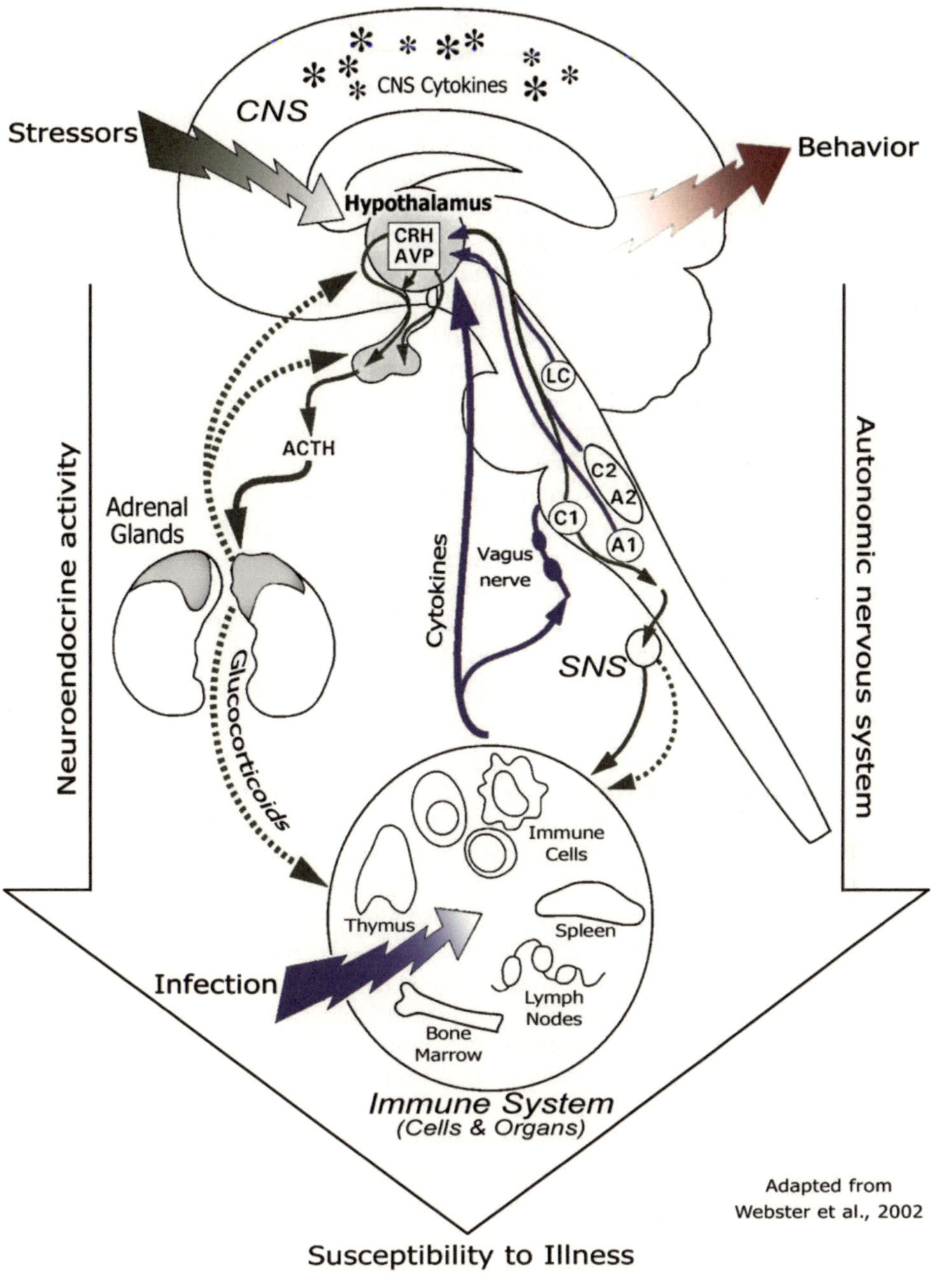


Fig. 1. Diagram of the routes of communication between the brain and immune system, including the HPA axis, sympathetic nervous system, and cytokine feedback to the brain.

Since this chapter focuses on the effects of stress on the immune response, we will pay special attention to the neuroendocrine (hypothalamic-pituitary-adrenal, or HPA axis) and vegetative (sympathetic-adreno-medullary or SAM axis) pathways through which this relationship is established.

### 2.1 The neuroendocrine pathway, the hypothalamic-pituitary-adrenal axis (HPA)

The hypothalamic-pituitary-adrenal (HPA) axis is constituted by three main structures: the hypothalamus, the pituitary gland and the adrenal glands. The sensorial activation signals converge in the paraventricular nucleus (PVN) of the hypothalamus, where they stimulate the synthesis and release of adrenocorticotropin-releasing hormone (CRH) and other neuropeptides. The axons of these neurons extend to the outer layer of the median eminence, where they release their neurosecretary products into the hypophyseal portal system, triggering the synthesis and release of ACTH by corticotropic cells of the anterior pituitary gland. The fast release of ACTH reaches the adrenal glands, where it stimulates the synthesis and release of glucocorticoids. The activation of the HPA axis also triggers the activation of the set of opioid peptides, which are thought to play a key immunomodulatory role, and as well as ß-endorphin, derived from pro-opiomelanocortin (POMC), whose synthesis and release is activated by CRH and which seems to affect the IS, modulating the effects of glucocorticoids in the immune function and the activation of natural killer cells (NK cells) Other peptides from the family of endogenous opioids, such as encephalins and dynorphins, are also involved in the modulation of the immune response (Carr et al., 1990).
Other pituitary hormones, such as vasopressin or the group formed by prolactin, growth hormone and somatostatin, as well as other neurotransmitters and neuropeptides, seem also to have immunomodulatory effects (Jessop, 2002)
Finally, glucocorticoids (GCs) are one of the most secreted hormones in the stress response and the object of special attention in numerous research projects which have highlighted the important role that they play in the regulation of the immune response (Besedovsky & del Rey, 2007).

### 2.2 The neurovegetative pathway, the sympathetic-adreno-medullary axis (SAM)

The activation of the SAM axis involves the activation of the sympathetic nervous system, which in turn triggers the secretion of norepinephrine (NE) by the sympathetic nerve endings and the secretion of epinephrine (E) and NE by the adrenal medulla.
The SAM axis innervates all the primary and secondary lymphoid organs in both animals and humans (S. Y. Felten & Felten, 1991), providing catecholamines with the physical space they require to modulate many immune parameters (Oberbeck, 2006). The local secretion of NE from nerve endings and the secretion of E and NE into the blood stream enable them to influence not only innervated organs and tissues, but also other cells of the immune system. For this reason, the SAM axis provides a regulation and integration channel between the CNS and the IS. Specifically, noradrenergic fibers have been found to exist in both primary lymphoid organs, including the thymus and bone marrow, and secondary organs, including the spleen, lymph nodes and the mucosa-associated lymphoid tissue. Evidence has also been found of the existence of adrenergic receptors in immune cells (such as T and B lymphocytes), in natural killer cells (NK cells) and in macrophages (Benschop et al., 1997). Finally, it has also been found that lymphocytes are able to synthesize catecholamines, and that these in turn may act both autocrinally and paracrinally. The effects of E and NE in target cells are mediated by receptor-ligand interactions. There are two types of receptors, as

well as catecholamines, alpha adrenergic receptors (αAR) and beta adrenergic receptors (βAR), which are expressed specifically in accordance with the tissue and which have different degrees of affinity (Biber et al., 2006).

The regulatory effect of catecholamines on the immune system cells has been widely studied. It has been shown that catecholamines inhibit the activity of those cells associated with the innate immune response, and may either increase or inhibit the activity of cells associated with the adaptive immune response. Through adrenergic receptors, mainly β2-adrenergic receptors (β2AR), NE is able to regulate the immune responses of antigens, influencing clonal expansion, the production of cytokines and/or the response capacity of certain cells, altering the expression of receptors, changing the balance between T and B cells and increasing or inhibiting the inflammation response and lymphocyte mobilization (Bellinger et al., 2008). Adrenergic agonists may modulate *in vitro* all aspects of the immune response during the initiation phase, the proliferation phase and the effector phase. Research has shown that, in addition to inhibiting mitogen-induced T cell proliferation, the stimulation of β2ARs also inhibits the differentiation of T cells in type 1 T-helper cells (Th1), thus affecting early events which are involved in the initiation of the proliferation (Sanders et al., 1997).

The sympathetic nerve endings of the bone marrow are involved in regulating hematopoiesis. These endings respond to certain stressors which increase the concentration of NE, and may therefore affect the cell formation process. Diverse studies have shown that the function of noradrenergic innervation is to suppress the proliferation of thymocytes, while at the same time increasing their differentiation. The inhibition of T lymphocyte proliferation may be explained in part by the capacity of catecholamines to inhibit the expression of the interleukin-2 receptor (IL-2) and /or the production of this cytokine by activated T lymphocytes (Sanders et al., 1997). The increase in catecholamines affects B lymphocytes also. These lymphocytes complete their development in the bone marrow and possess β-adrenergic receptors (Whisler et al., 1992).

Like glucocorticoids, catecholamines have generally been considered immunosuppressants. However, evidence has been found indicating that, under normal physiological conditions or in conditions generated during situations of stress, catecholamines may influence the immune system in a much more complex way (Elenkov et al., 2000). This new approach may help explain some of the well-known yet often contradictory effects that occur as a result of the activation of the stress response and which affect the immune function.

## 3. Social stress and cancer

Since the first quarter of the 20th century, many epidemiological studies have been carried out on the effects of stress and other psychological variables on tumor development and growth in humans. The results suggest that stress and the ability to cope with it are related to both the incidence of cancer and survival time. These studies have generally be classed as retrospective, quasi-prospective and prospective. The majority of studies fall into the category of retrospective analysis, and reveal that the appearance of various forms of neoplasms are often preceded by stressful life events. Cancer appears more frequently than expected in people who have been widowed or who have gone through a divorce or separation (Hemminki & Li, 2003). Some authors have found a direct relationship in women between stressful life events and breast cancer (Forsen, 1991), although other authors have failed to find any such association (Priestman et al., 1985). These apparently contradictory results may be analyzed in more detail by taking into account the coping strategies employed in response to stress by the subjects in question. The concept of coping styles, i.e. the idea that both animals and humans adapt to adverse situations in different ways, and that the repercussions of these responses on health also differ, is an area of great scientific interest. This hypothesis has been corroborated by the results obtained in subsequent studies. Thus, an association has been found between the coping strategy adopted by breast cancer patients and the course of the disease (Lauver et al., 2007). It has also been observed that planning, positive coping and distraction are positive predictors of good health, while guilt has been found to be a negative predictor (Li & Lambert, 2007).

Quasi-prospective studies also support the idea that factors associated with life stressors are predictors of greater neoplasic development (Grossarth-Maticek et al., 1995). Cooper et al., (1989) found that although women diagnosed with breast cancer recounted fewer stressful life events, they tended to view them as more threatening (Cooper et al., 1989). Other authors have also found similar results. Price et al., (2001) observed that women who perceived a stressor as extremely threatening and who also lacked social and emotional/family support, were nine times more at risk of developing breast cancer (Price et al., 2001). These studies suggest that it is not the mere existence of life stressors in themselves that may affect our health and be associated with the development of cancer, but rather their specific impact on the individual. In accordance with these results, it has been found that individual differences in the type of coping strategy adopted may affect the health of women at serious risk from hereditary breast cancer (Pieterse et al., 2007).

Finally, in prospective studies, the effect of life stressors is fairly inconsistent. Some authors have found that the more intense the stressful life experience, the higher the recurrence rate of cancer and the shorter the survival time (Forsen, 1991); others, however, failed to find any such relationship (Surtees et al., 2010). Contradictory results have also been found in relation to cancer mortality rates in widows and widowers (Martikainen & Valkonen, 1996), as well as in connection with the relationship between social support and neoplasic progression (Maunsell et al., 1995)

In addition to life stressors, certain personality traits and, again, certain coping strategies (particularly the concept of emotional repression) have also been the subjects of much attention (Eysenck, 2000; Segerstrom, 2003). Specifically, studies involving patients with malignant melanomas indicate that personality type predicts neither recurrence nor survival time (Canada et al., 2005). However, a greater progression of the disease was found in patients who claimed to have accepted their illness or who expressed feelings of impotence/desperation (Temoshok et al., 1985) and a positive relationship was observed between the manifestation of active coping strategies and a higher survival rate (Fawzy et al., 1993).

### 3.1 Physiological response to stress and cancer

The biological mechanisms which underlie the effects of stress on cancer have yet to be fully explained, and their clinical significance for human diseases has yet to be clarified. A number of studies involving both humans and animals suggest that stress may influence the growth and behavior of tumor cells, either directly, through central nervous system mediators, or through the neuroendocrine regulation of the immune response to the tumor.

The former involves the effects of stress-released hormones on the tumor cells themselves or on their cellular microenvironment. Research carried out on animals has shown that stress may foster angiogenesis through the release of catecholamines, which though beta-adrenergic mechanisms trigger an increase in tumor vascularization (Tasker et al., 2006).

Hormones such as NE, which are linked to the activation of the SNS, foster angiogenesis in human tumors, increasing the levels of vascular endothelial growth factor (VEGF) through beta-adrenergic mechanisms (S. K. Lutgendorf et al., 2003). Norepinephrine also fosters various steps which are essential to tumor metastasis development, such as migration and invasion (Masur et al., 2001). Glucocorticoids regulate a wide variety of glucocorticoid-receptor-mediated cellar processes, activating or repressing target genes. Recent experimental studies carried out *in vitro* and *in vivo* have demonstrated that as well as inducing apoptosis in lymphocytes, glucocorticoid hormones also activate the survival of genes which protect cancer cells from the effects of chemotherapy (Wu et al., 2004). Glucocorticoids may also activate oncoviruses and inhibit anti-tumor and anti-viral cellular immune responses. Moreover, glucocorticoids such as cortisol may function in synergy with catecholamines to facilitate cancer growth (Nakane et al., 1990). It is therefore plausible that stressful situations characterized by increased levels of catecholamines and cortisol (such as uncontrollable stress, for example) may have a greater impact on cancer-related processes.

Stress affects the levels and expression of other hormones also, such as prolactin (which increases with stress) and oxytocin and dopamine (which decrease with stress). Prolactin may foster cell growth and survival in breast tumors and other tumor cells (Clevenger et al., 2003). Oxytocin inhibits the growth of epithelial tumor cells (such as those in the endometrium and the breast), as well as of cells of neural or medullar origin; however, this hormone has a stimulatory effect on the growth of trophoblastic and endothelial tumors (Pequeux et al., 2004). For example, endogenous oxytocin has a dose-dependent mitogenic effect on small lung cancer cell lines, which is blocked by oxytocin receptor antagonists. Dopamine, which inhibits the growth of various types of malignant tumors, blocks VEGF-induced angiogenesis both *in vitro* and *in vivo* (Basu et al., 2001). For a review of the physiological mechanisms through which stress influences angiogenesis and tumor development, see Antoni, 2006 (Antoni et al., 2006).

Another pathway through which stress may influence neoplasic processes is neuroimmunomodulation. As described above (section 1), the HPA axis and the SAM axis are the two principal pathways through which stress may alter the immune activity. The section below analyzes the data found by studies involving both humans and animals regarding the effects of social stress on different immune parameters.

### 3.2 Stress and the Immune System

#### 3.2.1 Studies in humans

Studies carried out in humans have revealed that stress can strongly influence both innate (Redwine et al., 2003), and adaptive immunity (Sommerhoff et al., 2010). The studies in question also demonstrate that these effects are not always the same. Research conducted with medical students has shown that academic exams may trigger an increase in the number of neutrophils and platelets, and a decrease in the number of eosinophils, monocytes and basophils (Qureshi et al., 2002). The activation of the response to this type of stress has also been associated with a reduction in the number of natural killer (NK) cells (Isowa et al., 2004). Chronic social stress has been linked to an increase in neutrophils and a reduction in the number of B cells, cytotoxic T cells and NK cells (McKinnon et al., 1989), as well as to a drop in the cytotoxic capacity of NK cells (Irwin et al., 1988a).

It has also been found that social stressors may induce an immature phenotype of dendritic cells through the secretion of powerful neuroimmune mediators such as glucocorticoids, catecholamines and cytokines (Piemonti et al., 1999). Thus, patients receiving high doses of corticoids have been found to have significantly lower levels of dendritic cells in the blood. Also, it has been shown *in vitro* that glucocorticoids prevent the maturing and correct functioning of dendritic cells (Rozkova et al., 2006). However, other studies have found that certain types of stress may trigger the immunostimulation of the immune response, inducing an activation of dendritic cells and an increase in their effectiveness as antigen presenter cells (Saint-Mezard et al., 2003). Stress has also been found to affect proinflammatory cytokines (Segerstrom & Miller, 2004). The stress induced by caring for dementia patients may increase interleukin-6 (IL-6) levels by up to four times (Kiecolt-Glaser et al., 2003). In a sample of homeless people, Arranz et al. (2009) found a decrease in the migratory and phagocytic capacity of neutrophils, a lower proliferative capacity of lymphocytes, lower levels of interleukin-2 and a reduced activity of NK cells (Arranz et al., 2009). It has also been observed that stress triggers changes in the balance of different types of lymphocytes. In a comparative study involving patients suffering from chronic pain, those with high levels of emotional stress were found to have a lower response of Th1 cells (Kaufmann et al., 2007). In situations of academic stress, a drop has been observed in the production of cytokines by Th1 cells, accompanied by an increase in the number of cytokines released by type 2 T helper cells (Th2) (Marshall et al., 1998).

Fifty years ago, Rudolph H. Moos proposed that the development of rheumatoid arthritis (an autoimmune disease) was related to certain personality traits, such as perfectionism, self-sacrifice and conflict denial (Moos, 1964). As stated earlier, major differences exist in the way in which individuals perceive and respond to the same external and internal environmental stimuli. Individual differences in cognition, emotion and behavior also seem to play a potentially important role in the modulation of the IS. The results of research into the relationship between personality traits and the immune function are not clear enough to enable an association to be established between one type of personality and a higher or lower level of IS activity (Segerstrom & Miller, 2004). However, what has been observed is that individual differences in the anxiety level triggered by a stressful situation correlate with a significant drop in the cytotoxic capacity of NK cells, or with a drop in the total number of monocytes (Ironson et al., 1990; Jamner et al., 1988). It has also been found that affiliative motivation, as a personality dimension, increases immunoglobulin A (IgA) levels in saliva, and that those receiving greater social support also have higher IgA levels in saliva (Jemmott et al., 1983).

### 3.2.2 Studies in animals

The need to understand the relationship between stress and the IS in humans has prompted much interest in the study of the impact of social stress in animals, and in the development of different models for analyzing this impact. Social adaptation and social status are determining factors for the activation of the HPA and SAM axes (Cole et al., 2003). For this reason, social stress models are currently considered the best models available for studying the causes and mechanisms involved in the development of stress-related pathologies.

The immunomodulatory effects of social stress on innate and adaptive immunity in animals are described below.

In relation to innate immunity, as with studies involving humans, divergent results have been found depending on the immune parameter measured and, above all, the type and duration of the stress model applied. Thus, it has been observed that acute social stress may trigger an increase in the infiltration capacity of leucocytes in the immune activation zone and an increase in the number of macrophages and neutrophils (Bailey et al., 2007; Viswanathan et al.,

2005), while chronic social stress decreases the number, traffic and infiltration of leucocytes (Sutherland et al., 2006). It has also been observed that the prolongation of social stress results in an increase in interleukin 1β (IL-1β) levels in the hypothalamus (Barnum et al., 2008). This effect on proinflammatory interleukins is specific to the type of brain structure studied and the type of stress applied (Plata-Salaman et al., 2000).

As regards the adaptive immune response, it has been shown, for example, that chronic stress alters the balance of Th1 and Th2 lymphocytes (Frick et al., 2009). Social stress may also trigger a decrease in the proliferative capacity of splenic T lymphocytes and the proliferative capacity of NK cells (Beitia et al., 2005; Stefanski & Ben-Eliyahu, 1996).

Diverse studies coincide in asserting that the main mediators of the effects of stress on immunity, regardless of whether those effects are positive or negative, are glucocorticoid hormones and catecholamines (Besedovsky & Del Rey, 1996). Evidence also exists of the existence of different neuroendocrine responses associated with different coping strategies, which in turn have different immune consequences (Bartolomucci et al., 2001).

## 4. The effect of social stress on melanoma tumor development

In order to study the mechanisms involved in the relationship between social stress and melanoma tumor development in more detail, the following section outlines some of the work which has been carried out with animal models of social stress. Using different experimental tumor development models, these studies show that social stress significantly increases the development of tumor metastases (Stefanski & Ben-Eliyahu, 1996). An increase in B16 melanoma pulmonary metastasis development has also been observed (Fig. 2) in a mouse model for human melanoma applied to socially-stressed mice (Sa-Rocha et al., 2006; Vegas et al., 2006). The relationship of dominance/subordination which is necessarily established following social interaction between male mice has enabled researchers to observe that the stress to which the defeated or subordinate animals are subject triggers a significant increase in the development of B16 melanoma pulmonary metastasis.

These results suggest that an understanding of the general neurobiology of stress and the specific alterations associated with an imbalance in the HPA and SAM axes will likely lead to a clarification of the role of stress in disease, including neoplastic processes (Armaiz-Pena et al., 2009; Kiecolt-Glaser et al., 2002b). While some studies have shown the anti-tumor effect of glucocorticoids (Banciu et al., 2008b; Bhakoo et al., 1981b; Carlson et al., 2001). Arbiser et al., (1999), using both *in vitro* and *in vivo* assays, have found that CRH is able to enhance angiogenesis and stimulate epithelial tumor growth in the skin (Arbiser et al., 1999). Evidence also exists of a possible involvement of the SAM axis in tumor development. A number of studies have shown that sympathetic ganglionic blockade, adrenal demedullation or the administration of a nonselective beta-blocker either ameliorated or attenuated tumor metastases induced by social stress (Ben-Eliyahu et al., 2000; Shakhar & Ben-Eliyahu, 1998; Stefanski & Ben-Eliyahu, 1996), and increased resistance to B16 melanoma tumor development (Hasegawa & Saiki, 2002).

Similarly, in our laboratory we have found that blocking the neuroendocrine response through the administration of antalarmin (a corticotropin-releasing factor receptor antagonist) or nadolol (a beta-adrenergic antagonist), results in fewer and smaller pulmonary metastatic foci in subjects exposed to acute social stress, confirming the involvement of both the HPA axis and the SAM axis in the effects of social stress on melanoma tumor development (Fig. 3).

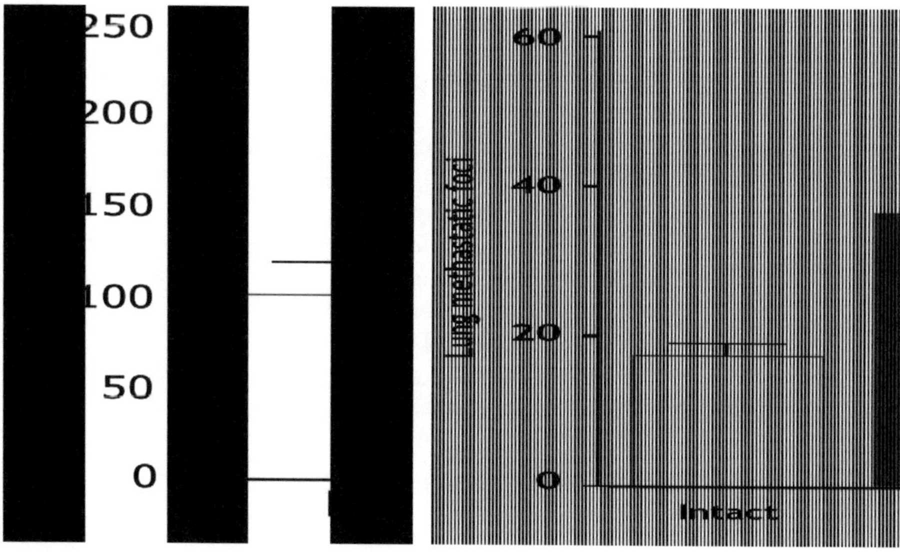


Fig. 2. (a) Effects of social stress on melanoma tumor development. (a) Number of metastasis in the lung of dominant (D) and submissive (S) mice counted 14 days after B16F10 ($2\times10^5$) tumor cell inoculation into their tail vein (Sa-Rocha et al., 2006). (b) Mean (GSE) pulmonary metastatic foci numbers in intact, handled control and stressed mice groups, inoculated with B16F10 murine melanoma cells, 21 days after inoculation (Vegas et al., 2006). $^*p<0.05$; $^{**}p<0.001$.

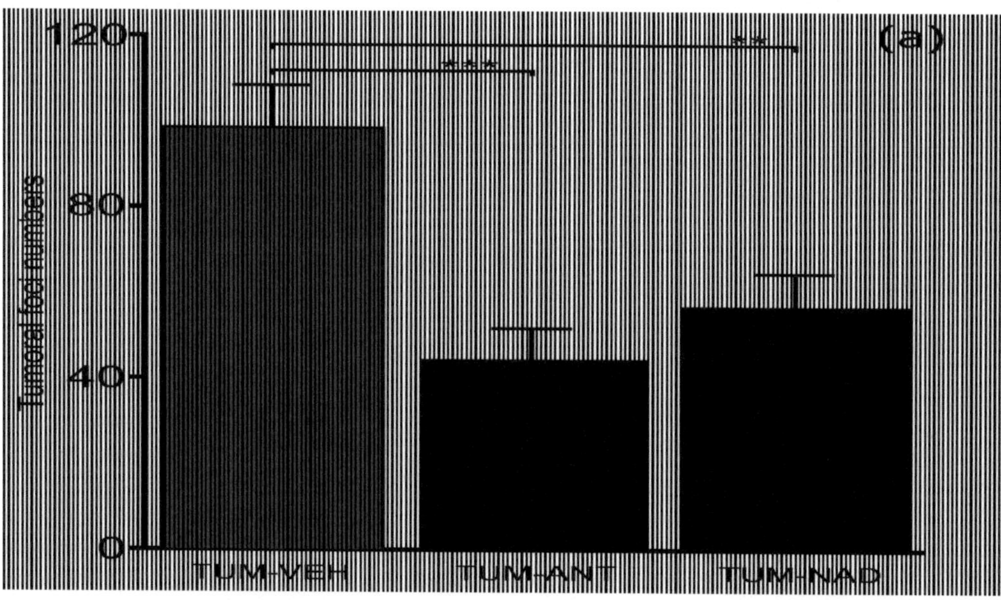


Fig. 3. Mean (±SE) tumor development (foci and area) in stressed mice inoculated with B16F10 melanoma cells, 21 days after inoculation (Vegas et al., 2009). $^*p < 0.05$, $^{**}p < 0.01$, $^{***}p < 0.0001$.

Diverse studies have shown that glucocorticoid receptors are widely expressed in normal and transformed melanocytes (Bhakoo et al., 1981a). Although some authors have found that glucocorticoid-based therapy appears to protect against melanoma incidence (Banciu et al., 2008a; Bhakoo et al., 1981b), the effect of GC on melanoma development is controversial (Arbiser et al., 1999; Chaudhuri et al., 1982). The results obtained in our laboratory do little to help clarify this point, since we observed a similar reduction in pulmonary metastatic development in both animals with lower levels of corticosterone (Antalarmin Group) and in animals with high levels of this hormone (Nadolol Group). However, it is possible that glucocorticoids may affect tumor development indirectly, through other mechanisms, or that the activation of the HPA axis may affect melanoma tumor development through mechanisms that are independent from the release of glucocorticoids.

Moreover, melanoma cells also express adrenergic receptors (alpha and beta) which may be activated by the catecholamines secreted in response to social stress. In this sense, Yang et al. (2009) found that the catecholamine stress hormone, norepinephrine, may influence tumor progression by modulating the expression of factors implicated in angiogenesis and metastasis (Yang et al., 2009).

Our results also indicate a clear involvement of the sympathetic pathway in melanoma tumor development, since blocking beta-adrenergic receptors resulted in a reduction of pulmonary metastases, as found also by other authors (Hasegawa & Saiki, 2002; Melamed et al., 2005; Stefanski & Ben-Eliyahu, 1996). The results of this study also suggest that the lower level of tumor development observed after blocking the HPA axis may also be due to indirect action on the sympathetic pathway, as other authors also point out (Gold & Chrousos, 2002), and that blocking CRH receptors may decrease the activity of both axes (Habib et al., 2000).

Different studies have indicated that the effects of neuroendocrine stress mediators on tumor development may be produced through their effects on the immune activity. There is a broad consensus regarding the idea that psychosocial stress affects parameters of the immune activity involved in tumor processes (Kiecolt-Glaser et al., 2002a, 2002b), and that the catecholamines released in response to stress act as important efferent immune modulators, often acting in concert with the activation of the HPA axis (Cunnick et al., 1990). Studies in animals have revealed that the intraventricular administration of CRH results in a suppression of NK activity which may be attenuated through peripheral adrenergic blocking (Irwin et al., 1988b; Tasker et al., 2006). The administration of Z-100, an immunomodulating agent, increases interferon *gamma* levels and reduces the development of B16F10 melanoma tumor metastases via the suppression of glucocorticoid-genesis (Oka et al., 2002). Nevertheless, a negative effect of stress on NK cell activity and tumor development has also been observed; this effect is independent of the reactivity of the HPA axis (Ben-Eliyahu & Shakhar, 2001). The increase of the aggressive potential of melanoma tumor cells observed by Yang et al. (2009) after the administration of NE is partly due at least to the fact that this catecholamine stimulates the production of VEGF, IL-8 and IL-6 (Yang et al., 2009). In this sense, the results obtained in our laboratory have shown that social stress reduces diverse parameters of the immune activity (proliferative response to Con-A, IL-2 and IL-12), and that this immunosuppression is accompanied by greater tumor development (Vegas et al., 2006). The data presented so far suggest that the course of melanoma tumor development may be affected by the hormones released during the stress response, either through the intervention of this response in the immune balance, or through other mechanisms capable of regulating the complex process of neoplastic development.

In the study of the possible effects of social stress on tumor development, it is important to bear in mind that the same adverse stimulus may not pose the same threat to all individuals, and that individuals respond to threats differently, from both a behavioral and physiological perspective. It has been observed that the neuroendocrine and immune changes produced by social stress in defeated subjects depend on the behavioral characteristics shown during social interactions (Sa-Rocha et al., 2006). Subjects which adopt different coping strategies (active or passive coping strategies) have different HPA and SAM activation patterns (Koolhaas et al., 2007). Previous studies in our laboratory show that social stress increases the pulmonary metastatic development of B16 melanoma, and point to a greater degree of tumor development in subjects which employ a more passive coping strategy in response to stress (Vegas et al., 2006). The coping strategies for social stress were obtained from an exhaustive analysis of the complete mouse ethogram developed by Brain et al. (1989), which covers 51 behavioral elements grouped into 11 broad categories: attack, threat, non-social exploration, social investigation, exploration from a distance, digging, body care, avoidance/flee, defense submission, sexual behavior and immobility.

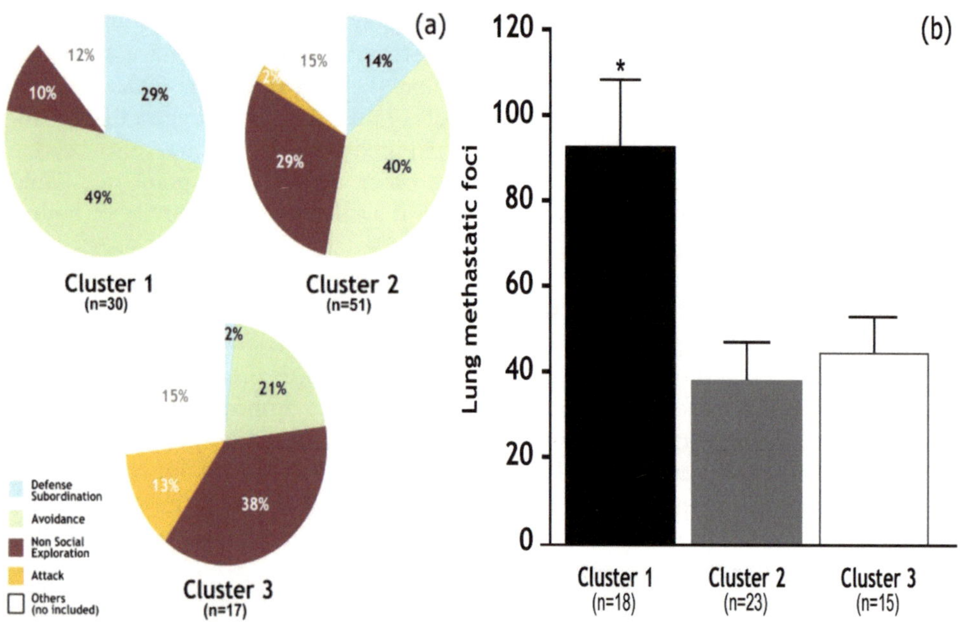


Fig. 4. (a) Mean percentages of the time allocated by mice inoculated with melanoma cells and subjected to the sensory contact stress protocol, to the behavioral categories that the discriminant analysis revealed to be most relevant in defining each cluster, namely: attack, defense/subordination, avoidance and non-social exploration. (b) Mean (GSE) pulmonary metastatic foci numbers in mice subjected to social stress and inoculated with B16F10 murine melanoma cells, belonging to each of the three clusters derived from the final cluster analysis, 21 days after inoculation (Vegas et al., 2006). *$P<0.05$.

Furthermore, these differences in HPA and SAM activation patterns have been shown to occur in conjunction with differences in the activation of monoaminergic pathways (Overli et al., 2001; Salome et al., 2006). One of the most interesting aspects of the impact of stress on the immune system or tumor development is the possible relevance of the individual behavioral characteristics exhibited by subjects in such situations (i.e. coping strategies). These differences in the physiological and behavioral coping styles adopted in response to stress may underlie differences in vulnerability to disease, including malignant melanoma (Azpiroz et al., 2008; Sajti et al., 2004; Stefanski & Ben-Eliyahu, 1996; Vegas et al., 2006). In this sense, recently in our laboratory we have demonstrated that individual differences in behavioral coping strategies are associated with unique alterations in the activation of the HPA and SAM axes and monoaminergic pathways. Thus, subjects from the active group had a lower level of HPA axis activity and a higher level of SAM axis activity, while subjects from the passive group were found to have a greater activation of the HPA axis and a lower activation of the SAM axis. Similarly, different coping strategies were observed to be associated with different levels of mRNA expression for serotonergic and dopaminergic synthetic enzymes (De Miguel et al., 2011). Taken together, these studies provide new evidence in favor of the idea that coping styles in response to social stress are involved in the determination of individual vulnerability to stress-related illnesses, such as malignant melanoma.

These studies, carried out in animals, indicate that social stress and coping strategies may have an effect on melanoma development, although the mechanisms involved in this relationship have yet to be determined. In humans, there are no studies to date which demonstrate this relationship. Nevertheless, later on is an outline of various studies focusing on the benefits of social intervention in cancer patients, particularly those suffering from melanoma.

## 5. The neurochemical and behavioral effects produced by melanoma tumor development

Since this relationship is bi-directional, the IS also sends messages to the CNS; this communication is carried out by proinflammatory cytokines, which are substances secreted by the peripheral immune cells (monocytes and macrophages) in response to infection or injury. The action of cytokines on the CNS affects both diverse physiological parameters and behavior (for a review see (Dantzer et al., 2001)). The series of behavioral changes associated with infection or injury are considered unspecific and are known as sickness behavior. They generally manifest themselves through a reduction in activity, a decrease in appetite, a loss of interest in social activities and an increase in tiredness. A number of different studies involving the peripheral or central administration of these cytokines have shown that mainly interleukin 1 (IL-1α and IL-1β), but also interleukin 6 (IL-6) and the tumor necrosis factor (TNF-α), are responsible (either directly or indirectly) for sickness behavior (Bluthe et al., 1994). In addition to behavioral changes, the immune response also provokes changes in the metabolism of the brain monoamines and the activation of the HPA axis. The result is an increase in the noradrenaline metabolism (NE) in different areas of the brain, particularly in the hypothalamus, as well as an increase in the serotonin metabolism (5HT) and, in some cases, the dopamine metabolism (DA) also (Dunn, 1992). The majority of the data regarding this type of behavioral and physiological changes have been obtained by means of virus inoculation, the administration of lipopolysaccharide endotoxins (LPS) or the central administration of IL-1, IL-2, IL-6, and TNF-α (Zalcman et al., 1994). Some studies have observed changes in the brain neurotransmitters produced in mice bearing tumors, that have been associated with hyperammonemia and reduced food intake (Chance et al., 2003). Chuluyan et al. (Chuluyan et al., 2000) found changes in the monoaminergic activity in different areas of the brain in mice inoculated with murine lymphoma cells, neoplasic line cells that do not induce an immune response. Few studies have focused on the behavioral and neurochemical effects produced by the activation of the immune system in situations of social stress. Cirulli et al. (Cirulli et al., 1998) found modifications in the agonistic behavior of young mice exposed to situations of conflict with adult mice following the peripheral administration of IL-1. We have studied the behavioral and neurochemical effects produced during the early phases of melanoma tumor development, under the most natural circumstances possible, i.e.. territorial aggression between male mice of the same species. Besides, the effects on the brain metabolism were analyzed in relation to the hypothalamus, by assessing the activity of 5HT and DA, and in relation to the striatum (SRT) by measuring the density of dopaminergic D2-receptors.

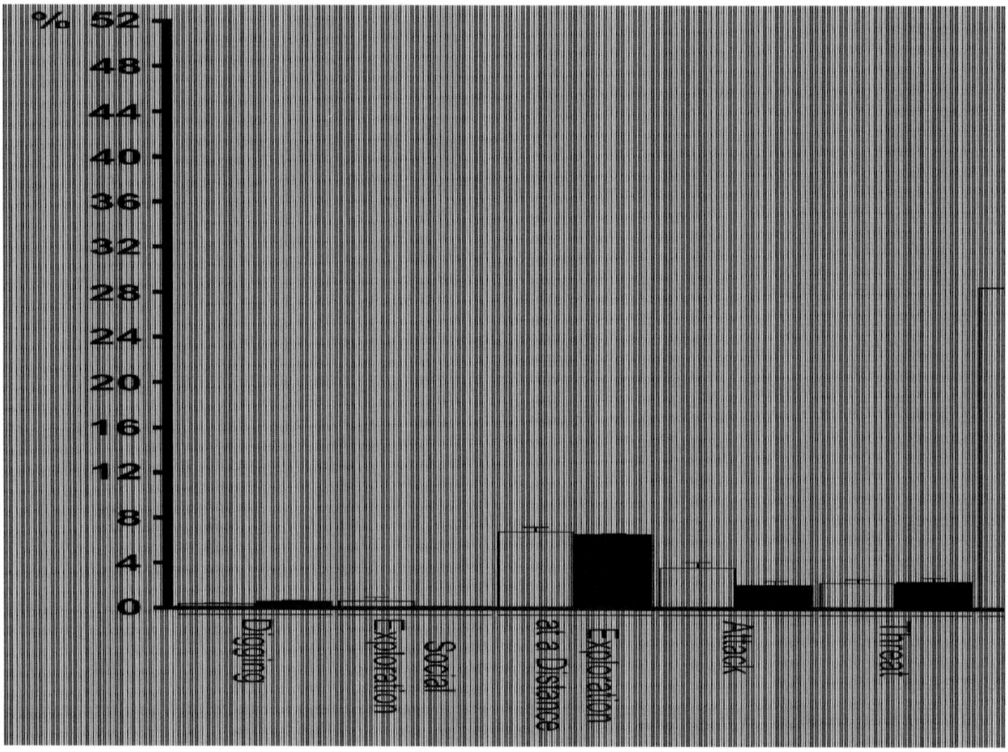


Fig. 5. Percentage of time (mean ±S.E.M.) dedicated to each of the behavioral categories, in male OF1 mice subjected to social stress, without tumoral inoculation ($n$ = 28) and with tumoral inoculation ($n$ = 28). (*) Tumor-bearing subjects vs. tumor-free control subjects (Vegas et al., 2004). * $P < 0.05$; *** $P < 0.001$.

After analyzing the behavioral data, we observed an effect of social stress in both inoculated and non-inoculated animals, in relation to 3 of the 11 behavioral categories analyzed (Fig. 5). We found that after a prior experience of defeat, a second confrontation with the dominant opponent resulted in a significant reduction in threat and non-social exploration behaviors, accompanied by an increase in fleeing. These results correspond with those found in other studies in which social stress was found to provoke a reduction in aggressive behavior and an increase in defensive and submissive behaviors (Albonetti & Farabollini, 1994). Although social stress was also found to have an effect on avoidance behavior, this was only true for non-inoculated animals. The fact that inoculated subjects demonstrated high levels of fleeing in the first confrontation (something which is a major characteristic of the behavior of these subjects and is discussed later on), may be the reason for our failure to observe a reduction in fleeing among the subjects in this group. To continue with the analysis of the behavioral results we observed that animals inoculated with B16 tumor cells demonstrated the same repertoire of behavior as untreated subjects submitted to social stress. Nevertheless, clear differences were found as regards the time dedicated to each of these behaviors, and an important change was observed in the confrontation strategy used. A significant increase was observed in avoidance behavior, coupled with a decrease in non-social exploration, defense-submission and immobility in inoculated subjects.

| Assays | Tumor-free subjects | | Tumor-bearing subjects | |
|---|---|---|---|---|
| | Non-stressed | Stressed | Non-stressed | Stressed |
| Catecholamines | | | | |
| DA† | 0.242 ± 0.008 | 0.256 ± 0.012 | 0.247 ± 0.008 | 0.287 ± 0.016 |
| DOPAC*** | 0.103 ± 0.005 | 0.124 ± 0.006 | 0.413 ± 0.112 | 0.287 ± 0.048 |
| DOPAC/DA ratio*** | 0.433 ± 0.031 | 0.485 ± 0.017 | 1.669 ± 0.464 | 1.002 ± 0.160 |
| 5HT*** | 2.425 ± 0.037 | 2.406 ± 0.065 | 1.656 ± 0.182 | 2.166 ± 0.151 |
| 5HIAA | 0.588 ± 0.007 | 0.672 ± 0.020 | 0.644 ± 0.024 | 0.647 ± 0.032 |
| 5HIAA/5HT ratio** | 0.243 ± 0.002 | 0.282 ± 0.012 | 0.479 ± 0.097 | 0.319 ± 0.030 |
| Cell proliferation | | | | |
| Con-A proliferation*** | 1.162 ± 0.112 | 1.192 ± 0.068 | 2.372 ± 0.197 | 2.360 ± 0.179 |
| PHA proliferation** | 1.456 ± 0.061 | 1.302 ± 0.030 | 1.512 ± 0.066 | 1.496 ± 0.049 |
| $D_2$-receptors* | 201.58 ± 27.63 | 161.35 ± 20.41 | 248.91 ± 26.34 | 241.64 ± 28.19 |

Table 1. Effects of tumoral inoculation and social stress on the physiological variables analyzed. Data are expressed as mean ± S.E.M. The interaction between these two factors was not significant in none of the analyzed variables. (Vegas et al., 2004); *tumor-bearing subjects vs. tumor-free subjects (*$P < 0.05$, **$P < 0.01$, ***$P < 0.001$); †non-stressed vs. stressed (†$P < 0.05$. * $P < 0.05$; *** $P < 0.001$).

Although sickness behavior is characterized by a drop in activity and a lack of interest in the subject's environment due to the effect of proinflammatory cytokines on the nervous system (Dantzer & Kelley, 1989), the behavior observed in this study failed to coincide exactly with this definition. The results revealed a drop in non-social exploration similar to that observed by other authors studying exploratory behavior in response to a new environment after the central or peripheral (Cirulli et al., 1998; Dunn, 1992; Spadaro & Dunn, 1990) administration of LPS, IL-1α, or IL-1β. However, has been postulated that sickness behavior should also be considered as the expression of an organized strategy that is vital for the survival of the organism; in this case, the sick individual will be capable of reorganizing his/her behavior depending on the consequences and internal and external circumstances to which he/she is exposed. This is similar to the way in which Zalcman et al. (Zalcman et al., 1998) interpret the behavioral activation observed in mice after the administration of IL-2 and IL-6. In the context of aggressive confrontation between rodents after the administration of IL-1, Cirulli et al. (Cirulli et al., 1998) observed a decrease in the aggressive components of agonistic behavior, although defensive elements such as upright submissive posture, crouching, or fleeing were not affected. Nevertheless, we should bear in mind that in our study, we observed a passive defensive behavior: avoidance. This behavior increased significantly in inoculated subjects and may form part of a defensive strategy against attack by opponents, characterized by lower energy expenditure and a reduced receipt of injury. These changes in the behavioral strategy of inoculated animals may be related to the increase in the density of D2-receptors in the striatum. The "up regulation" of these receptors indicates a decrease in the dopaminergic activity in this structure, which may be the cause of the reduced motor activity observed (Boehme & Ciaranello, 1981; Isovich et al., 2001). In light of these data, we can hypothesize that the behavioral effects observed in inoculated animals may be caused by an increase in the secretion of cytokines. This increase may in turn be the result of the activation of the immune system in response to the B16 melanoma tumoral antigens, which are recognized by the T lymphocytes (Houghton et al., 2001), or by cytokines produced by the tumor itself. The B16 melanoma tumor produces growth factors and cytokines (IL-1α, IL-6, TGF-β, OSM, TNF, and IFN) during the early phases of tumor development (Lazar-Molnar et al., 2000). Although we did not measure the interleukins, we did find evidence of immune activation upon observing a significant increase in the proliferative capacity of spleen monocytes in animals inoculated with tumor cells, in comparison with their non-inoculated counterparts (Table 1). The changes produced by the development of the B16 melanoma both in the hypothalamic monoaminergic activity and in the density of D2-receptors in the striatum may also be caused by the action of cytokines. Uomoto et al. (Uomoto et al., 1998) found a decrease in the DA turnover in the striatum, along with a decrease in the locomotive activity and a significant increase in plasmatic IL-6 levels in mice bearing colon-26 tumor cells. Although the effects of IL-2 on behavior have yet to be fully investigated, some studies point to a possible involvement of this cytokine in behavior modulated by the dopaminergic activity of the forebrain (Petitto et al., 1997). Furthermore, a significant increase was found in the turnover of both 5HT and DA in inoculated animals, both control subjects and those exposed to social stress. These results coincide with the increase in the 5HT and DA activity found in the hypothalamus of mice after various days of inoculation with lymphoma tumor cells (Chuluyan et al., 2000). Although it has been found that an acute defeat experience may produce an increase in the serotonergic activity in different areas of the brain, including the hypothalamus (Blanchard et al., 1993), in our study, social stress only produced a significant increase in the DA content, with the turnover of this catecholamine remaining unchanged. The administration of diverse interleukins provokes changes in the monoaminergic activity in mice in different areas of the brain. A number of studies using rodents have shown that the peripheral administration of diverse interleukins produces alterations in the 5HT, DA and NE activity in different areas of the brain (Connor et al., 1998). As regards the hypothalamus, various studies have found increases in the noradrenergic activity following the peripheral administration of IL-1 and IL-2 (Zalcman et al., 1994). In relation to the 5HT and DA activity, a number of authors have found an increase in the turnover of these two monoamines following the peripheral administration of IL-1 (Dunn, 1992), and in the PNV paraventricular nucleus following the peripheral administration of IL-1 and TNF-α (Brebner et al., 2000), might be in line with our results. Similarly, following the administration of IL-1 in the front hypothalamus in rats, Shintani et al. (Shintani et al., 1993) found that this interleukin acted directly on the hypothalamus in a dosage-dependent manner, increasing the release of NE, DA, and 5HT, as well as their metabolites. In light of all these data, we can conclude that tumor development produces behavioral changes, manifested mainly in a change in defensive strategy, and neurochemical changes when subjects are exposed to situations of intense social stress. These changes may be mediated by an increase in secretion of interleukins provoked by tumor development.

## 6. Psychosocial intervention and cancer progression

Over recent years, many researchers have tried to establish a link between psychosocial intervention and improvements in the condition of cancer patients. Although the psychological benefits of these interventions have been well documented, evidence exists both in favor of and against the assertion that they influence the course of the disease itself. Lutgendorf et al. (2010) analyzed this relationship by reviewing over 300 intervention studies carried out over the last 50 years (S.K. Lutgendorf et al., 2010). The majority of these studies involved breast cancer patients. The review analyzes the data obtained from studies which found a beneficial effect of different forms of psychosocial intervention (including relaxation and coping techniques) on patients' quality of life (Coyne et al., 2007; Spiegel, 2002). In this sense, the review highlights the ability of psychosocial interventions to alleviate pain and anxiety in metastatic breast cancer patients with the most severe symptoms (Goodwin et al., 2001) and to improve the quality of life, depressed mood, distress and social disorders of cancer patients (Andersen et al., 2007; Antoni et al., 2006).

More controversial is the question of whether psychosocial interventions can affect the progression of cancer and patients' chances of survival. In this sense, the studies conducted (all with powerful and rigorous methodologies) offer contradictory results. In three studies with varied methodologies focusing on psychosocial interventions with breast cancer patients, the authors found that either a reduced risk of disease recurrence or the survival rate increased (Andersen et al., 2008; Coyne et al., 2007). However, in two other studies, also involving women with metastatic breast cancer, here receiving expressive therapy, the authors failed to find any increase in survival (Kissane et al., 2007; Spiegel et al., 2007). Possible explanations for this divergence include differences in the status of the disease between patient populations and differences in the physiological effects produced by the various interventions (Andersen et al., 2004; Stefanek et al., 2009). It has also been suggested that the optimization of the neuroendocrine and immune status may require both psychological and pharmacological interventions, in order to fully mitigate the deleterious effects of the biology of stress on tumor growth and progression.

The most common psychological interventions in cancer cases include, among others, training in stress coping skills. The idea that this type of intervention may have a positive effect on psychological adaptation is becoming increasingly widely accepted. Aspects of this positive effect include neuroendocrine and immune changes, a drop in cortisol levels and an increase in lymphocyte proliferation, as well as an increase in cytokines (IL-1β, IL-2, etc.) (McGregor & Antoni, 2009). Other beneficial effects of psychological therapy on health should also be taken into consideration in the effort to halt the progression of the disease. It has been shown that psychological interventions trigger changes in health behavior, improve adherence to pharmacological treatment and may reduce the incidence of opportunistic infection both during and after a surgical procedure or adjuvant therapy (Andersen et al., 2004; Coyne et al., 2007; Pereira et al., 2003).

Studies carried out in this respect with malignant melanoma patients seem to support this theory (Fawzy et al., 2003; Fawzy et al., 1990; Fawzy & Fawzy, 1994; Fawzy et al., 1993). ). In these studies, recurrence and survival rate were studied in a group of 68 patients who had either been recently diagnosed or undergone a surgical procedure. Half of the sample group participated six times a week in group sessions which focused on social interaction, health education, stress management and coping skills. It was a randomized controlled experimental study. The Cox proportion hazards regression model was used to quantify the relationship between treatment and the outcomes adjusted by the covariates: age, sex,

Breslow depth, tumor site, baseline profile of Mood States Total Mood Disturbance, baseline active-behavioral coping, baseline natural killer cell activity and treatment. The stepwise procedure was used for covariate selection.

At six months, those patients who had participated in the support groups were found to be less depressed and more vigorous, and had developed better coping skills. They also had an increase in the number and function of NK lymphocytes in the blood, in comparison with their counterparts from the control group (Fawzy et al., 1990). Six years after the intervention, the same patients were studied again in relation to recurrence and death rates. Those patients who had participated in the intervention showed a trend towards a longer recurrence-free state and a statistically significant lower death rate. Finally, baseline affective distress and coping baseline were predictors for recurrence and survival (Fawzy et al., 1993).

The same authors then studied the effects of the intervention on the course of the disease in the same patients, 10 years after the treatment. In this univariate analysis, the survival and recurrence distributions for the intervention and control groups were estimated using the Kaplan-Meier method, and were tested for equality by the log-rank test. The multivariate analysis used the Cox proportional hazards regression model with the following prognostic factors: age, sex, Breslow depth, tumor size, and treatment status (i.e. intervention group vs control group). When analyzed as single covariates, the results obtained revealed that the differences between the intervention and control groups were not significant at the 10-year follow-up. However, being male and having a greater Breslow depth were predictive of poorer outcome. An analysis of multiple covariates also revealed that sex and Breslow depth were significant for survival. Furthermore, participation in the intervention was significant for survival. After adjusting for sex and Breslow depth, participation in the intervention remained significant for survival. The authors conclude that these results suggest that while the survival benefit of intervention weakens after the 5-to-6 year follow-up, participation in the intervention remains predictive of survival when the effects of other known prognosis indicators are statistically controlled (Fawzy et al., 2003).

## 7. Conclusion

Although the mechanisms through which psychosocial factors may affect the disease remain uncertain, and it is important to wait for the results of future replication studies, the results obtained to date suggest that this type of approach may be highly effective for exploring psychosocial influences on melanoma progression and highlight the urgent need to supplement both traditional and new medical therapies with a greater effort to ensure the psychosocial wellbeing of cancer patients.

## 8. Acknowledgments

This work was supported by the Project Grant of the Basque Government GIC07/19-238.

## 9. References

Albonetti, M. E., & Farabollini, F. (1994). Social stress by repeated defeat: effects on social behaviour and emotionality. *Behavioural Brain Research,* Vol.62, No.2, pp. 187-193, ISSN 0166-4328

Andersen, B. L., Farrar, W. B., Golden-Kreutz, D., Emery, C. F., Glaser, R., Crespin, T., et al. (2007). Distress reduction from a psychological intervention contributes to improved health for cancer patients. *Brain Behavior and Immunity,* Vol.21, No.7, pp. 953-961, ISSN 0889-1591.

Andersen, B. L., Farrar, W. B., Golden-Kreutz, D. M., Glaser, R., Emery, C. F., Crespin, T. R., et al. (2004). Psychological, behavioral, and immune changes after a psychological intervention: a clinical trial. *Journal of Clinical Oncology,* Vol.22, No.17, pp. 3570-3580, ISSN 0732-183X

Andersen, B. L., Yang, H. C., Farrar, W. B., Golden-Kreutz, D. M., Emery, C. F., Thornton, L. M., et al. (2008). Psychologic Intervention Improves Survival for Breast Cancer Patients A Randomized Clinical Trial. *Cancer,* Vol.113, No.12, pp. 3450-3458, ISSN 0008-543X.

Antoni, M. H., Lutgendorf, S. K., Cole, S. W., Dhabhar, F. S., Sephton, S. E., McDonald, P. G., et al. (2006). The influence of bio-behavioural factors on tumour biology: pathways and mechanisms. *Nat Rev Cancer,* Vol.6, No.3, pp. 240-248, ISSN 1474-175X .

Arbiser, J. L., Karalis, K., Viswanathan, A., Koike, C., Anand-Apte, B., Flynn, E., et al. (1999). Corticotropin-releasing hormone stimulates angiogenesis and epithelial tumor growth in the skin. *Journal of Investigative Dermatology,* Vol.113, No.5, pp. 838-842, ISSN 0022-202X .

Armaiz-Pena, G. N., Lutgendorf, S. K., Cole, S. W., & Sood, A. K. (2009). Neuroendocrine modulation of cancer progression. *Brain, Behavior, and Immunity,* Vol.23, No.1, pp. 10-15, ISSN 1090-2139.

Arranz, L., de Vicente, A., Munoz, M., & De la Fuente, M. (2009). Impaired immune function in a homeless population with stress-related disorders. *Neuroimmunomodulation,* Vol.16, No.4, pp. 251-260, ISSN 1423-0216

Azpiroz, A., De Miguel, Z., Fano, E., & Vegas, O. (2008). Relations between different coping strategies for social stress, tumor development and neuroendocrine and immune activity in male mice. *Brain, Behavior, and Immunity,* Vol.22, No.5, pp. 690-698, ISSN 1090-2139.

Bailey, M. T., Engler, H., Powell, N. D., Padgett, D. A., & Sheridan, J. F. (2007). Repeated social defeat increases the bactericidal activity of splenic macrophages through a Toll-like receptor-dependent pathway. *Am J Physiol Regul Integr Comp Physiol,* Vol.293, No.3, pp. R1180-1190, ISSN 0363-6119

Banciu, M., Fens, M. H., Storm, G., & Schiffelers, R. M. (2008a). Antitumor activity and tumor localization of liposomal glucocorticoids in B16 melanoma-bearing mice. *J Control Release,* Vol.127, No.2, pp. 131-136, ISSN 1873-4995

Banciu, M., Schiffelers, R. M., Metselaar, J. M., & Storm, G. (2008b). Utility of targeted glucocorticoids in cancer therapy. *J Liposome Res,* Vol.18, No.1, pp. 47-57, ISSN 1532-2394.

Barnum, C. J., Blandino, P., Jr., & Deak, T. (2008). Social status modulates basal IL-1 concentrations in the hypothalamus of pair-housed rats and influences certain features of stress reactivity. *Brain, Behavior, and Immunity,* Vol.22, No.4, pp. 517-527, ISSN 1090-2139

Bartolomucci, A., Palanza, P., Gaspani, L., Limiroli, E., Panerai, A. E., Ceresini, G., et al. (2001). Social status in mice: behavioral, endocrine and immune changes are context dependent. *Physiology and Behavior,* Vol.73, No.3, pp. 401-410

Basu, S., Nagy, J. A., Pal, S., Vasile, E., Eckelhoefer, I. A., Bliss, V. S., et al. (2001). The neurotransmitter dopamine inhibits angiogenesis induced by vascular permeability factor/vascular endothelial growth factor. *Nature Medicine,* Vol.7, No.5, pp. 569-574, ISSN 1078-8956

Beitia, G., Garmendia, L., Azpiroz, A., Vegas, O., Brain, P. F., & Arregi, A. (2005). Time-dependent behavioral, neurochemical, and immune consequences of repeated experiences of social defeat stress in male mice and the ameliorative effects of fluoxetine. *Brain, Behavior, and Immunity,* Vol.19, No.6, pp. 530-539, ISSN 0889-1591.

Bellinger, D. L., Millar, B. A., Perez, S., Carter, J., Wood, C., ThyagaRajan, S., et al. (2008). Sympathetic modulation of immunity: relevance to disease. *Cellular Immunology,* Vol.252, No.1-2, pp. 27-56, ISSN 1090-2163.

Ben-Eliyahu, S., & Shakhar, G. (2001). The impact of stress, catecholamines, and the menstrual cycle on NK activity and tumor development: from in vitro studies to biological significance. In R. Ader, N. Cohen & D. Felten (Eds.), *Psychoneuroimmunology,* Vol. 2, pp. 545-563, Academic Press, San Diego.

Ben-Eliyahu, S., Shakhar, G., Page, G. G., Stefanski, V., & Shakhar, K. (2000). Suppression of NK cell activity and of resistance to metastasis by stress: a role for adrenal catecholamines and beta-adrenoceptors. *Neuroimmunomodulation,* Vol.8, No.3, pp. 154-164

Benschop, R. J., Schedlowski, M., Wienecke, H., Jacobs, R., & Schmidt, R. E. (1997). Adrenergic control of natural killer cell circulation and adhesion. *Brain, Behavior, and Immunity,* Vol.11, No.4, pp. 321-332

Besedovsky, H. O., & Del Rey, A. (1996). Immune-neuro-endocrine interactions: facts and hypotheses. *Endocrine Reviews,* Vol.17, No.1, pp. 64-102

Besedovsky, H. O., & del Rey, A. (2007). Physiology of psychomeuroimmunology: A personal view. *Brain Behavior and Immunity,* Vol.21, No.1, pp. 34-44, ISSN 0889-1591.

Bhakoo, H. S., Milholland, R. J., Lopez, R., Karakousis, C., & Rosen, F. (1981a). High incidence and characterization of glucocorticoid receptors in human malignant melanoma. *Journal of the National Cancer Institute,* Vol.66, No.1, pp. 21-25, ISSN 0027-8874

Bhakoo, H. S., Paolini, N. S., Milholland, R. J., Lopez, R. E., & Rosen, F. (1981b). Glucocorticoid receptors and the effect of glucocorticoids on the growth of B16 melanoma. *Cancer Research,* Vol.41, No.5, pp. 1695-1701, ISSN 0008-5472

Biber, K., de Jong, E. K., van Weering, H. R., & Boddeke, H. W. (2006). Chemokines and their receptors in central nervous system disease. *Curr Drug Targets,* Vol.7, No.1, pp. 29-46, ISSN 1389-4501 .

Blalock, J. E., Smith, E. M., & Meyer, W. J. (1985). The pituitary-adrenocortical axis and the immune system. *Clinics in Endocrinology and Metabolism,* Vol.14, No.4, pp. 1021-1038

Blanchard, D. C., Sakai, R. R., McEwen, B., Weiss, S. M., & Blanchard, R. J. (1993). Subordination stress: behavioral, brain, and neuroendocrine correlates. *Behavioural Brain Research,* Vol.58, No.1-2, pp. 113-121

Bluthe, R. M., Pawlowski, M., Suarez, S., Parnet, P., Pittman, Q., Kelley, K. W., et al. (1994). Synergy between tumor necrosis factor alpha and interleukin-1 in the induction of sickness behavior in mice. *Psychoneuroendocrinology,* Vol.19, No.2, pp. 197-207, ISSN 0306-4530 .

Boehme, R. E., & Ciaranello, R. D. (1981). Dopamine receptor binding in inbred mice: strain differences in mesolimbic and nigrostriatal dopamine binding sites. *Proceedings of the National Academy of Sciences of the United States of America,* Vol.78, No.5, pp. 3255-3259

Brebner, K., Hayley, S., Zacharko, R., Merali, Z., & Anisman, H. (2000). Synergistic effects of interleukin-1beta, interleukin-6, and tumor necrosis factor-alpha: central monoamine, corticosterone, and behavioral variations. *Neuropsychopharmacology,* Vol.22, No.6, pp. 566-580

Canada, A. L., Fawzy, N. W., & Fawzy, F. I. (2005). Personality and disease outcome in malignant melanoma. *Journal of Psychosomatic Research,* Vol.58, No.1, pp. 19-27, ISSN 0022-3999

Carlson, K. W., Nawy, S. S., Wei, E. T., Sadee, W., Filov, V. A., Rezsova, V. V., et al. (2001). Inhibition of mouse melanoma cell proliferation by corticotropin-releasing hormone and its analogs. *Anticancer Research,* Vol.21, No.2A, pp. 1173-1179, ISSN 0250-7005 .

Carr, D. J., Radulescu, R. T., deCosta, B. R., Rice, K. C., & Blalock, J. E. (1990). Differential effect of opioids on immunoglobulin production by lymphocytes isolated from Peyer's patches and spleen. *Life Sciences,* Vol.47, No.12, pp. 1059-1069

Cirulli, F., De Acetis, L., & Alleva, E. (1998). Behavioral effects of peripheral interlukin-1 administration in adult CD-1 mice: specific inhibition of the offensive components of intermale agonistic behavior. *Brain Research,* Vol.791, pp. 308-312

Clevenger, C. V., Furth, P. A., Hankinson, S. E., & Schuler, L. A. (2003). The role of prolactin in mammary carcinoma. *Endocrine Reviews,* Vol.24, No.1, pp. 1-27, ISSN 0163-769X

Cole, S. W., Kemeny, M. E., Fahey, J. L., Zack, J. A., & Naliboff, B. D. (2003). Psychological risk factors for HIV pathogenesis: mediation by the autonomic nervous system. *Biological Psychiatry,* Vol.54, No.12, pp. 1444-1456, ISSN 0006-3223

Connor, T. J., Song, C., Leonard, B. E., Merali, Z., & Anisman, H. (1998). An assessment of the effects of central interleukin-1beta, -2, -6, and tumor necrosis factor-alpha administration on some behavioural, neurochemical, endocrine and immune parameters in the rat. *Neuroscience,* Vol.84, No.3, pp. 923-933

Cooper, C. L., Cooper, R., & Faragher, E. B. (1989). Incidence and perception of psychosocial stress: the relationship with breast cancer. *Psychological Medicine,* Vol.19, No.2, pp. 415-422

Coyne, J., Stefanek, M., & Palmer, S. (2007). Psychotherapy and survival in cancer: The conflict between hope and evidence. *Psychological Bulletin,* Vol.133, pp. 367-394

Cunnick, J. E., Lysle, D. T., Kucinski, B. J., & Rabin, B. S. (1990). Evidence that shock-induced immune suppression is mediated by adrenal hormones and peripheral beta-adrenergic receptors. *Pharmacology, Biochemistry and Behavior,* Vol.36, No.3, pp. 645-651, ISSN 0091-3057 .

Chance, W. T., Sheriff, S., Dayal, R., & Balasubramaniam, A. (2003). Refractory hypothalamic alpha-mSH satiety and AGRP feeding systems in rats bearing MCA sarcomas. *Peptides,* Vol.24, No.12, pp. 1909-1919

Chaudhuri, P. K., Das Gupta, T. K., Beattie, C. W., & Walker, M. J. (1982). Glucocorticoid-induced exacerbation of metastatic human melanoma. *Journal of Surgical Oncology,* Vol.20, No.1, pp. 49-52, ISSN 0022-4790

Chuluyan, H. E., Wolcott, R. M., Chervenak, R., & Dunn, A. J. (2000). Catecholamine, indoleamine and corticosteroid responses in mice bearing tumors. *Neuroimmunomodulation,* Vol.8, No.3, pp. 107-113

Dantzer, R., Bluthé, R. M., Castanon, N., Chauvet, N., Capuron, L., Goodall, G., et al. (2001). Cytokine Effects on Behavior. In A. R, D. L. Felten & N. Cohen (Eds.), *Psychoneuroimmunology,* Vol. 1, pp. 703-727, Academic Press, San Diego.

Dantzer, R., & Kelley, K. W. (1989). Stress and immunity: an integrated view of relationships between the brain and the immune system. *Life Sciences,* Vol.44, pp. 1995-2008

De Miguel, Z., Vegas, O., Garmendia, L., Arregi, A., Beitia, G., & Azpiroz, A. (2011). Behavioral coping strategies in response to social stress are associated with unique neuroendocrine, monoaminergic and immune response profiles in mice, *Behavioural Brain Research.*

Dunn, A. J. (1992). Endotoxin-induced activation of cerebral catecholamine and serotonin metabolism: comparison with interleukin-1. *Journal of Pharmacology and Experimental Therapeutics,* Vol.261, No.3, pp. 964-969

Elenkov, I. J., Wilder, R. L., Chrousos, G. P., & Vizi, E. S. (2000). The sympathetic nerve--an integrative interface between two supersystems: the brain and the immune system. *Pharmacological Reviews,* Vol.52, No.4, pp. 595-638

Eysenck, H. J. (2000). Personality as a risk factor in cancer and coronary heart disease. In D. T. Kenny, J. G. Carlson, F. J. McGuigan & J. L. Sheppard (Eds.), *Stress and health research and clinical applications,* pp. 291–318, Harwood Academic Publishers, Amsterdam, Países Bajos.

Fawzy, F. I., Canada, A. L., & Fawzy, N. W. (2003). Malignant melanoma: effects of a brief, structured psychiatric intervention on survival and recurrence at 10-year follow-up. *Archives of General Psychiatry,* Vol.60, No.1, pp. 100-103, ISSN 0003-990X

Fawzy, F. I., Cousins, N., Fawzy, N. W., Kemeny, M. E., Elashoff, R., & Morton, D. (1990). A structured psychiatric intervention for cancer patients. I. Changes over time in methods of coping and affective disturbance. *Archives of General Psychiatry,* Vol.47, No.8, pp. 720-725, ISSN 0003-990X

Fawzy, F. I., & Fawzy, N. W. (1994). A structured psychoeducational intervention for cancer patients. *General Hospital Psychiatry,* Vol.16, No.3, pp. 149-192

Fawzy, F. I., Fawzy, N. W., Hyun, C. S., Elashoff, R., Guthrie, D., Fahey, J. L., et al. (1993). Malignant melanoma. Effects of an early structured psychiatric intervention, coping, and affective state on recurrence and survival 6 years later. *Archives of General Psychiatry,* Vol.50, No.9, pp. 681-689

Felten, D. L., Felten, S. Y., Carlson, S. L., Olschowka, J. A., & Livnat, S. (1985). Noradrenergic and peptidergic innervation of lymphoid tissue. *Journal of Immunology,* Vol.135, No.2 Suppl, pp. 755s-765s

Felten, S. Y., & Felten, D. L. (1991). The innervation of lymphoid tissue. In R. Ader, D. L. Felten & N. Cohen (Eds.), *Psychoneuroimmunology,* Academic Press, San Diego.

Forsen, A. (1991). Psychosocial stress as a risk for breast cancer. *Psychotherapy and Psychosomatics,* Vol.55, No.2-4, pp. 176-185

Frick, L. R., Arcos, M. L., Rapanelli, M., Zappia, M. P., Brocco, M., Mongini, C., et al. (2009). Chronic restraint stress impairs T-cell immunity and promotes tumor progression in mice. *Stress,* Vol.12, No.2, pp. 134-143, ISSN 1607-8888

Gold, P. W., & Chrousos, G. P. (2002). Organization of the stress system and its dysregulation in melancholic and atypical depression: high vs low CRH/NE states. *Molecular Psychiatry,* Vol.7, No.3, pp. 254-275, ISSN 1359-4184 .

Goodwin, P. J., Leszcz, M., & Ennis, M. (2001). The effect of group psuchosocial support on survival in metastatic breast cancer. *New England Journal of Medicine,* Vol.345, pp. 1719-1726

Grossarth-Maticek, R., Eysenck, J. H., & Boyle, J. G. (1995). Method of test administration as a factor in test validity: the use of a personality questionnaire in the prediction of cancer and coronary heart disease. *Behaviour Research and Therapy,* Vol.33, No.6, pp. 705-710, ISSN IN.

Habib, K. E., Weld, K. P., Rice, K. C., Pushkas, J., Champoux, M., Listwak, S., et al. (2000). Oral administration of a corticotropin-releasing hormone receptor antagonist significantly attenuates behavioral, neuroendocrine, and autonomic responses to stress in primates. *Proceedings of the National Academy of Sciences of the United States of America,* Vol.97, No.11, pp. 6079-6084, ISSN 0027-8424 .

Hasegawa, H., & Saiki, I. (2002). Psychosocial stress augments tumor development through beta-adrenergic activation in mice. *Japanese Journal of Cancer Research,* Vol.93, No.7, pp. 729-735, ISSN 0910-5050 .

Hemminki, K., & Li, X. (2003). Lifestyle and cancer: effect of widowhood and divorce. *Cancer Epidemiology, Biomarkers and Prevention,* Vol.12, No.9, pp. 899-904

Houghton, A. N., Gold, J. S., & Blachere, N. E. (2001). Immunity against cancer: lessons learned from melanoma. *Current Opinion in Immunology,* Vol.13, pp. 134-140

Ironson, G., LaPerriere, A., Antoni, M., O'Hearn, P., Schneiderman, N., Klimas, N., et al. (1990). Changes in immune and psychological measures as a function of anticipation and reaction to news of HIV-1 antibody status. *Psychosomatic Medicine,* Vol.52, No.3, pp. 247-270

Irwin, M., Daniels, M., Risch, S. C., Bloom, E., & Weiner, H. (1988a). Plasma cortisol and natural killer cell activity during bereavement. *Biological Psychiatry,* Vol.24, No.2, pp. 173-178

Irwin, M., Hauger, R. L., Brown, M., & Britton, K. T. (1988b). CRF activates autonomic nervous system and reduces natural killer cytotoxicity. *American Journal of Physiology,* Vol.255, No.5 Pt 2, pp. R744-747, ISSN 0002-9513 .

Isovich, E., Engelmann, M., Landgraf, R., & Fuchs, E. (2001). Social isolation after a single defeat reduces striatal dopamine transporter binding in rats. *European Journal of Neuroscience,* Vol.13, No.6, pp. 1254-1256

Isowa, T., Ohira, H., & Murashima, S. (2004). Reactivity of immune, endocrine and cardiovascular parameters to active and passive acute stress. *Biological Psychology,* Vol.65, No.2, pp. 101-120, ISSN 0301-0511

Jamner, L. D., Schwartz, G. E., & Leigh, H. (1988). The relationship between repressive and defensive coping styles and monocyte, eosinophile, and serum glucose levels: support for the opioid peptide hypothesis of repression. *Psychosomatic Medicine,* Vol.50, No.6, pp. 567-575

Jemmott, J. B., 3rd, Borysenko, J. Z., Borysenko, M., McClelland, D. C., Chapman, R., Meyer, D., et al. (1983). Academic stress, power motivation, and decrease in secretion rate of salivary secretory immunoglobulin A. *Lancet,* Vol.1, No.8339, pp. 1400-1402

Jessop, D. S. (2002). Neuropeptides in the immune system: functional roles in health and disease. *Frontiers of Hormone Research,* Vol.29, pp. 50-68

Kaufmann, I., Eisner, C., Richter, P., Huge, V., Beyer, A., Chouker, A., et al. (2007). Lymphocyte subsets and the role of TH1/TH2 balance in stressed chronic pain patients. *Neuroimmunomodulation,* Vol.14, No.5, pp. 272-280, ISSN 1423-0216

Kiecolt-Glaser, J. K., McGuire, L., Robles, T. F., & Glaser, R. (2002a). Psychoneuroimmunology and psychosomatic medicine: back to the future. *Psychosomatic Medicine,* Vol.64, No.1, pp. 15-28

Kiecolt-Glaser, J. K., McGuire, L., Robles, T. F., & Glaser, R. (2002b). Psychoneuroimmunology: psychological influences on immune function and health. *Journal of Consulting and Clinical Psychology,* Vol.70, No.3, pp. 537-547

Kiecolt-Glaser, J. K., Preacher, K. J., MacCallum, R. C., Atkinson, C., Malarkey, W. B., & Glaser, R. (2003). Chronic stress and age-related increases in the proinflammatory cytokine IL-6. *Proceedings of the National Academy of Sciences of the United States of America,* Vol.100, No.15, pp. 9090-9095, ISSN 0027-8424

Kissane, D., B., G., & D., C. (2007). Supportive-expresive group therapy for women with metastatic breast cancer: Survival and psychosocial outcomes from a randomized controlled trial. *Psycho-Oncol,* Vol.16, pp. 277-286

Koolhaas, J. M., de Boer, S. F., Buwalda, B., & van Reenen, K. (2007). Individual variation in coping with stress: a multidimensional approach of ultimate and proximate mechanisms. *Brain, Behavior and Evolution,* Vol.70, No.4, pp. 218-226, ISSN 1421-9743.

Lauver, D. R., Connolly-Nelson, K., & Vang, P. (2007). Stressors and coping strategies among female cancer survivors after treatments. *Cancer Nursing,* Vol.30, No.2, pp. 101-111, ISSN 1538-9804

Lazar-Molnar, E., Hegyesi, H., Toth, S., & Falus, A. (2000). Autocrine and paracrine regulation by cytokines and growth factors in melanoma. *Cytokine,* Vol.12, No.6, pp. 547-554, ISSN 1043-4666 .

Li, J., & Lambert, V. A. (2007). Coping strategies and predictors of general well-being in women with breast cancer in the People's Republic of China. *Nurs Health Sci,* Vol.9, No.3, pp. 199-204, ISSN 1441-0745

Lutgendorf, S. K., Cole, S., Costanzo, E., Bradley, S., Coffin, J., Jabbari, S., et al. (2003). Stress-related mediators stimulate vascular endothelial growth factor secretion by two ovarian cancer cell lines. *Clinical Cancer Research,* Vol.9, No.12, pp. 4514-4521, ISSN 1078-0432

Lutgendorf, S. K., Sood, A. K., & Antoni, M. H. (2010). Host Factors and Cancer Progression: Biobehvioral Signaling Pathwaya and Interventions. *Journal of Clinical Oncology,* Vol.28, No.26, pp. 4094-4099

Marshall, G. D., Agarwal, S. K., Lloyd, C., Cohen, L., Henninger, E. M., & Morris, G. J. (1998). Cytokine dysregulation associated with exam stress in healthy medical students. *Brain, Behavior, and Immunity,* Vol.12, No.4, pp. 297-307

Martikainen, P., & Valkonen, T. (1996). Mortality after the death of a spouse: rates and causes of death in a large Finnish cohort. *American Journal of Public Health,* Vol.86, No.8 Pt 1, pp. 1087-1093

Masur, K., Niggemann, B., Zanker, K. S., & Entschladen, F. (2001). Norepinephrine-induced migration of SW 480 colon carcinoma cells is inhibited by beta-blockers. *Cancer Research,* Vol.61, No.7, pp. 2866-2869, ISSN 0008-5472.

Matzinger, P. (2002). The danger model: a renewed sense of self. *Science,* Vol.296, No.5566, pp. 301-305, ISSN 1095-9203.

Maunsell, E., Brisson, J., & Deschenes, L. (1995). Social support and survival among women with breast cancer. *Cancer,* Vol.76, No.4, pp. 631-637

McGregor, B. A., & Antoni, M. H. (2009). Psychological intervention and health outcomes among women treated for breast cancer: a review of stress pathways and biological mediators. *Brain, Behavior, and Immunity,* Vol.23, No.2, pp. 159-166, ISSN 1090-2139

McKinnon, W., Weisse, C. S., Reynolds, C. P., Bowles, C. A., & Baum, A. (1989). Chronic stress, leukocyte subpopulations, and humoral response to latent viruses. *Health Psychology,* Vol.8, No.4, pp. 389-402

Melamed, R., Rosenne, E., Shakhar, K., Schwartz, Y., Abudarham, N., & Ben-Eliyahu, S. (2005). Marginating pulmonary-NK activity and resistance to experimental tumor metastasis: suppression by surgery and the prophylactic use of a beta-adrenergic antagonist and a prostaglandin synthesis inhibitor. *Brain, Behavior, and Immunity,* Vol.19, No.2, pp. 114-126, ISSN 0889-1591 .

Moos, R. H. (1964). Personality Factors Associated with Rheumatoid Arthritis: A Review. *Journal of Chronic Diseases,* Vol.17, pp. 41-55

Nakane, T., Szentendrei, T., Stern, L., Virmani, M., Seely, J., & Kunos, G. (1990). Effects of IL-1 and cortisol on beta-adrenergic receptors, cell proliferation, and differentiation in cultured human A549 lung tumor cells. *Journal of Immunology,* Vol.145, No.1, pp. 260-266, ISSN 0022-1767

Oberbeck, R. (2006). Catecholamines: physiological immunomodulators during health and illness. *Current Medicinal Chemistry,* Vol.13, No.17, pp. 1979-1989, ISSN 0929-8673 .

Oka, H., Emori, Y., Sasaki, H., Shiraishi, Y., Yoshinaga, K., & Kurimoto, T. (2002). Anti-tumor mechanism of Z-100, an immunomodulatory Arabinomannan extracted from Mycobacterium tuberculosis strain Aoyama B, on pulmonary metastases of B16F10 melanoma: restoration of helper T cell responses via suppression of glucocorticoid-genesis. *Microbiology and Immunology,* Vol.46, No.5, pp. 343-351, ISSN 0385-5600 .

Overli, O., Pottinger, T. G., Carrick, T. R., Overli, E., & Winberg, S. (2001). Brain monoaminergic activity in rainbow trout selected for high and low stress responsiveness. *Brain, Behavior and Evolution,* Vol.57, No.4, pp. 214-224, ISSN 0006-8977

Pequeux, C., Keegan, B. P., Hagelstein, M. T., Geenen, V., Legros, J. J., & North, W. G. (2004). Oxytocin- and vasopressin-induced growth of human small-cell lung cancer is mediated by the mitogen-activated protein kinase pathway. *Endocr Relat Cancer,* Vol.11, No.4, pp. 871-885, ISSN 1351-0088

Pereira, D. B., Antoni, M. H., Danielson, A., Simon, T., Efantis-Potter, J., Carver, C. S., et al. (2003). Life stress and cervical squamous intraepithelial lesions in women with human papillomavirus and human immunodeficiency virus. *Psychosomatic Medicine,* Vol.65, No.3, pp. 427-434, ISSN 0033-3174.

Petitto, J. M., McCarthy, D. B., Rinker, C. M., Huang, Z., & Getty, T. (1997). Modulation of behavioral and neurochemical measures of forebrain dopamine function in mice by species-specific interleukin-2. *Journal of Neuroimmunology,* Vol.73, No.1-2, pp. 183-190

Piemonti, L., Monti, P., Allavena, P., Sironi, M., Soldini, L., Leone, B. E., et al. (1999). Glucocorticoids affect human dendritic cell differentiation and maturation. *Journal of Immunology,* Vol.162, No.11, pp. 6473-6481, ISSN 0022-1767 .

Pieterse, K., van Dooren, S., Seynaeve, C., Bartels, C. C., Rijnsburger, A. J., de Koning, H. J., et al. (2007). Passive coping and psychological distress in women adhering to regular breast cancer surveillance. *Psycho-Oncology,* Vol.16, No.9, pp. 851-858, ISSN 1057-9249

Plata-Salaman, C. R., Ilyin, S. E., Turrin, N. P., Gayle, D., Flynn, M. C., Bedard, T., et al. (2000). Neither acute nor chronic exposure to a naturalistic (predator) stressor influences the interleukin-1beta system, tumor necrosis factor-alpha, transforming growth factor-beta1, and neuropeptide mRNAs in specific brain regions. *Brain Research Bulletin,* Vol.51, No.2, pp. 187-193, ISSN 0361-9230

Price, M. A., Tennant, C. C., Butow, P. N., Smith, R. C., Kennedy, S. J., Kossoff, M. B., et al. (2001). The role of psychosocial factors in the development of breast carcinoma: Part II. Life event stressors, social support, defense style, and emotional control and their interactions. *Cancer,* Vol.91, No.4, pp. 686-697

Priestman, T. J., Priestman, S. G., & Bradshaw, C. (1985). Stress and breast cancer. *British Journal of Cancer,* Vol.51, No.4, pp. 493-498

Qureshi, F., Alam, J., Khan, M. A., & Sheraz, G. (2002). Effect of examination stress on blood cell parameters of students in a Pakistani medical college. *J Ayub Med Coll Abbottabad,* Vol.14, No.1, pp. 20-22, ISSN 1025-9589

Rassnick, S., Sved, A. F., & Rabin, B. S. (1994). Locus coeruleus stimulation by corticotropin-releasing hormone suppresses in vitro cellular immune responses. *Journal of Neuroscience,* Vol.14, No.10, pp. 6033-6040

Redwine, L., Snow, S., Mills, P., & Irwin, M. (2003). Acute psychological stress: effects on chemotaxis and cellular adhesion molecule expression. *Psychosomatic Medicine,* Vol.65, No.4, pp. 598-603, ISSN 1534-7796

Rozkova, D., Horvath, R., Bartunkova, J., & Spisek, R. (2006). Glucocorticoids severely impair differentiation and antigen presenting function of dendritic cells despite upregulation of Toll-like receptors. *Clinical Immunology,* Vol.120, No.3, pp. 260-271, ISSN 1521-6616

Sa-Rocha, V. M., Sa-Rocha, L. C., & Palermo-Neto, J. (2006). Variations in behavior, innate immunity and host resistance to B16F10 melanoma growth in mice that present social stable hierarchical ranks. *Physiology and Behavior,* Vol.88, No.1-2, pp. 108-115, ISSN 0031-9384

Saint-Mezard, P., Chavagnac, C., Bosset, S., Ionescu, M., Peyron, E., Kaiserlian, D., et al. (2003). Psychological stress exerts an adjuvant effect on skin dendritic cell functions in vivo. *Journal of Immunology,* Vol.171, No.8, pp. 4073-4080, ISSN 0022-1767

Sajti, E., Kavelaars, A., van Meeteren, N., Teunis, M., Gispen, W. H., & Heijnen, C. (2004). Tumor angiogenesis and metastasis formation are associated with individual differences in behavior of inbred Lewis rats. *Brain, Behavior, and Immunity,* Vol.18, No.6, pp. 497-504

Salome, N., Viltart, O., Lesage, J., Landgraf, R., Vieau, D., & Laborie, C. (2006). Altered hypothalamo-pituitary-adrenal and sympatho-adrenomedullary activities in rats bred for high anxiety: central and peripheral correlates. *Psychoneuroendocrinology,* Vol.31, No.6, pp. 724-735, ISSN 0306-4530

Sanders, V. M., Baker, R. A., Ramer-Quinn, D. S., Kasprowicz, D. J., Fuchs, B. A., & Street, N. E. (1997). Differential expression of the beta2-adrenergic receptor by Th1 and Th2 clones: implications for cytokine production and B cell help. *Journal of Immunology,* Vol.158, No.9, pp. 4200-4210, ISSN 0022-1767 .

Segerstrom, S. C. (2003). Individual differences, immunity, and cancer: lessons from personality psychology. *Brain, Behavior, and Immunity,* Vol.17, pp. S92-97

Segerstrom, S. C., & Miller, G. E. (2004). Psychological stress and the human immune system: a meta-analytic study of 30 years of inquiry. *Psychological Bulletin,* Vol.130, No.4, pp. 601-630, ISSN 0033-2909 .

Shakhar, G., & Ben-Eliyahu, S. (1998). In vivo beta-adrenergic stimulation suppresses natural killer activity and compromises resistance to tumor metastasis in rats. *Journal of Immunology,* Vol.160, No.7, pp. 3251-3258, ISSN 0022-1767 .

Shintani, F., Kanba, S., Nakaki, T., Nibuya, M., Kinoshita, N., Suzuki, E., et al. (1993). Interleukin-1 beta augments release of norepinephrine, dopamine, and serotonin in the rat anterior hypothalamus. *Journal of Neuroscience,* Vol.13, No.8, pp. 3574-3581

Sommerhoff, C. P., Avrutina, O., Schmoldt, H. U., Gabrijelcic-Geiger, D., Diederichsen, U., & Kolmar, H. (2010). Engineered cystine knot miniproteins as potent inhibitors of human mast cell tryptase beta. *Journal of Molecular Biology,* Vol.395, No.1, pp. 167-175, ISSN 1089-8638

Spadaro, F., & Dunn, A. J. (1990). Intracerebroventricular administration of interleukin-1 to mice alters investigatiion of stimuli in a novel environment. *Brain Behavior and Immunity,* Vol.4, pp. 308-322

Spiegel, D. (2002). Effects of psychotherapy on cancer survival. *Nature Reviews Cancer,* Vol.2, pp. 383-389

Spiegel, D., Butler, L. D., Giese-Davis, J., Koopman, C., Miller, E., DiMiceli, S., et al. (2007). Effects of supportive-expressive group therapy on survival of patients with metastatic breast cancer - A randomized prospective trial. *Cancer,* Vol.110, No.5, pp. 1130-1138, ISSN 0008-543X.

Stefanek, M. E., Palmer, S. C., Thombs, B. D., & Coyne, J. C. (2009). Finding What Is Not There Unwarranted Claims of an Effect of Psychosocial Intervention on Recurrence and Survival. *Cancer,* Vol.115, No.24, pp. 5612-5616, ISSN 0008-543X.

Stefanski, V., & Ben-Eliyahu, S. (1996). Social confrontation and tumor metastasis in rats: defeat and beta-adrenergic mechanisms. *Physiology and Behavior,* Vol.60, No.1, pp. 277-282

Surtees, P. G., Wainwright, N. W., Luben, R. N., Khaw, K. T., & Bingham, S. A. (2010). No evidence that social stress is associated with breast cancer incidence. *Breast Cancer Research and Treatment,* Vol.120, No.1, pp. 169-174, ISSN 1573-7217

Sutherland, M. A., Niekamp, S. R., Rodriguez-Zas, S. L., & Salak-Johnson, J. L. (2006). Impacts of chronic stress and social status on various physiological and performance measures in pigs of different breeds. *Journal of Animal Science,* Vol.84, No.3, pp. 588-596, ISSN 1525-3163

Tasker, J. G., Di, S., & Malcher-Lopes, R. (2006). Minireview: rapid glucocorticoid signaling via membrane-associated receptors. *Endocrinology,* Vol.147, No.12, pp. 5549-5556, ISSN 0013-7227 .

Temoshok, L., Heller, B. W., Sagebiel, R. W., Blois, M. S., Sweet, D. M., DiClemente, R. J., et al. (1985). The relationship of psychosocial factors to prognostic indicators in cutaneous malignant melanoma. *Journal of Psychosomatic Research,* Vol.29, No.2, pp. 139-153

Uomoto, M., Nishibori, M., Nakaya, N., Takeuchi, Y., Iwagaki, H., Tanaka, N., et al. (1998). Changes in Monoamine Turnover in the Brain of Cachectic Mice Bearing Colon-26 Tumor Cells. *Journal of Neurochemestry,* Vol.70, pp. 260-267, ISSN IN.

Vegas, O., Beitia, G., Sanchez-Martin, J. R., Arregi, A., & Azpiroz, A. (2004). Behavioral and neurochemical responses in mice bearing tumors submitted to social stress. *Behavioural Brain Research,* Vol.155, No.1, pp. 125-134

Vegas, O., Fano, E., Brain, P. F., Alonso, A., & Azpiroz, A. (2006). Social stress, coping strategies and tumor development in male mice: behavioral, neuroendocrine and immunological implications. *Psychoneuroendocrinology,* Vol.31, No.1, pp. 69-79, ISSN 0306-4530 .

Vegas, O., Garmendia, L., Arregi, A., Beitia, G., & Azpiroz, A. (2009). Effects of antalarmin and nadolol on the relationship between social stress and pulmonary metastasis development in male OF1 mice. *Behavioural Brain Research,* Vol.205, No.1, pp. 200-206, ISSN 1872-7549

Viswanathan, K., Daugherty, C., & Dhabhar, F. S. (2005). Stress as an endogenous adjuvant: augmentation of the immunization phase of cell-mediated immunity. *International Immunology,* Vol.17, No.8, pp. 1059-1069, ISSN 0953-8178

Weigent, D. A., & Blalock, J. E. (1987). Interactions between the neuroendocrine and immune systems: common hormones and receptors. *Immunological Reviews,* Vol.100, pp. 79-108

Whisler, R. L., Beiqing, L., Grants, I. S., & Newhouse, Y. G. (1992). Cyclic AMP modulation of human B cell proliferative responses: role of cAMP-dependent protein kinases in enhancing B cell responses to phorbol diesters and ionomycin. *Cellular Immunology,* Vol.142, No.2, pp. 398-415, ISSN 0008-8749 .

Wu, W., Chaudhuri, S., Brickley, D. R., Pang, D., Karrison, T., & Conzen, S. D. (2004). Microarray analysis reveals glucocorticoid-regulated survival genes that are associated with inhibition of apoptosis in breast epithelial cells. *Cancer Research,* Vol.64, No.5, pp. 1757-1764, ISSN 0008-5472 .

Yada, T., Misumi, I., Muto, K., Azuma, T., & Schreck, C. B. (2004). Effects of prolactin and growth hormone on proliferation and survival of cultured trout leucocytes. *General and Comparative Endocrinology,* Vol.136, No.2, pp. 298-306

Yang, E. V., Kim, S. J., Donovan, E. L., Chen, M., Gross, A. C., Webster Marketon, J. I., et al. (2009). Norepinephrine upregulates VEGF, IL-8, and IL-6 expression in human melanoma tumor cell lines: implications for stress-related enhancement of tumor progression. *Brain, Behavior, and Immunity,* Vol.23, No.2, pp. 267-275, ISSN 1090-2139

Zalcman, S., Green-Johnson, J. M., Murray, L., Wan, W., Nance, D. M., & Greenberg, A. H. (1994). Interleukin-2-induced enhancement of an antigen-specific IgM plaque-forming cell response is mediated by the sympathetic nervous system. *Journal of Pharmacology and Experimental Therapeutics,* Vol.271, No.2, pp. 977-982

Zalcman, S., Murray, L., Dick, D. G., Greenberg, A. H., & Nance, D. M. (1998). Interleukin-2 and -6 induce behvioral-activating effects in mice. *Brain Research,* Vol.811, pp. 111-121